Eating Behaviors, Body Composition and Neuro Vulnerability in Energy Metabolism Regulation

Eating Behaviors, Body Composition and Neuro Vulnerability in Energy Metabolism Regulation

Guest Editor

Paola Gualtieri

MDPI

Basel • Beijing • Wuhan • Barcelona • Belgrade • Novi Sad • Cluj • Manchester

Guest Editor
Paola Gualtieri
Department of Biomedicine and Prevention
University of Rome "Tor Vergata"
Rome
Italy

Editorial Office
MDPI AG
Grosspeteranlage 5
4052 Basel, Switzerland

This is a reprint of the Special Issue, published open access by the journal *Nutrients* (ISSN 2072-6643), freely accessible at: https://www.mdpi.com/journal/nutrients/special_issues/Eating_Behaviors_Body_Composition_Energy_Metabolism.

For citation purposes, cite each article independently as indicated on the article page online and as indicated below:

Lastname, A.A.; Lastname, B.B. Article Title. *Journal Name* **Year**, *Volume Number*, Page Range.

ISBN 978-3-7258-5365-6 (Hbk)
ISBN 978-3-7258-5366-3 (PDF)
https://doi.org/10.3390/books978-3-7258-5366-3

Contents

About the Editor

Paola Gualtieri

Paola Gualtieri is affiliated with the Tor Vergata University of Rome, where she serves as an Associate Professor of Nutrition and Food Science. Her research focuses on clinical nutrition, dietary interventions for chronic noncommunicable diseases, and the modulation of body composition and energy metabolism. She has a particular interest in omics sciences, including nutrigenetics, nutrigenomics, and metabolomics, applied to personalized nutrition and dietary management. Professor Gualtieri has participated in several research projects on nutrition and metabolism, contributing systematic reviews, original research articles, and Special Issues in high-impact journals.

Preface

This Reprint focuses on the interplay between dietary strategies, body composition, energy metabolism, and neurobehavioral mechanisms in human health. It aims to provide an updated synthesis of current research on the effects of nutrition on chronic noncommunicable diseases and eating disorders, integrating perspectives from clinical nutrition, neuroscience, and behavioral science.

The motivation for compiling this Reprint stems from the growing recognition that understanding eating behaviors and their physiological and neurological determinants is essential for effective prevention and treatment. While numerous studies have explored dietary models such as the Mediterranean diet, there is a need to examine their specific impact on body composition, metabolic regulation, neurobiological vulnerability, and gut microbiota.

This Reprint is addressed to researchers, clinicians, and healthcare professionals who are interested in translational nutrition, precision medicine, and the role of diet in modulating metabolic and neurobehavioral outcomes. By presenting a collection of original research and comprehensive reviews, it provides a resource for advancing both scientific understanding and clinical practice.

Paola Gualtieri
Guest Editor

nutrients MDPI

Editorial

Mediterranean Diet, Inflammation, and Neurovulnerability: Towards Personalized Nutritional Strategies

Paola Gualtieri *, Antonino De Lorenzo and Laura Di Renzo

Section of Clinical Nutrition and Nutrigenomics, Department of Biomedicine and Prevention, Tor Vergata University of Rome, Via Montpellier 1, 00133 Rome, Italy; delorenzo@uniroma2.it (A.D.L.); laura.di.renzo@uniroma2.it (L.D.R.)
* Correspondence: paola.gualtieri@uniroma2.it

The growing focus on the connection between eating behavior, body composition, and neuro-metabolic regulation reflects an urgent need to understand how nutrition impacts not only energy metabolism but also brain health. The Special Issue "Eating Behaviors, Body Composition and Neuro Vulnerability in Energy Metabolism Regulation" gathers publications addressing these topics through a multidimensional lens, emphasizing the necessity of an integrated and personalized approach.

Currently, there is a noticeable erosion of the Mediterranean Diet, which is well established as the most effective nutritional pattern to counteract chronic degenerative diseases [1–3].

Childhood obesity has been identified as a significant and widely recognized predictor of various cardiovascular risk factors in adulthood [4–6]. Numerous studies demonstrate that strong adherence to the Mediterranean Diet from early childhood is associated with a reduced likelihood of developing overweight and obesity in the short term during later childhood [7,8]. Although longitudinal studies investigating the effects of diet from childhood to adulthood are still lacking, following a Mediterranean Diet during adulthood over a 9-year period has been shown to confer long-term benefits on cardiovascular health [7]. Moreover, adherence to the Mediterranean Diet emerges as a key factor across different age groups. The Lookup 7+ project revealed that lower adherence to the Mediterranean pattern is associated with increased adiposity in elderly populations [9]. These findings support the idea that this dietary model promotes favorable cardiometabolic health, thereby reducing adipose tissue accumulation and future metabolic risk, and suggest that dietary quality from a young age has enduring effects on metabolic health [8,10,11].

In this context, combining school-based and family-oriented programs that include nutritional education and adequate physical activity has been shown to be effective in preventing childhood obesity, thus emphasizing the importance of early interventions in shaping healthy eating behaviors and maintaining healthy body composition in children [12].

Such preventive strategies are essential, as neurovulnerability in energy metabolism regulation arises from a complex interplay of genetic, molecular, and environmental factors, including neuro-endocrine dysfunction, neuroinflammation, and oxidative stress. These factors impair brain circuits responsible for appetite control and energy expenditure, favoring the development of metabolic disorders such as obesity and insulin resistance [13]. Promoting healthy lifestyle habits from a young age may help to strengthen the central nervous system's capacity to regulate energy homeostasis and reduce long-term metabolic risk.

Within this framework, psychiatric disorders, such as anorexia nervosa, are also implicated, where alterations in tryptophan metabolism via the kynurenine pathway appear to play a central role in the link between nutritional status, inflammation, and brain function [14]. These data strengthen the hypothesis of profound interdependence between nutrition, inflammation, and mental health.

In this scenario, it becomes essential to consider not only nutritional aspects but also neuro-metabolic health when defining prevention and treatment strategies. Personalized interventions that simultaneously target dietary balance, inflammation modulation, and neural function improvement could represent an effective pathway to counteract the progression of chronic metabolic diseases.

From this perspective, dietary personalization extends beyond macronutrient selection to include the integration of bioactive compounds and the modulation of inflammatory and oxidative processes, which are particularly relevant in specific clinical conditions [15].

The importance of nutritional personalization is highlighted by a pilot study on lipedema treatment, where a modified Mediterranean ketogenic diet combined with carboxytherapy led to clinical improvements and enhanced body composition [16]. Ketogenic diets are known for their effectiveness in promoting rapid weight loss by reducing carbohydrate intake and modulating energy metabolism. However, in chronic inflammatory conditions such as lipedema, a dietary approach incorporating anti-inflammatory components is more appropriate. For this reason, personalizing a ketogenic diet with a Mediterranean profile, integrating the beneficial effects of foods rich in bioactive compounds such as polyphenols, flavonoids, vitamins, and minerals, represents a promising strategy to modulate oxidative stress, reduce systemic inflammation, and improve endothelial function, thereby promoting more effective clinical and compositional outcomes [16].

In summary, the works collected in this Special Issue underscore the central role of nutrition in energy regulation and neuro-metabolic health. They reinforce the idea that adult metabolic trajectories are shaped during early life through dietary education and diet quality, even though the Mediterranean Diet is surprisingly uncommon among children living in the Mediterranean region itself [17] and should therefore be prioritized as a preventive policy strategy.

Furthermore, the findings support the efficacy of integrated and targeted interventions for complex pathological conditions. Evidence suggests that personalized nutritional approaches, tailored to age, pathophysiological conditions, and sociocultural contexts, represent a concrete pathway to promote well-being and prevention. The next challenge in nutrition research will be to combine clinical efficacy, sustainability, and accessibility. This Special Issue contributes to defining research directions and strategies that support stable metabolic function and promote long-term health through comprehensive and personalized approaches.

Conflicts of Interest: The authors declare no conflict of interest.

List of Contributions:

1. Fontes, T.; Rodrigues, L.; Ferreira-Pêgo, C. Comparison between Different Groups of Vegetarianism and Its Associations with Body Composition: A Literature Review from 2015 to 2021. *Nutrients* **2022**, *14*, 1853. https://doi.org/10.3390/nu14091853.
2. Dauty, M.; Menu, P.; Jolly, B.; Lambert, S.; Rocher, B.; Le Bras, M.; Jirka, A.; Guillot, P.; Pretagut, S.; Fouasson-Chailloux, A. Inpatient Rehabilitation during Intensive Refeeding in Severe Anorexia Nervosa. *Nutrients* **2022**, *14*, 2951. https://doi.org/10.3390/nu14142951.
3. Le, L.; Dang, L.; Wang, T.; Do, T.; Nguyen, D.; Hoang, T.; Pham, M.; Do, B.; Nguyen, H.; Tran, T.; et al. Osteoporosis Risk in Hemodialysis Patients: The Roles of Gender, Comorbidities, Biochemical Parameters, Health and Diet Literacy. *Nutrients* **2022**, *14*, 5122. https://doi.org/10.3390/nu14235122.
4. Alberts, C.; Owe-Larsson, M.; Urbanska, E. New Perspective on Anorexia Nervosa: Tryptophan-Kynurenine Pathway Hypothesis. *Nutrients* **2023**, *15*, 1030. https://doi.org/10.3390/nu15041030.

5. Arjona Garrido, Á.; Monserrat Hernández, M.; Checa Olmos, J. Healthy Eating in the Spanish University Community: A Case Study. *Nutrients* **2023**, *15*, 2053. https://doi.org/10.3390/nu15092053.
6. Lopes, S.; Fontes, T.; Menezes, R.; Rodrigues, L.; Ferreira-Pêgo, C. Mediterranean Diet Adherence and Its Relationship to Metabolic Markers and Body Composition in Portuguese University Students. *Nutrients* **2023**, *15*, 2330. https://doi.org/10.3390/nu15102330.
7. Thorsteinsdottir, S.; Bjarnason, R.; Eliasdottir, H.; Olafsdottir, A. Body Composition in Fussy-Eating Children, with and without Neurodevelopmental Disorders, and Their Parents, Following a Taste Education Intervention. *Nutrients* **2023**, *15*, 2788. https://doi.org/10.3390/nu15122788.
8. Clemente-Suárez, V.; Beltrán-Velasco, A.; Redondo-Flórez, L.; Martín-Rodríguez, A.; Yáñez-Sepúlveda, R.; Tornero-Aguilera, J. Neuro-Vulnerability in Energy Metabolism Regulation: A Comprehensive Narrative Review. *Nutrients* **2023**, *15*, 3106. https://doi.org/10.3390/nu15143106.
9. Cinelli, G.; Croci, I.; De Santis, G.; Chianello, I.; Miller, K.; Gualtieri, P.; Di Renzo, L.; De Lorenzo, A.; Tozzi, A.; Zanna, V. Adherence to a Mediterranean Diet, Body Composition and Energy Expenditure in Outpatients Adolescents Diagnosed with Anorexia Nervosa: A Pilot Study. *Nutrients* **2023**, *15*, 3223. https://doi.org/10.3390/nu15143223.
10. Di Renzo, L.; Gualtieri, P.; Zomparelli, S.; De Santis, G.; Seraceno, S.; Zuena, C.; Frank, G.; Cianci, R.; Centofanti, D.; De Lorenzo, A. Modified Mediterranean-Ketogenic Diet and Carboxytherapy as Personalized Therapeutic Strategies in Lipedema: A Pilot Study. *Nutrients* **2023**, *15*, 3654. https://doi.org/10.3390/nu15163654.
11. Shakoor, H.; Kizhakkayil, J.; Khalid, M.; Mahgoub, A.; Platat, C. Effect of Moderate-Intense Training and Detraining on Glucose Metabolism, Lipid Profile, and Liver Enzymes in Male Wistar Rats: A Preclinical Randomized Study. *Nutrients* **2023**, *15*, 3820. https://doi.org/10.3390/nu15173820.
12. Mela, V.; Agüera, Z.; Alvarez-Bermudez, M.; Martín-Reyes, F.; Granero, R.; Sánchez-García, A.; Oliva-Olivera, W.; Tomé, M.; Moreno-Ruiz, F.; Soler-Humanes, R.; et al. The Relationship between Depressive Symptoms, Quality of Life and miRNAs 8 Years after Bariatric Surgery. *Nutrients* **2023**, *15*, 4109. https://doi.org/10.3390/nu15194109.
13. Cacciatore, S.; Gava, G.; Calvani, R.; Marzetti, E.; Coelho-Júnior, H.; Picca, A.; Esposito, I.; Ciciarello, F.; Salini, S.; Russo, A.; et al. Lower Adherence to a Mediterranean Diet Is Associated with High Adiposity in Community-Dwelling Older Adults: Results from the Longevity Check-Up (Lookup) 7+ Project. *Nutrients* **2023**, *15*, 4892. https://doi.org/10.3390/nu15234892.

References

1. Jones, B.; Coe, S. Exploring the Role of Diet in Reducing Cancer Risk in UK Firefighters: Mediterranean Pattern and the Potential for Targeted Nutritional Strategies. *Nutr. Res. Rev.* **2025**, *28*, 1–45. [CrossRef]
2. Tehrani, S.D.; Ahmadi, A.R.; Sadeghi, N.; Keshani, M. The effects of the mediterranean diet supplemented with olive oils on pro-inflammatory biomarkers and soluble adhesion molecules: A systematic review and meta-analysis of randomized controlled trials. *Nutr. Metab.* **2025**, *22*, 52. [CrossRef]
3. Hu, F.B.; Drescher, G.; Trichopoulou, A.; Willett, W.C.; Martínez-González, M.A. Three decades of the Mediterranean diet pyramid: A narrative review of its history, evolution, and advances. *Am. J. Clin. Nutr.* **2025**, *122*, 17–28. [CrossRef] [PubMed]
4. Faienza, M.F.; Wang, D.Q.; Frühbeck, G.; Garruti, G.; Portincasa, P. The dangerous link between childhood and adulthood predictors of obesity and metabolic syndrome. *Intern. Emerg. Med.* **2016**, *11*, 175–182. [CrossRef] [PubMed]
5. Fraser, B.J.; Blizzard, L.; Tomkinson, G.R.; Dwyer, T.; Venn, A.J.; Magnussen, C.G. Added predictive value of childhood physical fitness to traditional risk factors for adult cardiovascular disease. *Eur. J. Prev. Cardiol.* **2025**, zwaf102. [CrossRef]
6. Umer, A.; Kelley, G.A.; Cottrell, L.E.; Giacobbi, P., Jr.; Innes, K.E.; Lilly, C.L. Childhood obesity and adult cardiovascular disease risk factors: A systematic review with meta-analysis. *BMC Public Health* **2017**, *17*, 683. [CrossRef]
7. Notario-Barandiaran, L.; Valera-Gran, D.; Gonzalez-Palacios, S.; Garcia-de-la-Hera, M.; Fernández-Barrés, S.; Pereda-Pereda, E.; Fernández-Somoano, A., Guxens, M.; Iñiguez, C.; Romaguera, D.; et al. High adherence to a mediterranean diet at age 4 reduces overweight, obesity and abdominal obesity incidence in children at the age of 8. *Int. J. Obes.* **2020**, *44*, 1906–1917.
8. George, E.S.; Gavrili, S.; Itsiopoulos, C.; Manios, Y.; Moschonis, G. Poor adherence to the Mediterranean diet is associated with increased likelihood of metabolic syndrome components in children: The Healthy Growth Study. *Public Health Nutr.* **2021**, *24*, 2823–2833. [CrossRef] [PubMed]

9. Cacciatore, S.; Gava, G.; Calvani, R.; Marzetti, E.; Coelho-Júnior, H.J.; Picca, A.; Esposito, I.; Ciciarello, F.; Salini, S.; Russo, A.; et al. Lower Adherence to a Mediterranean Diet Is Associated with High Adiposity in Community-Dwelling Older Adults: Results from the Longevity Check-Up (Lookup) 7+ Project. *Nutrients* **2023**, *15*, 4892. [CrossRef]
10. Vahid, F.; Wilk, P.; Bohn, T. Longitudinal effects of diet quality on healthy aging—Focus on cardiometabolic health: Findings from the Canadian longitudinal study on aging (CLSA). *Aging Clin. Exp. Res.* **2025**, *37*, 157. [CrossRef] [PubMed]
11. Kastorini, C.; Milionis, H.; Esposito, K.; Giugliano, D.; Goudevenos, J.A.; Panagiotakos, D.B. The Effect of Mediterranean Diet on Metabolic Syndrome and its Components: A Meta-Analysis of 50 Studies and 534,906 Individuals. *J. Am. Coll. Cardiol.* **2011**, *57*, 1299–1313. [CrossRef]
12. Marsigliante, S.; Ciardo, V.; Di Maglie, A.; My, G.; Muscella, A. Efficacy of school-based intervention programs in reducing overweight: A randomized trial. *Front. Nutr.* **2022**, *9*, 1001934. [CrossRef]
13. Clemente-Suárez, V.J.; Beltrán-Velasco, A.I.; Redondo-Flórez, L.; Martín-Rodríguez, A.; Yáñez-Sepúlveda, R.; Tornero-Aguilera, J.F. Neuro-Vulnerability in Energy Metabolism Regulation: A Comprehensive Narrative Review. *Nutrients* **2023**, *15*, 3106. [CrossRef] [PubMed]
14. Chen, Y.; Guillemin, G.J. Kynurenine pathway metabolites in humans: Disease and healthy States. *Int. J. Tryptophan Res.* **2009**, *2*, 1–19. [CrossRef]
15. Zhang, J.; Cianciosi, D.; Islam, M.O.; Zhang, L. Editorial: Intervention effects of food-derived polyphenols and bioactive peptides on chronic inflammation. *Front. Nutr.* **2024**, *11*, 1493706. [CrossRef]
16. Di Renzo, L.; Gualtieri, P.; Zomparelli, S.; De Santis, G.L.; Seraceno, S.; Zuena, C.; Frank, G.; Cianci, R.; Centofanti, D.; De Lorenzo, A. Modified Mediterranean-Ketogenic Diet and Carboxytherapy as Personalized Therapeutic Strategies in Lipedema: A Pilot Study. *Nutrients* **2023**, *15*, 3654. [CrossRef] [PubMed]
17. Denoth, F.; Scalese, M.; Siciliano, V.; Di Renzo, L.; De Lorenzo, A.; Molinaro, S. Clustering eating habits: Frequent consumption of different dietary patterns among the Italian general population in the association with obesity, physical activity, sociocultural characteristics and psychological factors. *Eat. Weight Disord.* **2016**, *21*, 257–268. [CrossRef] [PubMed]

nutrients

MDPI

Article

Lower Adherence to a Mediterranean Diet Is Associated with High Adiposity in Community-Dwelling Older Adults: Results from the Longevity Check-Up (Lookup) 7+ Project

Stefano Cacciatore [1], Giordana Gava [1], Riccardo Calvani [1,2,*], Emanuele Marzetti [1,2], Hélio José Coelho-Júnior [1], Anna Picca [2,3], Ilaria Esposito [1], Francesca Ciciarello [2], Sara Salini [2], Andrea Russo [2], Matteo Tosato [2] and Francesco Landi [1,2]

1 Department of Geriatrics, Orthopedics and Rheumatology, Università Cattolica del Sacro Cuore, L.go F. Vito 1, 00168 Rome, Italy; stefano.cacciatore01@icatt.it (S.C.); giordana.gava01@icatt.it (G.G.); emanuele.marzetti@policlinicogemelli.it (E.M.); coelhojunior@hotmail.com.br (H.J.C.-J.); ilaria.esposito1@unicatt.it (I.E.); francesco.landi@unicatt.it (F.L.)

2 Fondazione Policlinico Universitario "Agostino Gemelli" IRCCS, L.go A. Gemelli 8, 00168 Rome, Italy; picca@lum.it (A.P.); francesca.ciciarello@policlinicogemelli.it (F.C.); sara.salini@policlinicogemelli.it (S.S.); andrea.russo1@policlinicogemelli.it (A.R.); matteo.tosato@policlinicogemelli.it (M.T.)

3 Department of Medicine and Surgery, LUM University, SS100 km 18, 70100 Casamassima, Italy

* Correspondence: riccardo.calvani@unicatt.it; Tel.: +39-06-3015-8885

Abstract: High adiposity impacts health and quality of life in old age, owing to its association with multimorbidity, decreased physical performance, and frailty. Whether a high adherence to a Mediterranean diet (Medi-Diet) is associated with reduced body adiposity in older adults is unclear. The present study was conducted to assess the prevalence of high adiposity in a large sample of community-dwelling older adults. We also explored the relationship between whole-body adiposity estimated through relative fat mass (RFM) and Medi-Diet adherence. Data were obtained from the Longevity Check-up 7+ (Lookup7+) project database. RFM was estimated from anthropometric and personal parameters using a validated equation. RFM was categorized as high if $\geq$40% in women and $\geq$30% in men. Information on diet was collected using a food frequency questionnaire, while Medi-Diet adherence was assessed through a modified version of the Medi-Lite scoring system. Analyses were conducted in 2092 participants (mean age 73.1 $\pm$ 5.9 years; 53.4% women). Mean RFM was 39.6 $\pm$ 5.14% in women and 29.0 $\pm$ 3.6% in men. High adiposity was found in 971 (46.4%) participants and was more frequent in those with a low (54.2%) or moderate (46.4%) Medi-Diet adherence compared with the high-adherence group (39.7%, $p < 0.001$). Logistic regression indicated that older adults with high Medi-Diet adherence were less likely to have a high RFM. Other factors associated with a greater risk of having high adiposity were older age, female sex, and physical inactivity. Our findings support an association between healthy lifestyles, including a greater adherence to a Mediterranean-style diet, and lower body adiposity in older adults.

Keywords: aging; body composition; body fat; relative fat mass; nutrition; obesity; Medi-Lite; healthy diet; lifestyle; behavioral interventions

1. Introduction

Excessive fat accumulation is associated with negative health outcomes and is a public health concern at all life stages [1,2]. The World Health Organization estimates that the global prevalence of obesity has increased threefold since 1975, affecting more than 650 million individuals (13%) worldwide in 2016 [2]. According to the World Obesity Federation, more than half of the global population will be overweight or obese in the next 12 years [3]. Adipose tissue accumulation, infiltration, and dysfunction are responsible for endocrine, cardiometabolic, and functional alterations [4–6]. Body mass index (BMI) is the most used metric to assess adiposity in the general population. BMI values greater than 25 kg/m^2 and 30 kg/m^2 (which indicate overweight and obesity, respectively) are associated with ncreased morbidity and mortality [7,8]. However, recent evidence suggests that BMI may not possess sufficient sensitivity for identifying excess fat at the individual level [9,10]. Furthermore, the association between BMI-defined obesity and negative health outcomes in older adults is controversial. According to a recent systematic review, greater BMI values were negatively associated with short- and long-term all-cause mortality in older adults, especially in those with chronic diseases or facing an acute medical event. This counterintuitive finding could potentially be attributed to the lack of body composition information provided by BMI, as well as the weaker correlation between BMI and percentage of body mass or fat mass index [11]. Indeed, a meta-analysis of 32 studies comprising 31,968 individuals from 12 countries found that commonly used BMI cutoffs for diagnosing obesity failed to identify almost half of those with high adiposity as assessed by body composition reference techniques (e.g., dual energy X-ray absorptiometry (DXA), air-displacement plethysmography, hydrostatic weighing) [9].

The availability of reliable and easy-to-apply measures of body fat is particularly relevant to older adults, as aging is often accompanied by fat accumulation at the expenses of lean body mass [12]. Novel whole-body fat estimators based on anthropometric measures have been proposed and validated [13–15]. Among them, relative fat mass (RFM) is a simple equation based on the ratio of height to waist circumference that was developed by Woolcott and Bergman [15] using data from National Health and Nutrition Examination Survey (NHANES) 1999–2004 and 2005–2006. RFM proved to be more accurate than BMI for estimating whole-body adiposity and reducing obesity misclassification in adults of different ethnicities, especially among older individuals [15–17]. In the general population, a high RFM has been associated with incident cardiovascular disease and diabetes as well as mortality [18–21]. An RFM greater than 26% in men and equal to or greater than 38% in women was related with incident atrial fibrillation, heart failure, and coronary artery disease in middle-aged individuals from the Dutch Lifelines Cohort Study over a four-year follow-up. [18]. In the PREVEND (Prevention of Renal and Vascular End-Stage Disease) study, several indices of adiposity were evaluated as potential predictors of incident heart failure during 11 years of follow-up in community-dwelling adults [21]. When compared with other adiposity indices (i.e., body circumference index, weight-adjusted waist index, and body shape index), RFM had the strongest association with heart failure with either preserved or reduced ejection fraction [21]. In the PREVEND cohort, RFM was also associated with the incidence of type 2 diabetes [19], which was validated in two independent Dutch cohorts (i.e., Lifelines and Rotterdam cohorts) [19]. In adults with type 2 diabetes, RFM was negatively associated with trabecular bone score and exhibited the highest predictive value for the likelihood of damaged bone microarchitecture compared with insulin resistance indices and hormonal indicators [22]. Recent evidence from the Moli-sani study showed that participants in the highest RFM quartile had an increased mortality risk, which was mediated by forced expiratory volume in 1 s (FEV1) and blood glucose and cystatin C levels [20]. In older adults with obesity, RFM has shown to be sensitive to changes following a 12-month weight loss intervention based on exercise and energy restriction [23]. A remarkable agreement was observed between RFM and direct measures of adiposity by DXA or magnetic resonance imaging (MRI), particularly among old women [23].

Physical inactivity and unhealthy dietary habits are the main modifiable contributors to excess adiposity [24]. The Mediterranean diet (Medi-Diet) is considered a healthy dietary model [25,26], owing to its well-known beneficial effects on several chronic conditions, including cardiovascular diseases [27], type 2 diabetes mellitus [28], cognitive decline [29,30], sarcopenia [31], osteoporosis [32], osteoarthritis [33,34], as well as quality of life [35]. Medi-Diet is characterized by a high intake of cereals, vegetables, fruits, and legumes, a modest intake of milk and dairy products, and sporadic consumption of meat and animal fats [36,37]. Several studies have highlighted a possible role for Medi-Diet as a suitable strategy for preventing and/or managing obesity [38,39]. However, most of the available evidence was gathered in young or middle-aged individuals, while less is known on the effects of a Mediterranean diet on body adiposity in older adults [40–42]. Furthermore, no studies have explored the association between adherence to a Mediterranean diet and anthropometry-based indices of body adiposity in old individuals.

The aim of this study was to assess the prevalence of high adiposity estimated by RFM in a large sample of Italian community-dwelling older individuals and explore its association with adherence to a Medi-Diet.

2. Materials and Methods

The data used in this study were collected within the Longevity Check-up 7+ (Lookup 7+) project. For the present investigation, analyses were performed using data on participants 65 years or older. The Lookup 7+ survey is an ongoing cross-sectional study carried out by the Department of Geriatrics, Orthopedics, and Rheumatology at the Università Cattolica del Sacro Cuore and the Fondazione Policlinico Universitario "Agostino Gemelli" IRCCS in Rome, Italy. The complete description of the study protocol can be found in other sources [43,44]. Candidate participants are considered eligible if they are 18 years or older. Self-reported pregnancy, refusal to perform capillary blood testing for the measurement of total cholesterol and glycemia, and unwillingness or inability to provide a written informed consent are exclusion criteria. Participants are recruited in public places (such as shopping malls, pharmacies, and supermarkets) and events, as well as during health prevention campaigns. Cities of varying sizes are selected to obtain a complete geographic characterization of Italian mainland and major islands. Cities are categorized as small, with a population of less than 100,000 people, medium-sized, with a population ranging from 100,000 to 250,000 residents, and large, with a population exceeding 250,000 inhabitants. The selection of locations is determined according to the availability of potential volunteers who can be approached. To provide adequate representation of the sociodemographic characteristics of residents, in large cities (e.g., Rome, Milan, Naples, Genoa, Bologna, Catania), activities are carried out in different places. Before enrolling, every participant is required to provide a signed informed consent. The study protocol was authorized by the Ethics Committee of the Università Cattolica del Sacro Cuore (protocol no.: A.1220/CE/2011).

At each location, assessments take place within a quiet and socially distanced moveable medical booth. To ensure consistency, all assessments are conducted in a standardized sequence: lifestyle interview, measurement of blood pressure, measurement of body weight and height, capillary blood testing for total cholesterol and glycemia, physical performance tests. As previously reported [43], the average completion time for each visit is 12.8 ± 1.6 min, with no significant differences among age groups, sexes, or settings.

2.1. Anthropometry and Lifestyle Habits

A questionnaire on dietary and other lifestyle habits was administered by trained personnel to collect information on personal characteristics and modifiable risk factors for chronic diseases [44]. Body weight and height were measured using an analog column scale with integrated stadiometer. The BMI was computed as the square of height (in m^2) divided by body weight (in kg). An anthropometric tape was used to measure the participant's waist circumference (in cm) as they stood with their feet together, head straight, eyes forward, and their arms at their sides. The measurement was taken at the midpoint between the last floating rib and the highest point of the iliac crest. Two categories (i.e., active or past/never smoker) were used to define smoking status. Regular engagement in physical activity or exercise was operationalized as consistent participation in either structured or non-structured activities, with a frequency of at least two sessions per week, each lasting for a minimum of 30 min, over the course of the preceding year. Individuals who did not engage in any form of physical activity or did not meet the frequency and/or duration specified above were classified as physically inactive [45,46].

2.2. *Relative Fat Mass*

Woolcott and Bergman's equation [15] was used to estimate RFM, as follows:

$$\text{RFM} = 64 - \left(20 \times \frac{\text{height (cm)}}{\text{waist circumference (cm)}}\right) + (12 \times \text{sex}),$$

where sex = 0 for men and 1 for women.

High adiposity was operationalized as having RFM values ≥40% in women and ≥30% in men [47]. RFM cutoff values were established using cut points associated with a higher risk of all-cause mortality in the National Health and Nutrition Examination Survey (NHANES) 1999–2014 [47]. According to a receiver operating characteristic (ROC) analysis, RFM showed a high accuracy in discriminating adult individuals with DXA-defined obesity in both men and women (C-statistics = 0.91, 95% confidence interval: 0.91–0.92) [47].

2.3. *Adherence to a Mediterranean Diet and Daily Energy Intake*

Nutritional data were obtained using a simplified food frequency questionnaire (FFQ) [48]. The survey evaluated the frequency with which respondents consumed a specified portion size of 12 different foods on a weekly basis [49]. The food items explored were fish, meat and derivatives (e.g., cured meat), eggs, milk and dairy products (e.g., cheese, yogurt), pasta and bakery products (e.g., bread, pizza), rice, legumes, vegetables, and other cereals (e.g., oat, rye, spelt). The Italian standard portion reference was used to estimate portion size. Adherence to a Medi-Diet was determined through a modified version of the Medi-Lite scoring system [31,50,51]. The Medi-Lite score considers nine food categories. A score from 0 (lowest intake) to 2 (highest consumption) was assigned to food items usually included in a Medi-Diet (i.e., cereals, fruits, legumes, fish, and vegetables). For dietary categories not included in a typical Medi-Diet (e.g., meat and meat derivatives), 2 points were allocated to the lowest intake, 1 point to an intermediate consumption, and 0 points to the highest consumption. In the case of olive oil, 2 points were assigned for daily usage, 1 point for regular use, and 0 points for occasional consumption. Since alcohol use was not recorded, the corresponding item was not considered for the calculation of the Medi-Lite score. As a result, the maximum score achievable was 16 instead of 18. Details on Medi-Lite scoring have been published elsewhere [31]. A summary score of 8 points or lower indicated a low Medi-Diet adherence, a score ranging from 9 to 11 was classified as moderate adherence, and a score of 12 or higher indicated high Medi-Diet adherence.

Mean daily energy intake was calculated as the sum of calorie content of a standard portion of individual food items listed in the FFQ, divided by seven (the days of a week). Calculations were based on calorie values reported in the online database of the Italian Center for Research on Foods and Nutrition (CREA) [52].

2.4. *Statistical Analysis*

Personal and anthropometric characteristics of participants according to their Medi-Diet adherence were compiled using descriptive statistics. The normal distribution of continuous data was evaluated using the Kolmogorov–Smirnov test. Means ± standard deviations were used to summarize continuous variables, whereas categorical data were expressed as absolute frequencies and percentages of the total. Comparisons among categories of adherence to a Mediterranean diet (i.e., low, moderate, high) for continuous variables were performed by one-way analysis of variance (ANOVA), with Bonferroni's post hoc test as needed. Chi-square statistics with Bonferroni correction for multiple comparisons were used for categorical variables. Logistic regression models were employed to examine the relationship between adherence to a Medi-Diet and high adiposity. Initially, crude odds ratios were calculated together with their corresponding 95% confidence intervals. Afterward, logistic regression models were built with adjustments for age, sex, and other factors associated with high adiposity at univariate analysis. The R software version 4.2.3 R (Core Team, Vienna, Austria) was used for all analyses.

3. Results

A total of 4720 participants aged 65 years or older were recruited across Italy between 1 June 2015 and 31 January 2023. Of them, 2628 were excluded due to missing values in the variables of interests (2583 for waist circumference and 1638 for nutrition data). A final sample of 2092 participants was considered for the present investigation. Personal characteristics of excluded participants were not significantly different from those with complete data. The mean age of the study population was 73.1 ± 5.9 years and 1117 (53.4%) were women. Adherence to a Medi-Diet was low in 346 (19.7%) participants, moderate in 1198 (57.3%), and high in 481 (23.0%). Table 1 shows the main characteristics of participants categorized according to their adherence to a Medi-Diet. Individuals with a low Medi-Diet adherence were predominantly women and were more frequently active smokers than in the other two groups. Daily energy intake was higher in participants with high Medi-Diet adherence than in those with moderate or low adherence. BMI values and waist circumference were lower in participants with a high Medi-Diet adherence. Mean RFM was 39.6 ± 5.1% in women and 29.0 ± 3.6% in men and was significantly lower in individuals with a high Medi-Diet adherence. A high adiposity was found in 971 (46.4%) participants and was more frequent in those with a low or moderate Medi-Diet adherence than in the high-adherence group.

Table 1. Main characteristics of study participants according to their adherence to a Mediterranean diet.

	Total Sample (n = 2092)	Mediterranean Diet Adherence			p
		Low (n = 413)	Moderate (n = 1198)	High (n = 481)	
Age, years	73.1 (5.9)	73.1 (6.0)	73.2 (5.9)	73.1 (5.8)	0.929
Sex, female	1117 (53.4%)	240 (58.1%)	611 (51.0%) [a]	266 (55.3%)	0.028
Active smoking	315 (15.1%)	71 (17.2%)	189 (15.8%)	55 (11.4%) [a,b]	0.034
Physically active	1118 (53.4%)	203 (49.2%)	652 (54.4%)	263 (54.7%)	0.149
Energy intake, kcal/day	1410 (264)	1160 (244)	1410 (240) [a]	1586 (179) [a,b]	<0.001
Medi-Lite score	10.4 (1.9)	7.5 (0.8)	10.1 (0.8) [a]	12.8 (1.0) [a,b]	<0.001
BMI, kg/m^2	25.9 (3.93)	26.5 (4.11)	26.0 (3.79)	25.4 (4.03) [a,b]	<0.001
Waist circumference, cm					
Women	88.8 (12.1)	90.5 (11.8)	89.5 (12.4)	86.4 (11.6) [a,b]	<0.001
Men	98.9 (10.0)	101 (10.1)	98.9 (9.9) [a]	97.5 (10.1) [a]	0.002
RFM, %					
Women	39.6 (5.14)	40.6 (4.86)	40.0 (5.14)	38.5 (5.03) [a,b]	<0.001
Men	29.0 (3.58)	29.9 (3.35)	29.0 (3.57)	28.4 (3.66) [a,b]	<0.001
High adiposity	971 (46.4%)	224 (54.2%)	556 (46.4%) [a]	191 (39.7%) [a,b]	<0.001

Data are reported as absolute numbers (percentages) for categorical variables (sex, active smoking, physically active, high adiposity). Continuous variables are shown as means (standard deviations). Physically active: engaged in physical activity at least twice weekly, with each session lasting a minimum of 30 min, throughout the preceding year. High adiposity: relative fat mass ≥40% in women and ≥30% in men. [a] $p < 0.05$ vs. low adherence; [b] $p < 0.05$ vs. moderate adherence. Abbreviations: BMI, body mass index; RFM: relative fat mass.

In the unadjusted logistic regression model, both moderate and low Medi-Diet adherence were associated with a greater risk of high adiposity compared with high Medi-Diet adherence (Table 2).

The association remained significant after adjusting for age and sex (Model 1). After controlling for potential confounders (age, female sex, active smoking, daily energy intake, engagement in physical activity), moderate and low Medi-Diet adherence were independently associated with a greater risk of high adiposity (Model 2). Predictors of high adiposity were age and female sex in both Model 1 and Model 2 (Table 2). Engagement in physical activity was associated with a reduced risk of high adiposity in Model 2. No significant associations were found between high adiposity and daily energy intake or active smoking (Table 2).

Table 2. Unadjusted and adjusted association between adherence to a Mediterranean diet and high body adiposity.

Characteristics	Unadjusted OR (95% CI)	*p*	Model 1 OR (95% CI)	*p*	Model 2 OR (95% CI)	*p*
Adherence to Mediterranean diet						
High adherence	Reference (1.00)	-	Reference (1.00)	-	Reference (1.00)	-
Moderate adherence	1.31 (1.06–1.63)	0.013	1.34 (1.08–1.67)	0.008	1.36 (1.09–1.71)	0.007
Low adherence	1.80 (1.38–2.35)	<0.001	1.80 (1.38–2.35)	<0.001	1.85 (1.33–2.58)	<0.001
Age			1.03 (1.02–1.05)	<0.001	1.03 (1.01–1.04)	0.001
Sex, female			1.50 (1.26–1.78)	<0.001	1.47 (1.23–1.76)	<0.001
Active smoking					1.01 (0.78–1.29)	0.990
Daily energy intake					1.00 (0.99–1.01)	0.400
Physically active					0.48 (0.40–0.58)	<0.001

High body adiposity: relative fat mass $\geq$40% in women and $\geq$30% in men. Model 1: odds ratio adjusted for age and female sex; model 2: odds ratio adjusted for age, female sex, active smoking, and engagement in physical activity. Abbreviations: CI: confidence interval; OR: odds ratio.

4. Discussion

In the present study, we investigated the prevalence of high adiposity estimated by RFM in a large cohort of Italian older adults living in the community and explored its association with adherence to a Mediterranean-style dietary pattern. Participants with a high Medi-Diet adherence had a lower frequency of high adiposity than those with moderate or low adherence. In logistic regression models, a significant association between high adiposity and Medi-Diet adherence was found after adjusting for potential confounders. Older age and female sex were predictors of high adiposity, while engagement in physical activity was associated with lower odds of having high adiposity.

The role of Medi-Diet in the prevention of adipose tissue accumulation is well documented in the literature [38,53]. A large cross-sectional study in 3162 Spanish adults found a significantly lower risk of obesity in those with a higher Medi-Diet adherence [54]. The MEDiterranean Islands Study (MEDIS) demonstrated that a high adherence to a Mediterranean-style dietary pattern decreased the risk of obesity and obesity-related complications in 1190 old men and women from Greece and Cyprus [40]. Similar results were observed in a smaller sample of older adults from Cyprus [55]. The Prevention with Medi-Diet (PREDIMED)—Canarias Intervention Randomized Trial tested the effects of three dietary regimens (i.e., Medi-Diet plus extra virgin olive oil, Medi-diet plus nuts, and a low-fat diet without a fixed daily caloric intake) on body composition in 351 community-dwelling individuals aged 55 to 80 years with type 2 diabetes or at least three cardiovascular risk factors [56]. After one year of intervention, participants allocated to Medi-Diet regimens experienced significant reductions in body adiposity and excess weight that were not observed in those on a low-fat diet [56]. In all these studies, obesity and high adiposity were defined according to BMI values and direct measurements of body fat by bioimpedance analysis (BIA) or DXA, respectively. As mentioned earlier, BMI may not be sufficiently sensitive for identifying obesity [8,9], with high misclassification rates observed for commonly adopted BMI cutoff points. On the other hand, BIA and especially DXA may not be available in settings with limited resources.

The positive effects of Medi-Diet on body fat accumulation may arise from its high content in plant-based food and a low consumption of meat and dairy products [39]. While ultra-processed foods elicit a high glycemic load and lower satiety, legumes, fruit, vegetables, and whole grains provide a higher intake of dietary fiber and low-density energy, and induce greater satiety [57]. Satiety-inducing properties of fiber depend on different mechanisms, such as increased mastication time and gastric distension, and stimulation of the release of appetite-reducing hormones, including cholecystokinin, glucagon-like peptide 1, and peptide YY [39]. Olive oil and fish provide mono- and polyunsaturated fatty acids with anti-inflammatory and antioxidant properties [58]. Moreover, when compared with saturated fats, unsaturated fatty acids increase energy expenditure, fat oxidation, and diet-induced thermogenesis [59,60]. A regular use of olive oil is not associated with weight gain, despite being one of the most energy-dense foods [61,62]. Unexpectedly, participants with low Medi-Diet adherence had lower daily energy intake. This finding may be due to a selective underreporting of "unhealthy foods", such as those rich in carbohydrates and fats [63]. Energy underreporting is also more frequent in individuals living with obesity [64]. Vegetables, fruit, and fish instead tend to be reported to a similar extent by under-reporters and non-under-reporters [65].

Medi-Diet may also increase the diversity of gut microbiota and shape its composition toward an increase in probiotic species (e.g., Lactobacilli, Bifidobacteria) [66]. Such changes in the intestinal microbial ecosystem are associated with reduced inflammatory and oxidative status and amelioration in overall metabolic health [67]. The adoption of a Medi-Diet may also help manage obesity and high adiposity in older adults. Aged individuals are at increased risk of protein–energy malnutrition, which leads to weight loss and predisposes to negative health outcomes, including the development and/or worsening of sarcopenia and frailty [68]. Overweight and obesity have traditionally been considered protective in old age, as meta-analyses showed a lower mortality risk in healthy older adults in the overweight range [7,69,70]. A recent systematic review found a lower risk of short- (within 12 months) or long-term mortality (five years or more) in older adults living with overweight or obesity in 30 out of 58 studies [11]. The survival advantage was more evident in those with chronic diseases or experiencing an acute medical event as well in the oldest old [11]. In this regard, studies have shown that the risk of death and complications associated with excess body weight is greater in those aged 65–75 years than in younger adults but is lower in older individuals [71,72]. This phenomenon may be due to a "bottleneck" effect that leads a greater percentage of obese individuals to die early, while those who live longer may be the least compromised [73]. Alternatively, the "obesity paradox" might reflect greater robustness or higher reserves, and reduced risk of undernutrition [11]. However, the obesity paradox has been challenged by studies suggesting possible methodological errors and inaccurate assessments [74,75]. A meta-analysis by the Global BMI Mortality Collaboration conducted on data from 239 studies in four continents highlighted a consistent association of excess body weight with all-cause mortality [7]. Furthermore, as pointed out in a meta-analysis by Yuan et al. [76], obesity is associated with frailty as much as undernutrition, and high adiposity in older adults has been associated with higher inflammation levels and oxidative stress [77], metabolic abnormalities [78,79], worsening of sarcopenia and osteoporosis [77,80], poor physical performance [80,81], frailty [82], disability [83], and reduced quality of life [81,84]. On the other hand, the Medi-Diet has shown benefits on body adiposity [55], bone health [31,85], muscle mass and strength [31,86], as well as physical performance [29]. Moreover, adiposity is a key parameter in cardiovascular risk assessment. A systematic review by Kastorini et al. [87] found that the beneficial effects conveyed by a Medi-Diet on weight gain and obesity play a key role in protecting against coronary artery disease.

Although the present study reports interesting results, it has limitations that should be mentioned. First, the cross-sectional design prevents from drawing cause-and-effect conclusions between adherence to a Medi-Diet and body adiposity. Second, a substantial number of participants were excluded from the analysis because of incomplete data. Although efforts were made to maintain the duration of assessments within a reasonable length, participants were evaluated while attending social events or carrying out shopping activities. In several instances, participants decided to interrupt the assessment before all data could be collected. However, the main characteristics of participants with incomplete data did not significantly differ from those included in the analysis. This, together with the large sample size, limited the impact of participant exclusion on the robustness of results. Third, although current evidence indicates that the Woolcott and Bergman's equation provides reliable RFM estimates across ages and ethnicities, it is not a direct measure of body fat. Nevertheless, RFM was shown to be a reliable predictor of whole-body fat percentage measured by DXA [15]. Furthermore, RFM has recently been included in the

Moli-sani risk score [88], a validated algorithm to estimate the impact of modifiable risk factors on cardiovascular risk. Fourth, no data on alcohol consumption were collected. Fifth, data available in the Lookup 7+ database did not include information on disease conditions, medications, living arrangement, or socioeconomic status. Collection of a comprehensive personal and medical/drug history would significantly lengthen the assessments, rendering them unsuitable for the nontraditional contexts in which the research is conducted. This limitation, which is intrinsic to the Lookup 7+ survey, needs to be addressed in future studies specifically designed to evaluate the influence of personal and clinical variables on the association between dietary regimens and body adiposity. Sixth, virtually all participants were Caucasians; thereby, results may not be applicable to other ethnicities. Seventh, our study exclusively focused on older adults residing in the community. As a result, the implications and conclusions drawn from our findings may not be applicable to different contexts or populations. Eighth, there are several validated questionnaires available for evaluating adherence to the Medi-Diet. However, no single measure demonstrated clear superiority over others. Finally, the health benefits associated with the Medi-Diet are believed to be conveyed by a combination of nutritional factors as well as lifestyle and sociocultural influences, including engaging in regular physical activity, adequate rest, and conviviality [89]. Additional research is required to determine whether the Medi-Diet as a whole lifestyle pattern or its dietary components alone affect the risk of body fat accumulation.

5. Conclusions

The results obtained from this study indicate that there is a significant correlation between a higher Medi-Diet adherence and decreased levels of body adiposity in a large and relatively unselected sample of older adults residing in the community. Additional research is required to ascertain the possible impact of adopting a Mediterranean-style dietary pattern on general health and quality of life in older individuals.

Supplementary Materials: The following supporting information can be downloaded at: https://www.mdpi.com/article/10.3390/nu15234892/s1, Lookup 7+ Project Team Members.

Author Contributions: Conceptualization, S.C., R.C., E.M., F.L.; methodology, S.C., R.C., H.J.C.-J. and I.E.; validation, H.J.C.-J., A.P. and M.T.; investigation, G.G. and A.R.; writing—original draft preparation, S.C. and G.G.; writing—review and editing, F.C., S.S., R.C. and E.M.; funding acquisition, E.M. and F.L.; supervision, F.L. All authors have read and agreed to the published version of the manuscript.

Funding: This work was supported by the Università Cattolica del Sacro Cuore (D1.2020, D1.2022, and D1.2023) and the nonprofit research foundation "Centro Studi Achille e Linda Lorenzon" (N/A). The authors also acknowledge co-funding from Next Generation EU, in the context of the National Recovery and Resilience Plan, Investment PE8—Project Age-It: "Ageing Well in an Ageing Society". This resource was co-financed by the Next Generation EU (DM 1557 11.10.2022). The views and opinions expressed are only those of the authors and do not necessarily reflect those of the European Union or the European Commission. Neither the European Union nor the European Commission can be held responsible for them.

Institutional Review Board Statement: The study was conducted in accordance with the Declaration of Helsinki and approved by the Ethics Committee of the Università Cattolica del Sacro Cuore, Rome, Italy (protocol #A.1220/CE/2011; date of approval: 3 March 2014).

Informed Consent Statement: Informed consent was obtained from all subjects involved in the study.

Data Availability Statement: The data that support the findings of this study are available on request from the corresponding author. The data are not publicly available due to their containing information that could compromise the privacy of the research participants.

Acknowledgments: The authors recognized support by the Italian Ministry of Health (Ricerca Corrente 2023). We also thank Carni Sostenibili, Danone Italia, Errekappa, Ferrarini, Italfarmaco, Italia Longeva, IVSI, Laborest, Yakult, Marche Region, Nutricia, ProAction, Serenissima, and Novartis for their unconditional support to the organization of Lookup 7+ project events. Members of the Lookup 7+ project team are listed in the Supplementary Material.

Conflicts of Interest: The authors declare no conflict of interest.

References

1. WHO Regional Office for Europe. WHO European Regional Obesity Report 2022. Available online: https://apps.who.int/iris/handle/10665/353747 (accessed on 3 July 2023).
2. WHO: Obesity and Overweight. Available online: https://www.who.int/news-room/fact-sheets/detail/obesity-and-overweight (accessed on 21 April 2023).
3. World Obesity Federation. World Obesity Atlas 2023. Available online: https://s3-eu-west-1.amazonaws.com/wof-files/World_Obesity_Atlas_2023_Report.pdf (accessed on 16 November 2023).
4. De Lorenzo, A.; Romano, L.; Di Renzo, L.; Di Lorenzo, N.; Cenname, G.; Gualtieri, P. Obesity: A preventable, treatable, but relapsing disease. *Nutrition* **2020**, *71*, 110615. [CrossRef] [PubMed]
5. Fuster, J.J.; Ouchi, N.; Gokce, N.; Walsh, K. Obesity-induced changes in adipose tissue microenvironment and their impact on cardiovascular disease. *Circ. Res.* **2016**, *118*, 1786–1807. [CrossRef]
6. Hilton, T.N.; Tuttle, L.J.; Bohnert, K.L.; Mueller, M.J.; Sinacore, D.R. Excessive adipose tissue infiltration in skeletal muscle in individuals with obesity, diabetes mellitus, and peripheral neuropathy: Association with performance and function. *Phys. Ther.* **2008**, *88*, 1336–1344. [CrossRef] [PubMed]
7. Global BMI Mortality Collaboration; Di Angelantonio, E.; Bhupathiraju, S.; Wormser, D.; Gao, P.; Kaptoge, S.; Berrington de Gonzalez, A.; Cairns, B.J.; Huxley, R.; Jackson, C.L.; et al. Body-mass index and all-cause mortality: Individual-participant-data meta-analysis of 239 prospective studies in four continents. *Lancet* **2016**, *388*, 776–786. [CrossRef]
8. Kivimaki, M.; Strandberg, T.; Pentti, J.; Nyberg, S.T.; Frank, P.; Jokela, M.; Ervasti, J.; Suominen, S.B.; Vahtera, J.; Sipilä, P.N.; et al. Body-mass index and risk of obesity-related complex multimorbidity: An observational multicohort study. *Lancet Diabetes Endocrinol.* **2022**, *10*, 253–263. [CrossRef] [PubMed]
9. Okorodudu, D.O.; Jumean, M.F.; Montori, V.M.; Romero-Corral, A.; Somers, V.K.; Erwin, P.J.; Lopez-Jimenez, F. Diagnostic performance of body mass index to identify obesity as defined by body adiposity: A systematic review and meta-analysis. *Int. J. Obes.* **2010**, *34*, 791–799. [CrossRef] [PubMed]
10. Lahav, Y.; Kfir, A.; Gepner, Y. The paradox of obesity with normal weight; A cross-sectional study. *Front. Nutr.* **2023**, *10*, 1173488. [CrossRef]
11. Dramé, M.; Godaert, L. The obesity paradox and mortality in older adults: A systematic review. *Nutrients* **2023**, *15*, 1780. [CrossRef]
12. Baumgartner, R.N. Body composition in healthy aging. *Ann. N. Y. Acad. Sci.* **2000**, *904*, 437–448. [CrossRef]
13. Krakauer, N.Y.; Krakauer, J.C. A new body shape index predicts mortality hazard independently of body mass index. *PLoS ONE* **2012**, *7*, e39504. [CrossRef]
14. Moosaie, F.; Fatemi Abhari, S.M.; Deravi, N.; Karimi Behnagh, A.; Esteghamati, S.; Dehghani Firouzabadi, F.; Rabizadeh, S.; Nakhjavani, M.; Esteghamati, A. Waist-to-height ratio is a more accurate tool for predicting hypertension than waist-to-hip circumference and BMI in patients with type 2 diabetes: A prospective study. *Front. Public Health* **2021**, *9*, 726288. [CrossRef] [PubMed]
15. Woolcott, O.O.; Bergman, R.N. Relative fat mass (RFM) as a new estimator of whole-body fat percentage—A cross-sectional study in American adult individuals. *Sci. Rep.* **2018**, *8*, 10980. [CrossRef] [PubMed]
16. Senkus, K.; Crowe-White, K.; Locher, J.; Ard, J. Relative fat mass (RFM) as an estimate of total adiposity in older adults. *Curr. Dev. Nutr.* **2021**, *5* (Suppl. S2), 51. [CrossRef]
17. Woolcott, O.O.; Seuring, T. Temporal trends in obesity defined by the relative fat mass (RFM) index among adults in the United States from 1999 to 2020: A population-based study. *BMJ Open* **2023**, *13*, e071295. [CrossRef]
18. Zwartkruis, V.W.; Suthahar, N.; Idema, D.L.; Mahmoud, B.; van Deutekom, C.; Rutten, F.H.; van der Schouw, Y.T.; Rienstra, M.; de Boer, R.A. Relative fat mass and prediction of incident atrial fibrillation, heart failure and coronary artery disease in the general population. *Int. J. Obes.* **2023**. *online ahead of print*. [CrossRef]
19. Suthahar, N.; Wang, K.; Zwartkruis, V.W.; Bakker, S.J.L.; Inzucchi, S.E.; Meems, L.M.G.; Eijgenraam, T.R.; Ahmadizar, F.; Sijbrands, E.G.; Gansevoort, R.T.; et al. Associations of relative fat mass, a new index of adiposity, with type-2 diabetes in the general population. *Eur. J. Intern. Med.* **2023**, *109*, 73–78. [CrossRef]
20. Ghulam, A.; Gianfagna, F.; Bonaccio, M.; Costanzo, S.; Di Castelnuovo, A.; De Curtis, A.; Gialluisi, A.; Cerletti, C.; Donati, M.B.; de Gaetano, G.; et al. Association between BMI, RFM and mortality and potential mediators: Prospective findings from the Moli-sani study. *Int. J. Obes.* **2023**, *47*, 697–708. [CrossRef]
21. Suthahar, N.; Meems, L.M.G.; Withaar, C.; Gorter, T.M.; Kieneker, L.M.; Gansevoort, R.T.; Bakker, S.J.L.; van Veldhuisen, D.J.; de Boer, R.A. Relative fat mass, a new index of adiposity, is strongly associated with incident heart failure: Data from Prevend. *Sci. Rep.* **2022**, *12*, 147. [CrossRef]

22. Hayón-Ponce, M.; García-Fontana, B.; Avilés-Pérez, M.D.; González-Salvatierra, S.; Andújar-Vera, F.; Moratalla-Aranda, E.; Muñoz-Torres, M. Lower trabecular bone score in type 2 diabetes mellitus: A role for fat mass and insulin resistance beyond hyperglycaemia. *Diabetes Metab.* **2021**, *47*, 101276. [CrossRef]
23. Senkus, K.E.; Crowe-White, K.M.; Locher, J.L.; Ard, J.D. Relative fat mass assessment estimates changes in adiposity among female older adults with obesity after a 12-month exercise and diet intervention. *Ann. Med.* **2022**, *54*, 1160–1166. [CrossRef]
24. Biddle, S.J.H.; Garcia Bengoechea, E.; Pedisic, Z.; Bennie, J.; Vergeer, I.; Wiesner, G. Screen time, other sedentary behaviours, and obesity risk in adults: A review of reviews. *Curr. Obes. Rep.* **2017**, *6*, 134–147. [CrossRef]
25. Ferro-Luzzi, A.; Branca, F. Mediterranean diet, Italian-style: Prototype of a healthy diet. *Am. J. Clin. Nutr.* **1995**, *61*, 1338S–1345S. [CrossRef] [PubMed]
26. Boccardi, V.; Calvani, R.; Limongi, F.; Marseglia, A.; Mason, A.; Noale, M.; Rogoli, D.; Veronese, N.; Crepaldi, G.; Maggi, S. Consensus paper on the "executive summary of the international conference on Mediterranean diet and health: A lifelong approach" an Italian initiative supported by the Mediterranean Diet Foundation and the Menarini Foundation. *Nutrition* **2018**, *51–52*, 38–45. [CrossRef]
27. Russo, G.L.; Siani, A.; Fogliano, V.; Geleijnse, J.M.; Giacco, R.; Giampaoli, S.; Iacoviello, L.; Kromhout, D.; Lionetti, L.; Naska, A.; et al. The Mediterranean diet from past to future: Key concepts from the second "Ancel Keys" International Seminar. *Nutr. Metab. Cardiovasc. Dis.* **2021**, *31*, 717–732. [CrossRef] [PubMed]
28. Uusitupa, M.; Khan, T.A.; Viguiliouk, E.; Kahleova, H.; Rivellese, A.A.; Hermansen, K.; Pfeiffer, A.; Thanopoulou, A.; Salas-Salvadó, J.; Schwab, U.; et al. Prevention of type 2 diabetes by lifestyle changes: A systematic review and meta-analysis. *Nutrients* **2019**, *11*, 2611. [CrossRef]
29. Coelho-Junior, H.J.; Trichopoulou, A.; Panza, F. Cross-sectional and longitudinal associations between adherence to Mediterranean diet with physical performance and cognitive function in older adults: A systematic review and meta-analysis. *Ageing Res. Rev.* **2021**, *70*, 101395. [CrossRef]
30. Limongi, F.; Siviero, P.; Bozanic, A.; Noale, M.; Veronese, N.; Maggi, S. The effect of adherence to the Mediterranean diet on late-life cognitive disorders: A systematic review. *J. Am. Med. Dir. Assoc.* **2020**, *21*, 1402–1409. [CrossRef] [PubMed]
31. Cacciatore, S.; Calvani, R.; Marzetti, E.; Picca, A.; Coelho-Junior, H.J.; Martone, A.M.; Massaro, C.; Tosato, M.; Landi, F. Low adherence to Mediterranean diet is associated with probable sarcopenia in community-dwelling older adults: Results from the Longevity Check-Up (Lookup) 7+ project. *Nutrients* **2023**, *15*, 1026. [CrossRef]
32. Quattrini, S.; Pampaloni, B.; Gronchi, G.; Giusti, F.; Brandi, M.L. The Mediterranean diet in osteoporosis prevention: An insight in a peri- and post-menopausal population. *Nutrients* **2021**, *13*, 531. [CrossRef]
33. Veronese, N.; Stubbs, B.; Noale, M.; Solmi, M.; Luchini, C.; Smith, T.O.; Cooper, C.; Guglielmi, G.; Reginster, J.Y.; Rizzoli, R.; et al. Adherence to a Mediterranean diet is associated with lower prevalence of osteoarthritis: Data from the osteoarthritis initiative. *Clin. Nutr.* **2017**, *36*, 1609–1614. [CrossRef]
34. Veronese, N.; La Tegola, L.; Crepaldi, G.; Maggi, S.; Rogoli, D.; Guglielmi, G. The association between the Mediterranean diet and magnetic resonance parameters for knee osteoarthritis: Data from the Osteoarthritis Initiative. *Clin. Rheumatol.* **2018**, *37*, 2187–2193. [CrossRef] [PubMed]
35. Veronese, N.; Stubbs, B.; Noale, M.; Solmi, M.; Luchini, C.; Maggi, S. Adherence to the Mediterranean diet is associated with better quality of life: Data from the Osteoarthritis Initiative. *Am. J. Clin. Nutr.* **2016**, *104*, 1403–1409. [CrossRef]
36. Trichopoulou, A.; Lagiou, P. Healthy traditional Mediterranean diet: An expression of culture, history, and lifestyle. *Nutr. Rev.* **1997**, *55 Pt 1*, 383–389. [CrossRef] [PubMed]
37. Davis, C.; Bryan, J.; Hodgson, J.; Murphy, K. Definition of the Mediterranean diet; A literature review. *Nutrients* **2015**, *7*, 9139–9153. [CrossRef] [PubMed]
38. D'Innocenzo, S.; Biagi, C.; Lanari, M. Obesity and the Mediterranean diet: A review of evidence of the role and sustainability of the Mediterranean diet. *Nutrients* **2019**, *11*, 1306. [CrossRef] [PubMed]
39. Buckland, G.; Bach, A.; Serra-Majem, L. Obesity and the Mediterranean diet: A systematic review of observational and intervention studies. *Obes. Rev.* **2008**, *9*, 582–593. [CrossRef]
40. Tyrovolas, S.; Bountziouka, V.; Papairakleous, N.; Zeimbekis, A.; Anastassiou, F.; Gotsis, E.; Metallinos, G.; Polychronopoulos, E.; Lionis, C.; Panagiotakos, D. Adherence to the Mediterranean diet is associated with lower prevalence of obesity among elderly people living in Mediterranean islands: The MEDIS study. *Int. J. Food Sci. Nutr.* **2009**, *60* (Suppl. S6), 137–150. [CrossRef]
41. Estruch, R.; Martinez-Gonzalez, M.A.; Corella, D.; Salas-Salvado, J.; Fito, M.; Chiva-Blanch, G.; Fiol, M.; Gómez-Gracia, E.; Arós, F.; Lapetra, J.; et al. Effect of a high-fat Mediterranean diet on bodyweight and waist circumference: A prespecified secondary outcomes analysis of the PREDIMED randomised controlled trial. *Lancet Diabetes Endocrinol.* **2019**, *7*, e6–e17. [CrossRef]
42. Zelicha, H.; Kloting, N.; Kaplan, A.; Yaskolka Meir, A.; Rinott, E.; Tsaban, G.; Chassidim, Y.; Bluher, M.; Ceglarek, U.; Isermann, B.; et al. The effect of high-polyphenol Mediterranean diet on visceral adiposity: The DIRECT PLUS randomized controlled trial. *BMC Med.* **2022**, *20*, 327. [CrossRef]
43. Landi, F.; Calvani, R.; Picca, A.; Tosato, M.; Martone, A.M.; Ortolani, E.; Salini, S.; Pafundi, T.; Savera, G.; Pantanelli, C.; et al. Cardiovascular health metrics, muscle mass and function among Italian community-dwellers: The Lookup 7+ project. *Eur. J. Public Health* **2018**, *28*, 766–772. [CrossRef]

44. Landi, F.; Calvani, R.; Picca, A.; Tosato, M.; D'Angelo, E.; Martone, A.M.; Serafini, E.; Ortolani, E.; Savera, G.; Salini, S.; et al. Relationship between cardiovascular health metrics and physical performance in community-living people: Results from the Longevity check-up (Lookup) 7+ project. *Sci. Rep.* **2018**, *8*, 16353. [CrossRef] [PubMed]
45. Coelho-Júnior, H.J.; Calvani, R.; Picca, A.; Tosato, M.; Landi, F.; Marzetti, E. Engagement in aerobic exercise is associated with a reduced prevalence of sarcopenia and severe sarcopenia in Italian older adults. *J. Pers. Med.* **2023**, *13*, 655. [CrossRef]
46. Coelho-Junior, H.J.; Calvani, R.; Picca, A.; Cacciatore, S.; Tosato, M.; Landi, F.; Marzetti, E. Combined aerobic training and Mediterranean diet is not associated with a lower prevalence of sarcopenia in Italian older adults. *Nutrients* **2023**, *15*, 2693. [CrossRef] [PubMed]
47. Woolcott, O.O.; Bergman, R.N. Defining cutoffs to diagnose obesity using the relative fat mass (RFM): Association with mortality in NHANES 1999–2014. *Int. J. Obes.* **2020**, *44*, 1301–1310. [CrossRef] [PubMed]
48. Coelho-Junior, H.J.; Calvani, R.; Picca, A.; Tosato, M.; Savera, G.; Landi, F.; Marzetti, E. Protein intake is associated with blood pressure and cholesterol levels in Italian older adults: A cross-sectional study. *Metabolites* **2023**, *13*, 431. [CrossRef]
49. Landi, F.; Calvani, R.; Tosato, M.; Martone, A.M.; Picca, A.; Ortolani, E.; Savera, G.; Salini, S.; Ramaschi, M.; Bernabei, R.; et al. Animal-derived protein consumption is associated with muscle mass and strength in community-dwellers: Results from the Milan EXPO survey. *J. Nutr. Health Aging* **2017**, *21*, 1050–1056. [CrossRef]
50. Sofi, F.; Macchi, C.; Abbate, R.; Gensini, G.F.; Casini, A. Mediterranean diet and health status: An updated meta-analysis and a proposal for a literature-based adherence score. *Public Health Nutr.* **2014**, *17*, 2769–2782. [CrossRef]
51. Sofi, F.; Dinu, M.; Pagliai, G.; Marcucci, R.; Casini, A. Validation of a literature-based adherence score to Mediterranean diet: The Medi-lite score. *Int. J. Food Sci. Nutr.* **2017**, *68*, 757–762. [CrossRef]
52. CREA Centro di Ricerca Alimenti e Nutrizione. Available online: https://www.alimentinutrizione.it/ (accessed on 16 November 2023).
53. Bendall, C.L.; Mayr, H.L.; Opie, R.S.; Bes-Rastrollo, M.; Itsiopoulos, C.; Thomas, C.J. Central obesity and the Mediterranean diet: A systematic review of intervention trials. *Crit. Rev. Food Sci. Nutr.* **2018**, *58*, 3070–3084. [CrossRef]
54. Schröder, H.; Marrugat, J.; Vila, J.; Covas, M.I.; Elosua, R. Adherence to the traditional Mediterranean diet is inversely associated with body mass index and obesity in a Spanish population. *J. Nutr.* **2004**, *134*, 3355–3361. [CrossRef]
55. Panagiotakos, D.B.; Polystipioti, A.; Papairakleous, N.; Polychronopoulos, E. Long-term adoption of a Mediterranean diet is associated with a better health status in elderly people; A cross-sectional survey in Cyprus. *Asia Pac. J. Clin. Nutr.* **2007**, *16*, 331–337.
56. Alvarez-Perez, J.; Sanchez-Villegas, A.; Diaz-Benitez, E.M.; Ruano-Rodriguez, C.; Corella, D.; Martinez-Gonzalez, M.A.; Estruch, R.; Salas-Salvadó, J.; Serra-Majem, L.; PREDIMED Study Investigators. Influence of a Mediterranean dietary pattern on body fat distribution: Results of the PREDIMED-Canarias Intervention Randomized Trial. *J. Am. Coll. Nutr.* **2016**, *35*, 568–580. [CrossRef] [PubMed]
57. Fardet, A. Minimally processed foods are more satiating and less hyperglycemic than ultra-processed foods: A preliminary study with 98 ready-to-eat foods. *Food Funct.* **2016**, *7*, 2338–2346. [CrossRef] [PubMed]
58. Schroder, H. Protective mechanisms of the Mediterranean diet in obesity and type 2 diabetes. *J. Nutr. Biochem.* **2007**, *18*, 149–160. [CrossRef] [PubMed]
59. Krishnan, S.; Cooper, J.A. Effect of dietary fatty acid composition on substrate utilization and body weight maintenance in humans. *Eur. J. Nutr.* **2014**, *53*, 691–710. [CrossRef] [PubMed]
60. Monnard, C.R.; Dulloo, A.G. Polyunsaturated fatty acids as modulators of fat mass and lean mass in human body composition regulation and cardiometabolic health. *Obes. Rev.* **2021**, *22* (Suppl. S2), e13197. [CrossRef] [PubMed]
61. Sanchez-Villegas, A.; Bes-Rastrollo, M.; Martinez-Gonzalez, M.A.; Serra-Majem, L. Adherence to a Mediterranean dietary pattern and weight gain in a follow-up study: The SUN cohort. *Int. J. Obes.* **2006**, *30*, 350–358. [CrossRef]
62. Piers, L.S.; Walker, K.Z.; Stoney, R.M.; Soares, M.J.; O'Dea, K. Substitution of saturated with monounsaturated fat in a 4-week diet affects body weight and composition of overweight and obese men. *Br. J. Nutr.* **2003**, *90*, 717–727. [CrossRef]
63. Lafay, L.; Mennen, L.; Basdevant, A.; Charles, M.A.; Borys, J.M.; Eschwège, E.; Romon, M. Does energy intake underreporting involve all kinds of food or only specific food items? Results from the Fleurbaix Laventie Ville Santé (FLVS) study. *Int. J. Obes. Relat. Metab. Disord.* **2000**, *24*, 1500–1506. [CrossRef]
64. Heitmann, B.L.; Lissner, L. Dietary underreporting by obese individuals—Is it specific or non-specific? *BMJ* **1995**, *311*, 986–989. [CrossRef]
65. Bingham, S.A.; Cassidy, A.; Cole, T.J.; Welch, A.; Runswick, S.A.; Black, A.E.; Thurnham, D.; Bates, C.; Khaw, K.T.; Key, T.J.; et al. Validation of weighed records and other methods of dietary assessment using the 24 h urine nitrogen technique and other biological markers. *Br. J. Nutr.* **1995**, *73*, 531–550. [CrossRef] [PubMed]
66. Barber, T.M.; Kabisch, S.; Pfeiffer, A.F.H.; Weickert, M.O. The effects of the Mediterranean diet on health and gut microbiota. *Nutrients* **2023**, *15*, 2150. [CrossRef] [PubMed]
67. Merra, G.; Noce, A.; Marrone, G.; Cintoni, M.; Tarsitano, M.G.; Capacci, A.; De Lorenzo, A. Influence of Mediterranean diet on human gut microbiota. *Nutrients* **2020**, *13*, 7. [CrossRef]
68. Calvani, R.; Picca, A.; Coelho-Junior, H.J.; Tosato, M.; Marzetti, E.; Landi, F. Diet for the prevention and management of sarcopenia. *Metabolism* **2023**, *146*, 155637. [CrossRef] [PubMed]
69. Winter, J.E.; MacInnis, R.J.; Wattanapenpaiboon, N.; Nowson, C.A. BMI and all-cause mortality in older adults: A meta-analysis. *Am. J. Clin. Nutr.* **2014**, *99*, 875–890. [CrossRef] [PubMed]

70. Flegal, K.M.; Kit, B.K.; Orpana, H.; Graubard, B.I. Association of all-cause mortality with overweight and obesity using standard body mass index categories: A systematic review and meta-analysis. *JAMA* **2013**, *309*, 71–82. [CrossRef] [PubMed]
71. Calle, E.E.; Thun, M.J.; Petrelli, J.M.; Rodriguez, C.; Heath, C.W., Jr. Body-mass index and mortality in a prospective cohort of U.S. adults. *N. Engl. J. Med.* **1999**, *341*, 1097–1105. [CrossRef]
72. Harris, T.; Cook, E.F.; Garrison, R.; Higgins, M.; Kannel, W.; Goldman, L. Body mass index and mortality among nonsmoking older persons. The Framingham Heart Study. *JAMA* **1988**, *259*, 1520–1524. [CrossRef]
73. Stevens, J.; Cai, J.; Pamuk, E.R.; Williamson, D.F.; Thun, M.J.; Wood, J.L. The effect of age on the association between body-mass index and mortality. *N. Engl. J. Med.* **1998**, *338*, 1–7. [CrossRef]
74. Banack, H.R.; Stokes, A. The 'obesity paradox' may not be a paradox at all. *Int. J. Obes.* **2017**, *41*, 1162–1163. [CrossRef]
75. Bosello, O.; Vanzo, A. Obesity paradox and aging. *Eat. Weight Disord.* **2021**, *26*, 27–35. [CrossRef] [PubMed]
76. Yuan, L.; Chang, M.; Wang, J. Abdominal obesity, body mass index and the risk of frailty in community-dwelling older adults: A systematic review and meta-analysis. *Age Ageing* **2021**, *50*, 1118–1128. [CrossRef] [PubMed]
77. Aguirre, L.; Napoli, N.; Waters, D.; Qualls, C.; Villareal, D.T.; Armamento-Villareal, R. Increasing adiposity is associated with higher adipokine levels and lower bone mineral density in obese older adults. *J. Clin. Endocrinol. Metab.* **2014**, *99*, 3290–3297. [CrossRef] [PubMed]
78. de Oliveira, C.C.; Roriz, A.K.; Ramos, L.B.; Gomes Neto, M. Indicators of adiposity predictors of metabolic syndrome in the elderly. *Ann. Nutr. Metab.* **2017**, *70*, 9–15. [CrossRef]
79. Wannamethee, S.G.; Shaper, A.G.; Morris, R.W.; Whincup, P.H. Measures of adiposity in the identification of metabolic abnormalities in elderly men. *Am. J. Clin. Nutr.* **2005**, *81*, 1313–1321. [CrossRef] [PubMed]
80. Ma, Y.; Zhang, W.; Han, P.; Kohzuki, M.; Guo, Q. Osteosarcopenic obesity associated with poor physical performance in the elderly Chinese community. *Clin. Interv. Aging* **2020**, *15*, 1343–1352. [CrossRef]
81. Forhan, M.; Gill, S.V. Obesity, functional mobility and quality of life. *Best Pract. Res. Clin. Endocrinol. Metab.* **2013**, *27*, 129–137. [CrossRef]
82. Falsarella, G.R.; Gasparotto, L.P.; Barcelos, C.C.; Coimbra, I.B.; Moretto, M.C.; Pascoa, M.A.; Ferreira, T.C.; Coimbra, A.M. Body composition as a frailty marker for the elderly community. *Clin. Interv. Aging.* **2015**, *10*, 1661–1666. [CrossRef]
83. Cawthon, P.M.; Fox, K.M.; Gandra, S.R.; Delmonico, M.J.; Chiou, C.F.; Anthony, M.S.; Caserotti, P.; Kritchevsky, S.B.; Newman, A.B.; Goodpaster, B.H.; et al. Clustering of strength, physical function, muscle, and adiposity characteristics and risk of disability in older adults. *J. Am. Geriatr. Soc.* **2011**, *59*, 781–787. [CrossRef]
84. Mikkola, T.M.; Kautiainen, H.; von Bonsdorff, M.B.; Salonen, M.K.; Wasenius, N.; Kajantie, E.; Eriksson, J.G. Body composition and changes in health-related quality of life in older age: A 10-year follow-up of the Helsinki Birth Cohort Study. *Qual. Life Res.* **2020**, *29*, 2039–2050. [CrossRef]
85. Savanelli, M.C.; Barrea, L.; Macchia, P.E.; Savastano, S.; Falco, A.; Renzullo, A.; Scarano, E.; Nettore, I.C.; Colao, A.; Di Somma, C. Preliminary results demonstrating the impact of Mediterranean diet on bone health. *J. Transl. Med.* **2017**, *15*, 81. [CrossRef] [PubMed]
86. Jennings, A.; Mulligan, A.A.; Khaw, K.T.; Luben, R.N.; Welch, A.A. A Mediterranean diet is positively associated with bone and muscle health in a non-Mediterranean region in 25,450 men and women from EPIC-Norfolk. *Nutrients* **2020**, *12*, 1154. [CrossRef] [PubMed]
87. Kastorini, C.M.; Milionis, H.J.; Goudevenos, J.A.; Panagiotakos, D.B. Mediterranean diet and coronary heart disease: Is obesity a link?—A systematic review. *Nutr. Metab. Cardiovasc. Dis.* **2010**, *20*, 536–551. [CrossRef] [PubMed]
88. Di Castelnuovo, A.; Bonaccio, M.; Costanzo, S.; De Curtis, A.; Persichillo, M.; Panzera, T.; Bracone, F.; Baldassarre, D.; Roncaglioni, M.C.; Baviera, M.; et al. The Moli-sani risk score, a new algorithm for measuring the global impact of modifiable cardiovascular risk factors. *Int. J. Cardiol.* **2023**, *389*, 131228. [CrossRef]
89. Apolzan, J.W.; Venditti, E.M.; Edelstein, S.L.; Knowler, W.C.; Dabelea, D.; Boyko, E.J.; Pi-Sunyer, X.; Kalyani, R.R.; Franks, P.W.; Srikanthan, P.; et al. Long-term weight loss with metformin or lifestyle intervention in the Diabetes Prevention Program Outcomes Study. *Ann. Intern. Med.* **2019**, *170*, 682–690. [CrossRef]

nutrients

MDPI

Article

The Relationship between Depressive Symptoms, Quality of Life and miRNAs 8 Years after Bariatric Surgery

Virginia Mela [1,2,3,4,†], Zaida Agüera [4,5,6,†], Maria D. Alvarez-Bermudez [1,3,4], Flores Martín-Reyes [1,7], Roser Granero [4,6,8], Ana Sánchez-García [1,3,4], Wilfredo Oliva-Olivera [1,3,4], Monica Tomé [9], Francisco J. Moreno-Ruiz [10], Rocío Soler-Humanes [11], Jose L. Fernández-Serrano [11], Pilar Sánchez-Gallegos [12], Jose M. Martínez-Moreno [12], Raquel Sancho-Marín [12], Fernando Fernández-Aranda [4,6,13,14], Eduardo García-Fuentes [1,7,15,*], Francisco J. Tinahones [1,2,3,4,*] and Lourdes Garrido-Sánchez [1,3,4]

1 Instituto de Investigación Biomédica de Málaga y Plataforma en Nanomedicina-IBIMA Plataforma BIONAND, 29590 Malaga, Spain; virginia.mela@ibima.eu (V.M.); mar17alv@gmail.com (M.D.A.-B.); floresmarey@hotmail.com (F.M.-R.); anasanchez-alozaina@hotmail.com (A.S.-G.); oliva_olivera@hotmail.com (W.O.-O.); lourgarrido@gmail.com (L.G.-S.)
2 Department of Medicine and Dermatology, Faculty of Medicine, University of Malaga, 29010 Malaga, Spain
3 Unidad de Gestión Clínica de Endocrinología y Nutrición, Hospital Universitario Virgen de la Victoria, 29010 Malaga, Spain
4 CIBER Fisiopatología de la Obesidad y Nutrición (CIBERObn), Instituto Salud Carlos III, 28029 Madrid, Spain; zaguera@ub.edu (Z.A.); roser.granero@uab.cat (R.G.); ffernandez@bellvitgehospital.cat (F.F.-A.)
5 Departament d'Infermeria de Salut Pública, Salut Mental i Maternoinfantil, Escola d'Infermeria, Facultat de Medicina i Ciències de la Salut, Universitat de Barcelona, 08036 Barcelona, Spain
6 Psychoneurobiology of Eating and Addictive Behaviors Group, Neurosciences Programme, Bellvitge Biomedical Research Institute (IDIBELL), 08908 Barcelona, Spain
7 Unidad de Gestión Clínica de Aparato Digestivo, Hospital Universitario Virgen de la Victoria, 29010 Malaga, Spain
8 Department of Psychobiology and Methodology, Autonomous University of Barcelona, 08193 Barcelona, Spain
9 Unidad de Gestión Clínica de Endocrinología y Nutrición, Hospital Regional Universitario de Málaga, 29009 Malaga, Spain; montome@hotmail.com
10 Unidad de Gestión Clínica de Cirugía General y Digestiva, Hospital Regional Universitario de Málaga, 29010 Malaga, Spain; javier.morenoruiz@gmail.com
11 Unidad de Gestión Clínica de Cirugía General y Digestiva, Hospital Universitario Virgen de la Victoria, 29010 Malaga, Spain; rocioshumanes@hotmail.com (R.S.-H.); jlfserrano@telefonica.net (J.L.F.-S.)
12 Department of Surgical Specialities, Biochemistry and Immunology, Faculty of Medicine, University of Malaga, 29010 Malaga, Spain; pilars@uma.es (P.S.-G.); jmmartinezm@uma.es (J.M.M.-M.); raquelsanchomarin@gmail.com (R.S.-M.)
13 Department of Psychiatry, University Hospital of Bellvitge, 08907 Barcelona, Spain
14 Department of Clinical Sciences, School of Medicine and Health Sciences, University of Barcelona, 08907 Barcelona, Spain
15 CIBER Enfermedades Hepáticas y Digestivas (CIBERehd), Instituto Salud Carlos III, 28029 Madrid, Spain
* Correspondence: edugf1@gmail.com (E.G.-F.); fjtinahones@hotmail.com (F.J.T.)
† These authors contributed equally to this work.

Abstract: (1) Background: There are conflicting results on whether weight loss after bariatric surgery (BS) might be associated with quality of life (QoL)/depressive symptomatology. We aim to determine whether BS outcomes are associated with QoL/depressive symptomatology in studied patients at the 8-year follow-up after BS, as well as their relationship with different serum proteins and miRNAs. (2) Methods: A total of 53 patients with class III obesity who underwent BS, and then classified into "good responders" and "non responders" depending on the percentage of excess weight lost (%EWL) 8 years after BS (%EWL $\geq$ 50% and %EWL < 50%, respectively), were included. Basal serum miRNAs and different proteins were analysed, and patients completed tests to evaluate QoL/depressive symptomatology at 8 years after BS. (3) Results: The good responders group showed higher scores on SF-36 scales of physical functioning, role functioning—physical, role functioning—emotional, body pain and global general health compared with the non-responders. The expression of hsa-miR-101-3p, hsa-miR-15a-5p, hsa-miR-29c-3p, hsa-miR-144-3p and hsa-miR-19b-3p were lower in non-responders. Hsa-miR-19b-3p was the variable associated with the response to BS in a logistic regression model.

(4) Conclusions: The mental health of patients after BS is limited by the success of the intervention. In addition, the expression of basal serum miRNAs related to depression/anxiety could predict the success of BS.

Keywords: bariatric surgery; class III obesity; quality of life; depressive symptoms; miRNAs

1. Introduction

The prevalence of obesity has tripled worldwide in recent decades [1]. Among all treatment options, bariatric surgery (BS) is the most effective, not only in reducing body weight but also in decreasing the risk of developing obesity-related comorbidities [2,3]. Roux-en-Y gastric bypass (RYGB) and biliopancreatic diversion (BPD) promote weight loss through malabsorption of ingested calories and are more effective in terms of losing weight compared with sleeve gastrectomy (SG) [3,4]. BS is considered a successful intervention when the outcome of the surgery is the loss of ≥50% of the percentage of excess weight (%EWL), which is related to decreasing the risk of developing obesity-related diseases [5]. This index is widely used, even in recent studies [6–10], including reviews on this topic [11–13], to analyse the efficacy of bariatric surgery on weight loss. However, there is still a high percentage of failure (up to 50%), since the efficacy of the procedure depends on many factors, such as type of procedure, age, sex and ethnic background [14]. For example, a recent study showed that SG was associated with a higher risk of weight non-response, measured by the %EWL, compared with gastric bypass in a total of 60,426 individuals [6]. This lack of response to different types of bariatric procedures (such as SG), primary vertical banded gastroplasty and gastric band procedures, leads in many cases to the consideration of a reconversion. Revisional RYGB is commonly employed to revise bariatric procedures due to insufficient WL or weight recurrence. However, despite this, only one third of all the patients undergoing revisional surgery had a sufficient %EWL after 2 years compared with primary RYGB [11].

Obesity is often accompanied by psychological distress and decreased quality of life (QoL) [15]. Depression and anxiety are commonly comorbid conditions in patients with obesity, mainly in those enrolled in BS procedures [16]. Most of the literature shows that BS has been shown to improve the QoL [17,18]. It is well known that psychosocial and psychiatric factors are predictors of BS outcome [19]. However, it is so far unclear which factors best predict a successful BS and in what way they act. While some studies found that presurgical depression may act as a predictor of greater weight loss after BS as measured by the %EWL [20], others, in contrast, revealed a negative association between depression and a favourable outcome at the 2-year follow-up [21]. These conflicting results highlight the need to explore this issue further. Most of the studies on this topic show a positive effect of BS on the psychological state of these patients, since after BS, they recover physical, mental and social functions [17]. In this context, the BS outcome could be associated with QoL or depressive symptomatology. However, there is a limited amount of research on long-term outcomes in terms of weight loss, resolution of co-morbidities and QoL after BS. In a previous study, RYGB was shown to lead to positive results regarding the %EWL and improved QoL at more than 10 years follow-up [10]. However, post-intervention improvements in QoL diminished over time and were dependent on the %EWL [7].

Because obesity or its perception is psychologically stressful [22], obesity is also a chronic psychological stressor exaggerating stress-dependent psychoimmune–neuroendocrine network dysfunction [23]. Depression could be linked to obesity through different physiological pathways including metabolic and mood regulation via adipokines, the autonomic nervous system and different hormones, which are linked by the hypothalamic–pituitary–adrenal axis and immuno-inflammatory function [24]. One interesting fact is the relation between different cytokines and the depression state. Some cytokines, such as IL-1β, IL-6 and tumour necrosis factor-α (TNF-α) appear to be involved in the onset and progression of depression [25]. Cytokines, such as interferon-γ (IFNγ), C-reactive protein (CRP) and IL-6, increase with chronic stress [26], correlate with the severity of depression [27] and predict cognitive changes in depression [28]. Cytokines can enter the brain through the blood–brain barrier and affect the neuron function and neuroactive molecule production, which are associated with depression [29]. Neuroinflammation could be the link between obesity and depression, as obesity leads to a low-grade inflammation state, at least in animals [30]. Increased inflammatory cytokines in the brain and in serum, such as CRP, and soluble cell-adhesion molecules IL-6, IL-1β, TNF-α and NF-κB, would be involved in the susceptibility to depression in stressed obese mice [30]. However, other serum proteins related to adipose tissue have not been well studied and may be involved in the relationship between obesity and depression. Several studies suggest the involvement of white adipose tissue in the depression–neuroinflammatory pathways [31], which are a mix of adipocytes, immune, vascular stromal and nervous cells.

Other systemic molecules that could be linked to obesity, including mental health aspects, are the so-called "miRNAs". miRNAs can regulate gene expression by post-transcriptional repression of their mRNA targets. miRNAs have been studied in relation to different pathologies, including obesity and depression [32,33]. Recent systematic reviews identified different circulatory miRNAs that were dysregulated in depression, most of them upregulated, such as miR-451a and miR-124-3p [32,34]. Moreover, other upregulated miRNAs, such as miR-34a-5p, appear to be susceptible to the action of 7-chlorokynurenic acid (7-CTKA), a potential and rapid antidepressant [32]. Other systematic reviews on circulatory obesity-related miRNAs found that most of them were also upregulated, such as miR-26b-5p and miR-30d-5p [33]. Some of these miRNAs could be associated with the mental health of patients 8 years after BS. However, to our knowledge, there are no studies analysing the profile of circulating miRNAs associated with depression in obesity 8 years after BS.

Therefore, in the present study, we aimed at achieving the following objectives: (a) to determine whether BS outcome is associated with QoL or depressive symptomatology in the studied patients at the 8-year follow-up after BS and (b) to analyse the relationship between different serum proteins and miRNAs and mental health and BS outcome.

2. Material and Methods

2.1. Participants

Ninety patients with class III obesity (BMI > 40 kg/m^2), who were scheduled for BS at the "Virgen de la Victoria University Hospital" and "Regional University Hospital" in Malaga between 2010 to 2013, were invited to participate in the present retrospective study. Participants were divided into 2 groups based on the surgical procedure: RYGB and BPD (both restrictive and malabsorptive techniques) (n = 41) vs. SG (restrictive technique) (n = 49). Among these 90 patients, only those who completed psychometric tests at the 8-year follow-up after the intervention were included in this study (n = 53), namely, 36 patients who underwent RYGB or BPD and 17 who underwent SG. In addition, these patients (n = 53) were classified according to their BS outcome into two groups: "good responders" (GR) (n = 30) vs. "non-responders" (NR) (n = 23). This classification was assessed by measuring the percentage of excess weight lost (%EWL) 8 years after BS. We assessed %EWL as 100 × (preoperative weight—weight at the time of evaluation)/(preoperative weight—weight corresponding to BMI = 25 kg/m^2) [35]. The different patterns of weight loss were defined based on the EWL Reinhold criteria modified by Christou et al. [36]. The patients with %EWL > 50% at the follow-up were considered GR. On the other hand, patients with %EWL < 50% at the follow-up were considered NR. The percentage of GR and NR did not significantly vary between groups of included and excluded patients.

The following sociodemographic data were obtained from patients: sex, age, medical history and drug consumption. All patients underwent standardized anthropometric and biochemical examinations. The percentage of total weight loss (%TWL) was calculated as (Initial Weight–Post-Operative Weight) × 100/Initial Weight [37]. Exclusion criteria included patients under 18 or over 60 years old, tobacco or alcohol abuse, psychiatric diseases, cardiovascular disease, acute inflammatory disease and antibiotic or probiotic treatment. The study was carried out in accordance with the Code of Ethics of the World Medical Association (Declaration of Helsinki). All participants gave their written informed consent, and the study was reviewed and approved by the Malaga Provincial Research Ethics Committee (Malaga, Spain).

2.2. Psychometric Instruments

All participants completed the following questionnaires only at 8 years after BS:

- The 36-item Short Form Health Survey (SF-36) [38]. The SF-36 is a valid and self-administered questionnaire that assesses eight dimensions of QoL: (1) Physical functioning (PF; 10 items), (2) Role functioning—Physical (RP; 4 items), (3) Body pain (BP; 2 items), (4) General health perception (GH; 5 items), (5) Vitality (VT; 4 items), (6) Social functioning (SF; 2 items), (7) Role functioning—Emotional (RE; 3 items) and (8) Mental health (MH; 5 items). Each domain is scored from 0 to 100, with greater scores indicating better perceived QoL (physical or mental health conditions). Excellent internal consistency was found in the study sample (Cronbach's $\alpha = 0.96$ for the total scale).
- Beck Depression Inventory (BD-II) [39]. This is a 21-item self-reported questionnaire that assesses the severity of depression symptoms. The total score can range from 0 to 63, with higher scores indicative of more severe depression symptoms. The clinical cut-off scores were classified as follows: no depression (0–13), mild depression (14–19), moderate depression (20–28) and severe depression (29 or more). In the current sample, total scores showed an excellent internal consistency (Cronbach's $\alpha = 0.96$).

2.3. Biochemical Data

Blood samples at baseline and 8 years after BS were collected after 12 h fasting. Serum was aliquoted and immediately stored at −80 °C. Serum glucose, cholesterol, triglycerides and HDL were analysed using an Advia Chemistry XPT autoanalyzer (Siemens Healthcare Diagnostics, Malvern, PA, USA). The LDL was calculated using the Friedewald equation. Serum insulin levels were measured via immunoassay using an ADVIA Centaur autoanalyzer (Siemens Healthcare Diagnostics, Malvern, PA, USA). Serum proteins, such as adhesion molecules (L-selectin, PECAM, ICAM-1, VCAM-1), metalloproteinases (MMP3, MMP9), growth factors (VEGF-A VEGF-D), adipokines (adiponectin, leptin), macrophage-related proteins (CD14, CD44, MBL, LVYE1) and other proteins (lactoferrin, elafin, NGAL, NRP1, PAI-1, RANTES) were analysed using ProcartaPlex immunoassay kit (Thermo Fisher Scientific Inc., Rockford, IL, USA) at baseline and 8 years after BS.

2.4. miRNAs Sequencing

Total RNA with an enhanced miRNA enrichment was extracted from baseline serum samples using the Maxwell® 16 miRNA Tissue Kit (Promega, Madison, WI, USA). Total RNA concentration was measured using the Qubit® RNA Assay Kit in the Qubit® 3.0 Flurometer (Thermo Fisher Scientific Inc., Waltham, MA, USA). RNA integrity was assessed using the RNA Nano 6000 Assay Kit with the Agilent Bioanalyzer 2100 system (Agilent Technologies, Santa Clara, CA, USA). For next-generation sequencing (NGS), small RNA transcripts were converted into barcoded cDNA libraries using 400–500 ng of RNA per sample as input material for the small RNA library. Sequencing libraries were generated using NEBNext Multiplex Small RNA Library Prep Set for Illumina (NEB, MA) following the manufacturer's instructions. Individual libraries, prepared with unique indexes, were pooled and subjected to the Illumina sequencing pipeline, passing through clonal cluster generation on sequencing-by-synthesis 1 × 50–75 pb single-end reads on the NextSeq 550 (Illumina Inc., San Diego, CA, USA). From the total miRNAs obtained in the massive sequencing, we selected those miRNAs that related with depression and anxiety for this study according to previous studies [32,40,41]. To do so, we listed all miRNAs that were commented on in three studies referenced in our bibliography [32,40,41]. On the other hand, we had another list with miRNAs obtained through massive sequencing with detectable expression. These two miRNA lists were overlapped, obtaining the shared miRNAs. These shared miRNAs are the 19 miRNAs included in our study: hsa-miR-101-3p, hsa-miR-144-3p, hsa -miR-144-5p, hsa-miR15a-5p, hsa-miR-197-3p, hsa-miR-19a-3p, hsa-miR-19b-3p, hsa-miR-21-5p, hsa-miR-221-3p, hsa-miR-26b-5p, hsa-miR-29c-3p, hsa-miR-30a-5p, hsa-miR-30d-5p, hsa-miR335-5p, hsa-miR-484, hsa-miR-7704, hsa-miR-92b-3p, hsa-miR-338-3p and hsa-miR-338-5p.

2.5. Statistical Analysis

Results are expressed as mean values ± standard deviation (SD). After testing the normal distribution of continuous variables via the Shapiro–Wilk test, we applied logarithmic transformation as needed to ensure normality of skewed variables. Student's t-test was performed to assess the differences between two independent means. Differences in the variables within the same group, before and after BS, were analysed by repeated-measures ANOVA. The comparison of quantitative variables of depressive symptoms and QoL between the groups was based on analysis of variance adjusted for the patients' sex, age and BMI (ANCOVA). In addition, the effect size of the mean comparisons was estimated with the standardized Cohen's d coefficient ($|d| > 0.20$ was considered low, $|d| > 0.5$ was considered moderate and $|d| > 0.8$ was considered high) [42]. The level of significance was set at $p < 0.05$ for the main effects and the interaction. Relationships between clinical and metabolic data, different serum proteins or miRNA expression with the psychometric test results were analysed via Spearman's correlation test. All statistical analyses were performed using SPSS statistical software 26.0 (SPSS Inc., Chicago, IL, USA).

3. Results

3.1. Characteristics of Participants

Differences in clinical and metabolic variables before and 8 years after BS between the RYGB/BPD and SG groups are summarized in Table 1. Patients with poorer metabolic control and gastroesophageal reflux disease underwent RYGB/BPD. BS improved most of the anthropometric and biochemical variables in both experimental groups (Table 1).

Table 1. Clinical and metabolic variables for each bariatric surgery type, before (white rows) and 8 years after (grey rows) the intervention.

	RYGB/BPD	SG	*p*-Value
n (male/female)	41 (6/35)	49 (9/40)	0.64
Age at the time of surgery (years)	42.4 ± 9.8	44.3 ± 9	0.34
%EWL	58.5 ± 36.6	52.8 ± 25.7	0.071
%TWL	30.1 ± 13.4	24.7 ± 12.1	0.003
BMI (kg/m^2)	50.1 ± 7.8	48.6 ± 7.6	0.03
	34.8 ± 7.3 ***	36.1 ± 6.1 ***	0.66
Waist (cm)	133.7 ± 15.5	130.5 ± 15.1	0.05
	103.3 ± 18.1 ***	104.2 ± 15.5 ***	0.74
Hip (cm)	145.8 ± 17.2	144.5 ± 12.3	0.17
	117.4 ± 17 ***	121.5 ± 12.5 ***	0.27
Waist/hip ratio	0.93 ± 0.15	0.9 ± 0.09	0.53
	0.87 ± 0.09 *	0.86 ± 0.09 *	0.26
SBP (mmHg)	138.5 ± 19.8	133 ± 17.6	0.23
	118 ± 16.1 ***	130.9 ± 23.6	0.002
DBP (mmHg)	82.9 ± 12.4	80.8 ± 9	0.42
	67.7 ± 9.3 ***	72 ± 12.6 ***	0.02

Table 1. *Cont.*

	RYGB/BPD	SG	*p*-Value
Glucose (mg/dl)	111.9 ± 44.1	97.9 ± 27	0.01
	81.4 ± 9.9 ***	84.1 ± 9 ***	0.45
Insulin (mg/dl)	20.8 ± 11.7	15.9 ± 12.1	0.03
	7.8 ± 6.1 ***	9.9 ± 5.3 ***	0.10
HOMA-IR	6.2 ± 5	4.1 ± 3.4	0.003
	1.65 ± 1.6 ***	2.12 ± 1.3 ***	0.15
Triglycerides (mg/dl)	136.9 ± 89	118.6 ± 53.8	0.17
	87.6 ± 35.4 ***	89.8 ± 40.5 ***	0.62
Cholesterol (mg/dl)	190.2 ± 41.8	178 ± 34.7	0.16
	164.1 ± 40.2	197.6 ± 39.4	<0.001
HDL-c (mg/dl)	46.3 ± 14.4	44.3 ± 13.7	0.47
	61.9 ± 16.9 ***	66.8 ± 16.5 ***	0.18
LDL-c (mg/dl)	113.5 ± 31.2	110.6 ± 33.6	0.92
	84.5 ± 31.1 ***	112.3 ± 32.6	<0.001

Data are means ± SD. %EWL, percentage of excess weight lost; %TWL, percentage of total weight loss; BMI, body mass index; SBP, systolic blood pressure; DBP, diastolic blood pressure; HDL-c, high-density lipoprotein cholesterol; LDL-c, low-density lipoprotein cholesterol. *p*-value column represents the *p*-value between types of bariatric surgery. The significant effect of time (basal vs. 8 years after bariatric surgery) is represented as * $p < 0.05$ and *** $p < 0.005$.

Table 2 summarizes clinical and biochemical characteristics of patients classified by their response 8 years after BS (GR and NR). At baseline, significant differences were only found in terms of insulin and HOMA-IR, with the GR group showing higher values than the NR group. The GR group showed better anthropometric and metabolic values after BS than the NR group.

Table 2. Clinical and metabolic variables split by good responders vs. non-responders to bariatric surgery, before (white rows) and 8 years after (grey rows) bariatric surgery.

	Good Responders	Non-Responders	*p*-Value
n (male/female)	60 (9/51)	30 (6/24)	0.55
Type of surgery (RYGB-BPD/SG)	60 (28/32)	30 (12/18)	0.35
Age at the time of surgery (years)	42.5 ± 10.2	45.3 ± 7.5	0.19
%EWL	71.0 ± 14.7	23.0 ± 34.8	<0.001
%TWL	33.8 ± 7.3	13.8 ± 12.6	<0.001
BMI (kg/m^2)	48.8 ± 6.7	50 ± 9.3	0.55
	32.2 ± 4.6 ***	42.2 ± 4.9 ***	<0.001
Waist (cm)	132.2 ± 15.7	131.6 ± 14.6	0.87
	98.1 ± 15.9 ***	116.3 ± 12.2 ***	<0.001
Hip (cm)	145.9 ± 13	143.57 ± 17.6	0.49
	112.8 ± 12.1 ***	132.7931 ± 11.3 **	<0.001
Waist/hip ratio	0.91 ± 0.1	0.94 ± 0.2	0.34
	0.85 ± 0.09 ***	0.9 ± 0.1	0.48
SBP (mmHg)	135.4 ± 19.2	134.6 ± 18.1	0.87
	116.6 ± 15.7 ***	140 ± 23.7	<0.001
DBP (mmHg)	81.8 ± 10.7	79.6 ± 9.1	0.38
	67.1 ± 10.4 ***	75.4 ± 11.2	0.005

Table 2. *Cont.*

	Good Responders	Non-Responders	p-Value
Glucose (mg/dl)	108.1 ± 41.7	97 ± 19.9	0.11
	81 ± 6.9 ***	87.2 ± 12.4 **	0.02
Insulin (mg/dl)	20.5 ±13.8	14.5 ± 7.3	0.05
	7.6 ± 5.8 ***	11.5 ± 4.9 *	0.003
HOMA-IR	5.9 ± 5	3.6 ± 2.2	0.01
	1.6 ± 1.5 ***	2.5 ± 1.3 *	0.004
Triglycerides (mg/dl)	134.2 ± 78.7	112.9 ±55.4	0.20
	79.2 ± 29.7 ***	108.5 ± 46 **	0.004
Cholesterol (mg/dl)	184.9 ± 40.9	180.5 ± 33.7	0.61
	181.2 ± 44.5	185.6 ± 41.3	0.72
HDL-c (mg/dl)	44.8 ± 13.6	45.3 ± 14.7	0.95
	66.6 ± 17.9 ***	59.9 ± 13.4 ***	0.05
LDL-c (mg/dl)	110.9 ± 34.4	113.7 ± 29.2	0.68
	99.2 ±35.1 *	103.6 ±33.5 *	0.52

Data are means ± SD. %EWL, percentage of excess weight lost; %TWL, percentage of total weight loss; BMI, body mass index; SBP, systolic blood pressure; DBP, diastolic blood pressure; HDL-c, high-density lipoprotein cholesterol; LDL-c, low-density lipoprotein cholesterol. p-value column represents the p-value between types of bariatric surgery. The significant effect of time (basal vs. 8 years after bariatric surgery) is represented as * $p < 0.05$, ** $p < 0.01$ and *** $p < 0.005$.

3.2. Quality of Life and Depression at 8-Year Follow-Up after BS

No statistically significant differences were found between the two groups of BS techniques (RYGB/BPD and SG) in neither the level of depression (BDI-II), nor any of the perceived QoL scales (SF-36). Table 3 includes the ANCOVA (adjusted for sex, age and BMI) comparing SF-36 and BDI-II scores between the two groups based on their outcome (GR vs. NR). The GR group showed higher scores on the SF-36 scales of physical functioning ($p = 0.039$), role functioning—physical ($p = 0.008$), role functioning—emotional ($p = 0.013$) and body pain ($p = 0.029$), as well as higher scores on the global general health ($p = 0.020$), than the NR group. Analyses of the depression state did not show statistically significant differences between the NR and GR groups, although a trend was observed (Supplementary Figure S1).

Table 3. Comparison of depressive symptoms and quality of life based on the bariatric surgery outcome: ANCOVA adjusted by sex, age and BMI.

	Good Responders (n = 30)		Non-Responders (n = 23)			
	Mean	*SD*	*Mean*	*SD*	p	$\vert d \vert$
SF-36 Physical functioning	72.32	26.95	54.07	27.95	**0.039** *	**0.66** †
SF-36 Role—physical	74.71	40.97	37.52	42.80	**0.008** *	**0.89** †
SF-36 Body pain	59.63	20.80	43.27	24.48	**0.029** *	**0.72** †
SF-36 General health	70.97	23.29	59.75	22.15	0.129	**0.51** †
SF-36 Vitality	49.93	25.19	40.06	22.85	0.187	0.41
SF-36 Social functioning	82.04	23.21	65.12	28.51	0.054	**0.65** †
SF-36 Role—emotional	84.02	39.65	51.28	43.25	**0.013** *	**0.79** †
SF-36 Mental health	59.79	24.39	53.57	26.10	0.449	0.25
SF-36 Global general health	69.24	22.63	51.39	24.68	**0.020** *	**0.75** †
BDI-II Total	12.44	13.52	22.44	15.91	**0.040** *	**0.68** †

Note. SD: standard deviation. * Bold: significant comparison. † Bold: effect size in the mild to large range.

3.3. Association between Serum Protein Levels before and after Surgery vs. Psychological Variables

Since the relation between different adipocytokines and psychological variables have not been well studied in relation to the mental well-being of patients with class III obesity, these proteins were analysed at baseline and 8 years after BS (Figure 1). No significant correlations were found between psychometric tests results and the levels of different basal proteins (before BS) (Figure 1A). Figure 1B shows the heatmap of the correlations between protein levels 8 years after BS and the mental health of the patients. The Fatigue/Energy measurement positively correlated with CD14 and MMP3 (p = 0.012 and p = 0.048, respectively), whereas it negatively correlated with leptin (p = 0.025). Emotional well-being negatively correlated with leptin (p = 0.023) and ICAM-1 (p = 0.048), and positively with NRP1 (p = 0.038). Social functioning positively correlated with MBL (p = 0.023) and NRP1 (p = 0.046), and negatively with LYVE1 (p = 0.038). Pain measurement positively correlated with CD14 levels (p = 0.039), and negatively with ICAM-1 levels (p = 0.031).

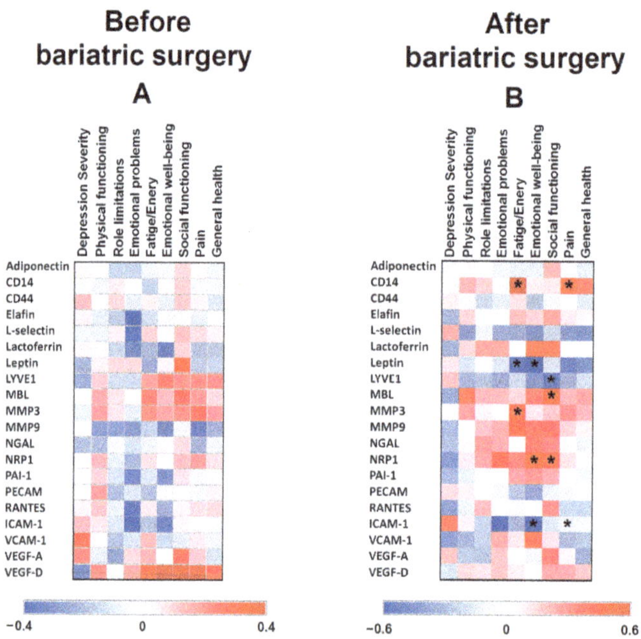

Figure 1. Heat maps representing associations between SF-36 and BDI-II scores vs. serum protein levels in patients with class III obesity before (**A**) and 8 years after bariatric surgery (**B**). The Spearman correlation is displayed on a colour scale from blue (negative correlation) to red (positive correlation). * Significant correlations ($p < 0.05$).

3.4. Association between Serum Protein Levels before and after Surgery vs. Bariatric Surgery Outcome

When these basal proteins were analysed according to BS outcome (Figure 2A), only leptin and MMP3 showed differences between the GR and NR groups, with the lowest levels in the NR group (p = 0.028 and p = 0.009, respectively). Figure 2B shows the heatmap of correlations between protein levels before BS and the %EWL of patients. Only MMP3 (p = 0.292) and NRP1 (p = 0.291) positively correlated with the %EWL of patients. Figure 2C shows the differences between the GR and NR groups in different protein levels 8 years after BS. Adiponectin (p = 0.001), ICAM-1 (p = 0.017), CD44 (p = 0.001) and NRP1 (p = 0.041) levels were lower in the NR group compared with the GR group, whereas the VEGF-D level was higher (p = 0.045). Figure 2D shows the heatmap of the correlations between protein levels 8 years after BS and the %EWL of patients. Adiponectin (p = 0.436), CD44

($p = 0.469$), MBL ($p = 0.392$), MMP3 ($p = 0.379$) and ICAM-1 ($p = 0.310$) positively correlated with the %EWL of patients.

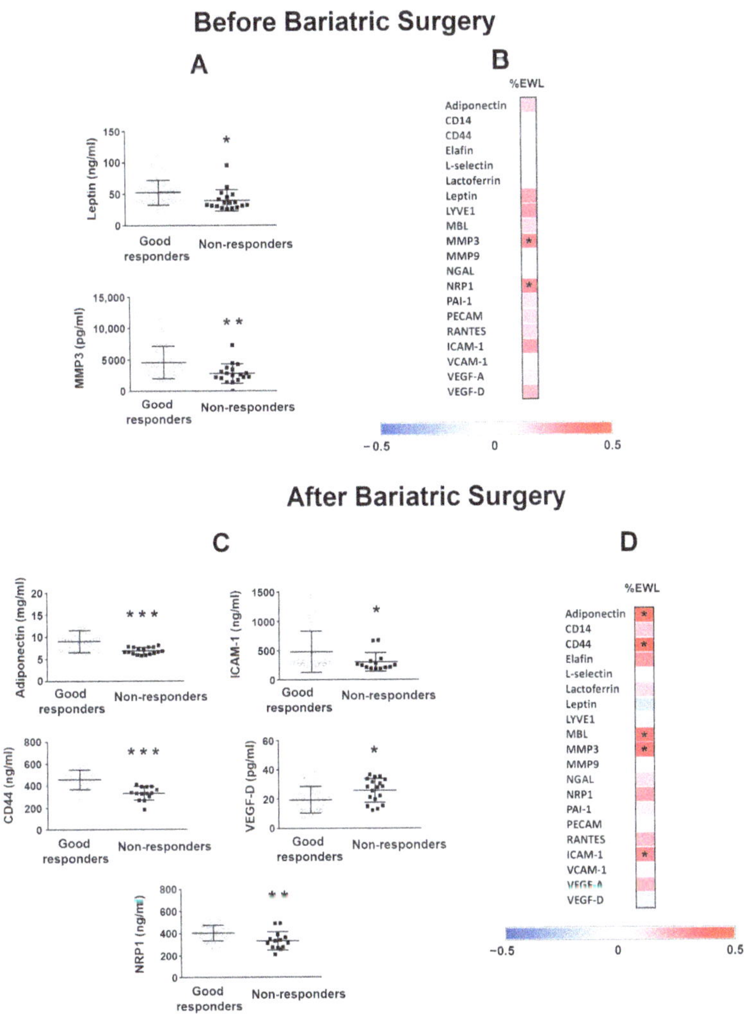

Figure 2. Levels of different proteins in patients with class III obesity before and 8 years after bariatric surgery. (**A**) Levels of basal serum leptin and MMP3 in patients with class III obesity classified depending on their outcome after bariatric surgery (good responders vs. non-responders). Data are expressed as the mean ± SD. Statistical significance is expressed as: * $p < 0.05$; ** $p < 0.01$. (**B**) The heat map represents the associations between basal serum protein levels and the percentage of excess weight lost (%EWL) 8 years after bariatric surgery. * Significant correlations ($p < 0.05$). (**C**) Levels of serum adiponectin, ICAM-1, CD44, VEGF-D and NRP1 in patients with class III obesity 8 years after bariatric surgery classified depending on their outcome after bariatric surgery (good responders vs. non-responders). Data are expressed as the mean ± SD. Statistical significance is expressed as: * $p < 0.05$; ** $p < 0.01$; *** $p < 0.001$. (**D**) The heat map represents the associations between serum proteins levels 8 years after bariatric surgery vs. %EWL 8 years after bariatric surgery. * Significant correlations ($p < 0.05$). The Spearman correlation is displayed on a colour scale from blue (negative correlation) to red (positive correlation).

3.5. *miRNA Levels as a Biomarker Predictor of Intervention Success in Patients with Class III Obesity*

Figure 3A shows different depression/anxiety-related miRNAs at basal levels obtained from serum samples from both groups (GR and NR).

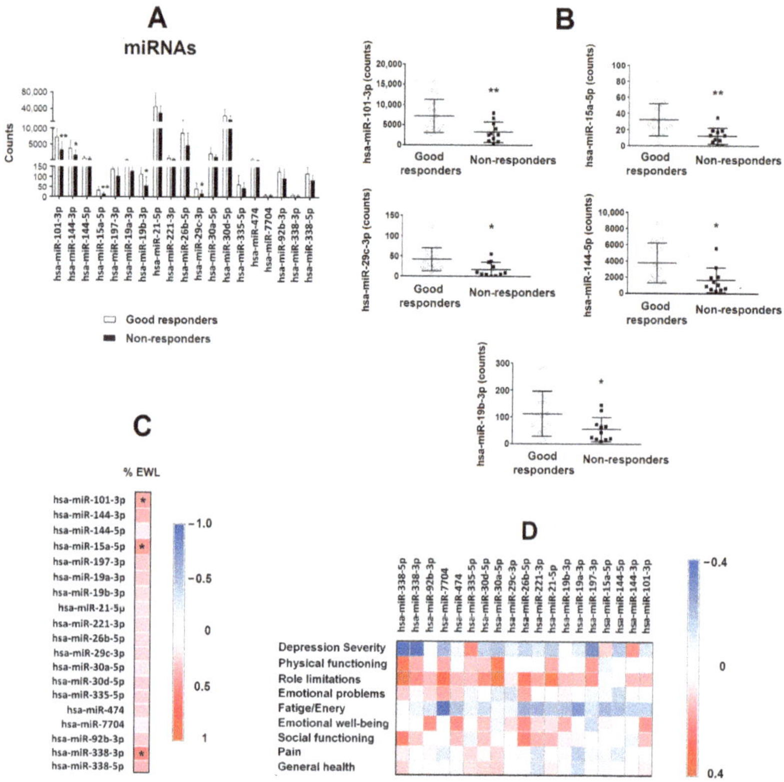

Figure 3. Serum miRNA levels as a predictive biomarker of bariatric surgery success in patients with class III obesity. (**A**) Different miRNAs related to depression and anxiety were evaluated by sequencing in the serum of patients with class III obesity before they underwent bariatric surgery. Patients were classified depending on their outcome after bariatric surgery (good responders vs. non-responders). Data are expressed as the mean ± SD. * $p < 0.05$; ** $p < 0.01$. (**B**) Levels of basal serum hsa-miR-101-3p, hsa-miR-15a-5p, hsa-miR-19b-3p, hsa-miR-29c-3p and hsa-miR-144-5p in patients with class III obesity, classified depending on their outcome after bariatric surgery (good responders vs. non-responders). Data are expressed as the mean ± SD. * $p < 0.05$; ** $p < 0.01$. (**C**) The heat map represents the associations between basal serum miRNAs levels and the percentage of excess weight lost (%EWL) 8 years after bariatric surgery. * Significant correlations ($p < 0.05$). (**D**) The heat map represents the association between basal serum miRNA levels and SF-36 and BDI-II scores. The Spearman correlation is displayed on a colour scale from blue (negative correlation) to red (positive correlation).

Lower levels of hsa-miR-101-3p ($p = 0.008$), hsa-miR-15a-5p ($p = 0.005$), hsa-miR-29c-3p ($p = 0.016$), hsa-miR-144-3p ($p = 0.018$) and hsa-miR-19b-3p ($p = 0.046$) were found in the NR group compared with the GR group (Figure 3B). No significant changes were found on the rest of miRNAs analysed. The heatmap (Figure 3C) shows the correlations between miRNAs at basal level and the %EWL of the patients. The %EWL was positively correlated with hsa-miR-101-3p ($p = 0.040$), hsa-miR-15a-5p ($p = 0.022$) and hsa-miR-338-3p ($p = 0.003$).

The variable that was associated with the response to BS (good responders = 0 and non-responders = 1) in a logistic regression model was hsa-miR-19b-3p ($\beta = 0.019$, $p = 0.041$, OR = 1.019, 95% IC = 1.001–1.037) after adjusting for sex, BMI and the other four miRNAs (hsa-miR-101-3p, hsa-miR-15a-5p, hsa-miR-29c-3p, hsa-miR-144-3p and hsa-miR-19b-3p).

To analyse the association between those basal miRNAs and the mental health of patients 8 years after BS, correlations were performed between miRNAs and the results of the different psychometric tests (Figure 3D). No significant associations were found.

4. Discussion

In this study, we sought to determine whether the %EWL is associated with QoL or depressive symptomatology in patients with class III obesity at the 8-year follow-up after BS, as well as its possible association with different serum proteins and miRNAs. The GR group showed higher scores on the SF-36 scales of physical functioning, role functioning—physical, role functioning—emotional and body pain, as well as higher scores on global general health, than the NR group. On the other hand, different adipocytokines showed significant correlations with patients' mental health and the %EWL 8 years after BS. In addition, the levels of several proteins were lower in the NR group at baseline and 8 years after BS. Moreover, different miRNAs were lower in the NR group, with hsa-miR-19b-3p being the miRNA most closely associated with the response to BS.

There are many studies focusing on the mental health of patients with obesity and how it changes after BS. The interesting contribution of this study is to analyse the data according to the percentage of weight loss instead of an analysis by surgical approach. Patients with a favourable outcome at the 8-year follow-up showed greater improvement in depression severity and in most of the QoL domains (such as physical functioning, role—physical, body pain, role—emotional, global general health and global index of QoL) than those with a poor outcome. These findings reinforce the fact that a successful BS can yield not only weight loss and stabilization of metabolic parameters, but also mental health and social improvements [16–18,43]. These results suggest that success in BS is associated with the recovery of daily activities that were previously physically and mentally limited, recovery and participation in social activities, less interference of pain with activities and household responsibilities, improvement of mood state and depressive symptoms and, in general, with a better perception of patients' own level of health and QoL. Likewise, in the group with poor outcome, the frustration of not achieving BS success and meeting weight loss expectations could also accentuate their psychological distress and poor perception of QoL. However, it seems that all findings follow the same path, suggesting that the improvement in QoL and depressive symptoms depends on the outcome of the BS.

In obesity, the presence of chronic low-grade systemic inflammation is well known. Some pro-inflammatory cytokines are associated with depression [25]. However, there are other serum proteins that are less studied and secreted by adipose tissue, which may also be associated with the regulation of inflammation, directly or indirectly, and other processes involved in mechanisms underlying depression. In the present study, different serum proteins were lower in the NR group compared with the GR group, mainly after BS. Moreover, most of those proteins positively correlated with the mental health of patients after BS. One interesting fact is the increased level of VEGF-D 8 years after the intervention in the NR group, who were the ones with the worst results in the psychometric tests. This angiogenic factor is elevated in the serum of overweight and obese individuals [44]. In obesity development, it has been shown that VEGF-D could be released in order to ameliorate the adipose tissue inflammation [44]. The higher level of VEGF-D found in the NR group could be due to an inadequate weight loss, per se. Regarding NRP1, the NR group showed lower levels than the GR group, and the correlation with the emotional well-being and social functioning was positive, which can explain why the NR group performed worse in the psychometric tests. This protein seems to protect against obesity and metabolic syndrome [45]. Another interesting fact was the decrease in adiponectin levels found in the NR compared with the GR group, since these have been related to atypical depression [46]. On the other hand, ICAM-1 is a pro-inflammatory molecule, which might be a useful biomarker for depression associated with vascular inflammation. This protein was negatively associated with emotional well-being. This is consistent with the hypothesis that depression can be secondary to vascular inflammation [47]. Together, our results show a group of proteins with different functions, some of them not clearly associated with the regulation of obesity, which seem to be associated with a favourable outcome at the 8-year follow-up. However, further in-depth investigations into their role in the regulation of weight and mental well-being of these patients are needed.

We were also able to identify a group of proteins, some of the above and others such as CD14, leptin, MBL and MMP3, which could be used as an indirect biomarker of mental illnesses, and which link different aspects of inflammation with the results of psychometric tests. CD14 is a surface antigen, which participates in the innate immune response to bacterial lipopolysaccharide. In this context, serum MBL is an important element in the innate immune system and recognizes the mannose and *N*-acetylglucosamine of a wide range of microbial microorganisms. These proteins would increase the systemic inflammation in response to different microbial components and may lead to neuroinflammation in the central nervous system [48]. This neuroinflammation is also induced by MMP3, an endogenous neuronal activator of microglia [49]. Also, plasma leptin has been negatively correlated, as in our case, with symptoms of anxiety and depression [50].

Regarding miRNAs, they were analysed to understand their predictive ability in patients with obesity undergoing different surgical approaches. Some studies show similarities with our data. For instance, hsa-miRNA-144-5p was downregulated in the NR group, who showed a higher percentage of depression. This has been also found in depressive patients compared with healthy individuals [51]. Looking at the miRNA serum expression per group of patients, most of them presented lower values in the NR vs. GR group, which may also explain the worse performance of this group during psychometric tests and their non-response to the intervention 8 years after. A previous study showed that lower levels of mRNAs were found in patients with depression [41]. The relationship between depression and obesity is reciprocal [18]. In this context, the significant miRNAs found in our study that are related to depression/anxiety could also be associated with the regulation of obesity. For example, several miRNAs, such as miR-144-5p, miR-15a-5p and miR-29c-3p, are associated with a response to a low-fat diet and with several metabolic processes, including glucose and lipid metabolism, adipocyte development and adipose tissue physiology, inflammatory pathways and weight gain [52]. Moreover, hsa-miR-15a-5p binds to CCND1 [53], which is a molecule regulated by FTO [54], a gene identified as a risk gene for obesity. Regarding hsa-miR-19b-3p, its expression changed after bariatric surgery, suggesting an association with the weight loss [55]. In our study, we have found that has-mir-19b-3p was the miRNA more closely associated with a good response 8 years after BS. Serum miR-19b-3p upregulation was found to inhibit the lipopolysaccharide-induced expression of pro-inflammatory cytokines IL-6 and TNF-α [56]. Another study found that miR-19b-3p attenuated the inflammatory injury [57], and that the upregulation of circulating miR-19b-3p suppressed fibrogenesis in the liver by regulating inflammation [58]. The interesting contribution of our study is the finding that most of these miRNAs could be used as predictors of the response to BS in a non-invasive way, which is the main goal of the personalized medicine approach, and more specifically, we could suggest that miR-19b-3p, an miRNA related to depression/anxiety, would be involved in achieving a good response to BS.

The main limitation of this retrospective study is the lack of psychometric tests before BS, which would be interesting to have had in order to know if depressive symptoms observed in the non-responders group were already present before BS and if therefore, these patients did not achieve a positive response after BS. Moreover, the number of participants is quite limited, so results should be further validated in additional cohorts of patients. Overall, although some caution should be exercised with the results obtained, they can give us preliminary information of some relevance. Another limitation of the study is the non-use of the %TWL instead of the %EWL to classify patients. In this study, we wanted to show whether the loss of excess weight needed to be considered normal weight can be related to QoL/depression, miRNAs related to the latter pathology or adipocytokines. The perception that obesity is still present or that one's weight is in the normal range (BMI greater than or equal to 18.5 to 24.9 kg/m^2), and not only the amount of weight loss, is of great importance for the state of depression [14]. In this regard, it is true that recent guidelines recommend the use of the %TWL [59] because this index seems to be less influenced by the baseline BMI during short-term follow-ups after SG and RYGB [60]. However, to date, there are no perfect indices for reporting weight loss outcomes after BS that are completely independent of the baseline BMI. When the %EWL is used, patients with a lower BMI have significantly "better" weight loss outcomes [60]. However, from 9 months after surgery, results using the %TWL have shown a significant trend of better outcomes for patients with higher BMI, especially in the case of RYGB [60]. Furthermore, the cut-off point for the %TWL is unclear, with some studies using 20% [61–64] and others using 25% [65–67]. A comparison of the obtained results relating to QoL/depression, miRNAs and adipocytokines with these two indices, %EWL vs. %TWL, is not the aim of the present study. This needs to be further analysed in other studies and with a larger number of participants. On the other hand, recent studies show that the information provided by body composition techniques for determining body fat percentage, such as bioelectrical impedance analysis, dual-energy X-ray absorptiometry, plethysmography or magnetic resonance imaging [68], may be more relevant than that provided by BMI. These new techniques make it possible to detect the presence of a condition with important functional implications, consisting of the simultaneous presence of excess adiposity and a deficit in skeletal muscle mass and function (sarcopenia), which is defined as sarcopenic obesity [69,70]. This medical condition is highly correlated with an increased risk of obesity-related comorbidities [69] and is associated with increased mortality [71]. However, there are hardly any studies using these techniques to analyse body composition and QoL in long-term follow-up of patients undergoing BS [72].

5. Conclusions

Taking into consideration all this information, we can outline two main conclusions. First, the mental health of the individual after BS is limited by the success of the intervention. Second, we showed that the expression of basal serum miRNAs related to depression/anxiety could predict the success of bariatric surgery in patients with class III obesity. Further investigation would be appropriate to assess whether these proteins and miRNAs before bariatric surgery could indicate whether class III obesity could lead to symptoms of depression/anxiety.

Supplementary Materials: The following supporting information can be downloaded at: https://www.mdpi.com/article/10.3390/nu15194109/s1, Figure S1: Pie charts representing the severity of depression at 8-year follow-up after bariatric surgery in percentage out of the total number of patients (good responders vs. non-responders groups).

Author Contributions: V.M., Z.A., M.D.A.-B., R.G., F.M.-R., A.S.-G., W.O.-O., M.T., F.J.M.-R., R.S.-H., J.L.F.-S., P.S.-G., J.M.M.-M., R.S.-M., F.F.-A., E.G.-F., F.J.T. and L.G.-S.: investigation, M.D.A.-B., A.S.-G., R.S.-H. and W.O.-O.: Data curation; V.M., Z.A. and R.G.: formal analysis. V.M., F.M.-R., E.G.-F. and L.G.-S.: Metodology; F.J.T., E.G.-F., F.F.-A. and L.G.-S.: Conceptualization and resources; F.J.T., E.G.-F. and L.G.-S.: Supervision; V.M., Z.A., E.G.-F. and L.G.-S.: writing—review and editing draft. All authors have read and agreed to the published version of the manuscript.

Funding: This study has been co-funded by UMA20-FEDERJA-144 (Malaga University, Malaga, Spain), PI-0194-2017 (Consejeria de Salud y Familia, Junta de Andalucia, Spain) and FEDER funds ("A way to make Europe"). L.G.-S. and E.G.-F. are supported by the Nicolas Monardes program from the Consejería de Salud de Andalucía (Spain) (C-0028-2018, RC-005-2020, respectively). VM and W.O.-O. are supported by a grant from the Consejería de Transformación Económica, Industria, Conocimiento y Universidades de Junta de Andalucía (Spain) (DOC_00288 and DOC_01095, respectively). F.M.-R. is supported by a grant from the ISCIII (Spain) ("PFIS" program, FI19/00189).

Institutional Review Board Statement: The study was conducted in accordance with the Declaration of Helsinki and approved by the Malaga Provincial Research Ethics Committee of the Biomedical Research Institute of Malaga (IBIMA) (protocol code PI-0194-2017 (1 February 2018)).

Informed Consent Statement: Informed consent was obtained from all subjects involved in the study.

Data Availability Statement: The data presented in this study are available on request from the corresponding author. The data are not publicly available due to ethical reasons.

Acknowledgments: CIBER Fisiopatología de la Obesidad y Nutrición (CIBEROBN) and CIBER Enfermedades Hepáticas y Digestivas (CIBERehd) are ISCIII projects (Spain).

Conflicts of Interest: The authors declare that they have no conflict of interest.

References

1. World Health Organization, Updated 9 June 2021. Available online: https://www.who.int/news-room/fact-sheets/detail/obesity-and-overweight (accessed on 25 May 2022).
2. Golzarand, M.; Toolabi, K.; Farid, R. The bariatric surgery and weight losing: A meta-analysis in the long- and very long-term effects of laparoscopic adjustable gastric banding, laparoscopic Roux-en-Y gastric bypass and laparoscopic sleeve gastrectomy on weight loss in adults. *Surg. Endosc.* **2017**, *31*, 4331–4345. [CrossRef] [PubMed]
3. Closs, C.; Ackerman, M.; Masson, W.; Lobo, M.; Molinero, G.; Lavalle-Cobo, A.; Béliard, S.; Mourre, F.; Valéro, R.; Nogueira, J.P. Effectiveness of Roux-en-Y Gastric Bypass vs. Sleeve Gastrectomy on Lipid Levels in Type 2 Diabetes: A Meta-analysis. *J. Gastrointest. Surg.* **2022**, *26*, 1575–1584. [CrossRef] [PubMed]
4. Di Lorenzo, N.; Antoniou, S.A.; Batterham, R.L.; Busetto, L.; Godoroja, D.; Iossa, A.; Carrano, F.M.; Agresta, F.; Alarçon, I.; Azran, C.; et al. Clinical practice guidelines of the European Association for Endoscopic Surgery (EAES) on bariatric surgery: Update 2020 endorsed by IFSO-EC, EASO and ESPCOP. *Surg. Endosc.* **2020**, *34*, 2332–2358. [CrossRef] [PubMed]
5. Buchwald, H.; Avidor, Y.; Braunwald, E.; Jensen, M.D.; Pories, W.; Fahrbach, K.; Schoelles, K. Bariatric surgery: A systematic review and meta-analysis. *JAMA* **2004**, *292*, 1724–1737. [CrossRef] [PubMed]
6. Axer, S.; Szabo, E.; Näslund, I. Non-response After Gastric Bypass and Sleeve Gastrectomy-the Theoretical Need for Revisional Bariatric Surgery: Results from the Scandinavian Obesity Surgery Registry. *Obes. Surg.* **2023**, *33*, 2973–2980. [CrossRef] [PubMed]
7. Riedel, O.; Braitmaier, M.; Dankhoff, M.; Hornschuch, M.; Klein, M.; Zachariassen, W.; Hoyer, J. Quality of life in bariatric patients up to twelve years after surgery—Results from a nationwide retrospective cohort study. *Obes. Res. Clin. Pract.* **2023**, *17*, 353–360. [CrossRef] [PubMed]
8. Lammert, M.; Medawar, E.; Hartmann, H.; Grasser, L.; Dietrich, A.; Fenske, W.; Horstmann, A. Distinct adaptations of endocrine and cognitive functions may contribute to high variability in long-term weight loss outcome after bariatric surgery. *Physiol. Behav.* **2023**, *269*, 114279. [CrossRef] [PubMed]
9. Grönroos, S.; Helmiö, M.; Juuti, A.; Tiusanen, R.; Hurme, S.; Löyttyniemi, E.; Ovaska, J.; Leivonen, M.; Peromaa-Haavisto, P.; Mäklin, S.; et al. Effect of Laparoscopic Sleeve Gastrectomy vs Roux-en-Y Gastric Bypass on Weight Loss and Quality of Life at 7 Years in Patients with Morbid Obesity: The SLEEVEPASS Randomized Clinical Trial. *JAMA Surg.* **2021**, *156*, 137–146. [CrossRef]
10. Askari, A.; Dai, D.; Taylor, C.; Chapple, C.; Halai, S.; Patel, K.; Mamidanna, R.; Munasinghe, A.; Rashid, F.; Al-Taan, O.; et al. Long-Term Outcomes and Quality of Life at More than 10 Years After Laparoscopic Roux-en-Y Gastric Bypass Using Bariatric Analysis and Reporting Outcome System (BAROS). *Obes. Surg.* **2020**, *30*, 3968–3973. [CrossRef]
11. Hany, M.; Zidan, A.; Sabry, K.; Ibrahim, M.; Agayby, A.S.S.; Aboelsoud, M.R.; Torensma, B. How Good is Stratification and Prediction Model Analysis Between Primary and Revisional Roux-en-Y Gastric Bypass Surgery? A Multi-center Study and Narrative Review. *Obes. Surg.* **2023**, *33*, 1431–1448. [CrossRef]
12. Suh, H.R.; Mui, J.; Cheng, E.; Liu, D.; Sun, S.L.; Loi, K.; Magdy, M.; Gagner, M. Outcomes of single anastomosis duodeno ileal bypass and single anastomosis stomach ileal bypass for type II diabetes: A systematic review. *Expert. Rev. Endocrinol. Metab.* **2023**, *18*, 337–346. [CrossRef] [PubMed]
13. Ali, M.; Wang, Y.; Ji, J.; Wang, W.; Wang, D. One Anastomosis Gastric Bypass Versus Sleeve Gastrectomy for Obesity: A Systemic Review and Meta-analysis. *J. Gastrointest. Surg.* **2023**. [CrossRef] [PubMed]
14. Admiraal, W.M.; Celik, F.; Gerdes, V.E.; Dallal, R.M.; Hoekstra, J.B.; Holleman, F. Ethnic differences in weight loss and diabetes remission after bariatric surgery: A meta-analysis. *Diabetes. Care.* **2012**, *35*, 1951–1958. [CrossRef] [PubMed]
15. Calderone, A.; Calabro, P.F.; Lippi, C.; Jaccheri, R.; Vitti, J.; Santini, F. Psychopathological Behaviour and Cognition in Morbid Obesity. *Recent. Pat. Endocr. Metab. Immune. Drug. Discov.* **2017**, *10*, 112–118. [CrossRef] [PubMed]
16. Luppino, F.S.; de Wit, L.M.; Bouvy, P.F.; Stijnen, T.; Cuijpers, P.; Penninx, B.W.; Zitman, F.G. Overweight, obesity, and depression: A systematic review and meta-analysis of longitudinal studies. *Arch. Gen. Psychiatry.* **2010**, *67*, 220–229. [CrossRef] [PubMed]
17. Sierżantowicz, R.; Ładny, J.R.; Lewko, J. Quality of Life after Bariatric Surgery-A Systematic Review. *Int. J. Environ. Res. Public. Health.* **2022**, *19*, 9078. [CrossRef] [PubMed]

18. Małczak, P.; Mizera, M.; Lee, Y.; Pisarska-Adamczyk, M.; Wysocki, M.; Bała, M.M.; Witowski, J.; Rubinkiewicz, M.; Dudek, A.; Stefura, T. Quality of Life After Bariatric Surgery-a Systematic Review with Bayesian Network Meta-analysis. *Obes. Surg.* **2021**, *31*, 5213–5223. [CrossRef] [PubMed]
19. Wimmelmann, C.L.; Dela, F.; Mortensen, E.L. Psychological predictors of mental health and health-related quality of life after bariatric surgery: A review of the recent research. *Obes. Res. Clin. Pract.* **2014**, *8*, e314–e324. [CrossRef]
20. Averbukh, Y.; Heshka, S.; El-Shoreya, H.; Flancbaum, L.; Geliebter, A.; Kamel, S.; Pi-Sunyer, F.X.; Laferrère, B. Depression score predicts weight loss following Roux-en-Y gastric bypass. *Obes. Surg.* **2003**, *13*, 833–836. [CrossRef]
21. Aguera, Z.; García-Ruiz-de-Gordejuela, A.; Vilarrasa, N.; Sanchez, I.; Baño, M.; Camacho, L.; Granero, R.; Jiménez-Murcia, S.; Virgili, N.; Lopez-Urdiales, R.; et al. Psychological and Personality Predictors of Weight Loss and Comorbid Metabolic Changes After Bariatric Surgery. *Eur. Eat. Disord. Rev.* **2015**, *23*, 509–516. [CrossRef]
22. Atlantis, E.; Baker, M. Obesity effects on depression: Systematic review of epidemiological studies. *Int. J. Obes.* **2008**, *32*, 881–891. [CrossRef]
23. Roberts, R.E.; Duong, H.T. Does major depression affect risk for adolescent obesity? *J. Affect Disord.* **2015**, *186*, 162–167. [CrossRef] [PubMed]
24. Patist, C.M.; Stapelberg, N.J.C.; Du Toit, E.F.; Headrick, J.P. The brain-adipocyte-gut network: Linking obesity and depression subtypes. *Cogn. Affect Behav. Neurosci.* **2018**, *18*, 1121–1144. [CrossRef] [PubMed]
25. Raison, C.L.; Capuron, L.; Miller, A.H. Cytokines sing the blues: Inflammation and the pathogenesis of depression. *Trends. Immunol.* **2006**, *27*, 24–31. [CrossRef] [PubMed]
26. Stapelberg, N.J.C.; Neumann, D.L.; Shum, D.H.K.; McConnell, H.; Hamilton-Craig, I. From physiome to pathome: A systems biology model of major depressive disorder and the psycho-immune-neuroendocrine network. *Curr. Psychiatry Rev.* **2015**, *11*, 32–62. [CrossRef]
27. Elovainio, M.; Aalto, A.M.; Kivimäki, M.; Pirkola, S.; Sundvall, J.; Lönnqvist, J.; Reunanen, A. Depression and C-reactive protein: Population-based Health 2000 Study. *Psychosom. Med.* **2009**, *71*, 423–430. [CrossRef] [PubMed]
28. Gimeno, D.; Kivimäki, M.; Brunner, E.J.; Elovainio, M.; De Vogli, R.; Steptoe, A.; Kumari, M.; Lowe, G.D.; Rumley, A.; Marmot, M.G.; et al. Associations of C-reactive protein and interleukin-6 with cognitive symptoms of depression: 12-year follow-up of the Whitehall II study. *Psychol. Med.* **2009**, *39*, 413–423. [CrossRef]
29. Serna-Rodríguez, M.F.; Bernal-Vega, S.; de la Barquera, J.A.O.; Camacho-Morales, A.; Pérez-Maya, A.A. The role of damage associated molecular pattern molecules (DAMPs) and permeability of the blood-brain barrier in depression and neuroinflammation. *J. Neuroimmunol.* **2022**, *371*, 577951. [CrossRef]
30. Wang, Y.; Xu, J.; Liu, Y.; Li, Z.; Li, X. TLR4-NF-κB Signal Involved in Depressive-Like Behaviors and Cytokine Expression of Frontal Cortex and Hippocampus in Stressed C57BL/6 and ob/ob Mice. *Neural. Plast.* **2018**, *2018*, 7254016. [CrossRef]
31. Ouakinin, S.R.S.; Barreira, D.P.; Gois, C.J. Depression and Obesity: Integrating the Role of Stress, Neuroendocrine Dysfunction and Inflammatory Pathways. *Front. Endocrinol.* **2018**, *9*, 431. [CrossRef]
32. Ferrua, C.P.; Giorgi, R.; da Rosa, L.C.; do Amaral, C.C.; Ghisleni, G.C.; Pinheiro, R.T.; Nedel, F. MicroRNAs expressed in depression and their associated pathways: A systematic review and a bioinformatics analysis. *J. Chem. Neuroanat.* **2019**, *100*, 101650. [CrossRef] [PubMed]
33. Ortiz-Dosal, A.; Rodil-García, P.; Salazar-Olivo, L.A. Circulating microRNAs in human obesity: A systematic review. *Biomarkers* **2019**, *24*, 499–509. [CrossRef] [PubMed]
34. Rasheed, M.; Asghar, R.; Firdoos, S.; Ahmad, N.; Nazir, A.; Ullah, K.M.; Li, N.; Zhuang, F.; Chen, Z.; Deng, Y. A Systematic Review of Circulatory microRNAs in Major Depressive Disorder: Potential Biomarkers for Disease Prognosis. *Int. J. Mol. Sci.* **2022**, *23*, 1294. [CrossRef] [PubMed]
35. De Hollanda, A.; Ruiz, T.; Jimenez, A.; Flores, L.; Lacy, A.; Vidal, J. Patterns of Weight Loss Response Following Gastric Bypass and Sleeve Gastrectomy. *Obes. Surg.* **2015**, *25*, 1177–1183. [CrossRef] [PubMed]
36. Christou, N.V.; Look, D.; Maclean, L.D. Weight gain after short- and long-limb gastric bypass in patients followed for longer than 10 years. *Ann. Surg.* **2006**, *244*, 734–740. [CrossRef]
37. Brethauer, S.A.; Kim, J.; el Chaar, M.; Papasavas, P.; Eisenberg, D.; Rogers, A.; Ballem, N.; Kligman, M.; Kothari, S.; ASMBS Clinical Issues Committee. Standardized outcomes reporting in metabolic and bariatric surgery. *Surg. Obes. Relat. Dis.* **2015**, *11*, 489–506. [CrossRef] [PubMed]
38. Ware, J.E., Jr.; Sherbourne, C.D. The MOS 36-item short-form health survey (SF-36). I. Conceptual framework and item selection. *Med. Care* **1992**, *30*, 473–483. [CrossRef] [PubMed]
39. Beck, A.T.; Epstein, N.; Brown, G.; Steer, R.A. An inventory for measuring clinical anxiety: Psychometric properties. *J. Consult. Clin. Psychol.* **1988**, *56*, 893–897. [CrossRef]
40. Dwivedi, Y. MicroRNAs in depression and suicide: Recent insights and future perspectives. *J. Affect Disord.* **2018**, *240*, 146–154. [CrossRef]
41. Wingo, T.S.; Yang, J.; Fan, W.; Canon, S.M.; Gerasimov, E.S.; Lori, A.; Logsdon, B.; Yao, B.; Seyfried, N.T.; Lah, J.; et al. Brain microRNAs associated with late-life depressive symptoms are also associated with cognitive trajectory and dementia. *NPJ Genom. Med.* **2020**, *5*, 6. [CrossRef]
42. Lachowicz, M.J.; Preacher, K.J.; Kelley, K. A novel measure of effect size for mediation analysis. *Psychol. Methods* **2018**, *23*, 244–261. [CrossRef] [PubMed]

43. Silha, J.V.; Krsek, M.; Sucharda, P.; Murphy, L.J. Angiogenic factors are elevated in overweight and obese individuals. *Int. J. Obes.* **2005**, *29*, 1308–1314. [CrossRef] [PubMed]
44. Chakraborty, A.; Barajas, S.; Lammoglia, G.M.; Reyna, A.J.; Morley, T.S.; Johnson, J.A.; Scherer, P.E.; Rutkowski, J.M. Vascular Endothelial Growth Factor-D (VEGF-D) Overexpression and Lymphatic Expansion in Murine Adipose Tissue Improves Metabolism in Obesity. *Am. J. Pathol.* **2019**, *189*, 924–939. [CrossRef] [PubMed]
45. Wilson, A.M.; Shao, Z.; Grenier, V.; Mawambo, G.; Daudelin, J.-F.; Dejda, A.; Pilon, F.; Popovic, N.; Boulet, S.; Parinot, C.; et al. Neuropilin-1 expression in adipose tissue macrophages protects against obesity and metabolic syndrome. *Sci. Immunol.* **2018**, *3*, eaan4626. [CrossRef] [PubMed]
46. Lamers, F.; Bot, M.; Jansen, R.; Chan, M.K.; Cooper, J.D.; Bahn, S.; Penninx, B.W.J.H. Serum proteomic profiles of depressive subtypes. *Transl. Psychiatry* **2016**, *6*, e851. [CrossRef] [PubMed]
47. Kalkman, H.O. The Association Between Vascular Inflammation and Depressive Disorder. Causality, Biomarkers and Targeted Treatment. *Pharmaceuticals* **2020**, *13*, 92. [CrossRef] [PubMed]
48. Suda, K.; Matsuda, K. How Microbes Affect Depression: Underlying Mechanisms via the Gut-Brain Axis and the Modulating Role of Probiotics. *Int. J. Mol. Sci.* **2022**, *23*, 1172. [CrossRef] [PubMed]
49. Connolly, C.; Magnusson-Lind, A.; Lu, G.; Wagner, P.K.; Southwell, A.L.; Hayden, M.R.; Björkqvist, M.; Leavitt, B.R. Enhanced immune response to MMP3 stimulation in microglia expressing mutant huntingtin. *Neuroscience* **2016**, *325*, 74–88. [CrossRef]
50. Fulton, S.; Décarie-Spain, L.; Fioramonti, X.; Guiard, B.; Nakajima, S. The menace of obesity to depression and anxiety prevalence. *Trends. Endocrinol. Metab.* **2022**, *33*, 18–35. [CrossRef]
51. Wang, X.; Sundquist, K.; Hedelius, A.; Palmer, K.; Memon, A.A.; Sundquist, J. Circulating microRNA-144-5p is associated with depressive disorders. *Clin. Epigenetics* **2015**, *7*, 69. [CrossRef]
52. Assmann, T.S.; Riezu-Boj, J.I.; Milagro, F.I.; Martínez, J.A. Circulating adiposity-related microRNAs as predictors of the response to a low-fat diet in subjects with obesity. *J. Cell. Mol. Med.* **2020**, *24*, 2956–2967. [CrossRef] [PubMed]
53. Yao, J.; Wang, Z.; Cheng, Y.; Ma, C.; Zhong, Y.; Xiao, Y.; Gao, X.; Li, Z. M2 macrophage-derived exosomal microRNAs inhibit cell migration and invasion in gliomas through PI3K/AKT/mTOR signaling pathway. *J. Transl. Med.* **2021**, *19*, 99. [CrossRef] [PubMed]
54. Hirayama, M.; Wei, F.Y.; Chujo, T.; Oki, S.; Yakita, M.; Kobayashi, D.; Araki, N.; Takahashi, N.; Yoshida, R.; Nakayama, H.; et al. FTO Demethylates Cyclin D1 mRNA and Controls Cell-Cycle Progression. *Cell Rep.* **2020**, *31*, 107464. [CrossRef] [PubMed]
55. Langi, G.; Szczerbinski, L.; Kretowski, A. Meta-Analysis of Differential miRNA Expression after Bariatric Surgery. *J. Clin. Med.* **2019**, *8*, 1220. [CrossRef]
56. Huimin, X.; Xiuwu, L.; Huaijun, N. Clinical significance of miR-19b-3p in patients with sepsis and its regulatory role in the LPS-induced inflammatory response. *Eur. J. Med. Res.* **2020**, *25*, 9.
57. Liang, D.; Dapeng, D.; Wenbo, W.; Zhengming, S.; Honghai, X.; Lipeng, G.; Xuanhui, W. MiR-19b-3p attenuates IL-1β induced extracellular matrix degradation and inflammatory injury in chondrocytes by targeting GRK6. *Mol. Cell Biochem.* **2019**, *459*, 205–214.
58. Lan, T.; Lim, C.; Yang, G.; Sun, Y.; Zhuang, L.; Ou, Y.; Li, H.; Wang, G.; Kisseleva, T.; Brenner, D.; et al. Sphingosine kinase 1 promotes liver fibrosis by preventing miR-19b-3p-mediated inhibition of CCR2. *Hepatology* **2018**, *68*, 1070–1086. [CrossRef]
59. Van Rijswijk, A.S.; van Olst, N.; Schats, W.; van der Peet, D.L.; van de Laar, A.W. What Is Weight Loss After Bariatric Surgery Expressed in Percentage Total Weight Loss (%TWL)? A Systematic Review. *Obes. Surg.* **2021**, *31*, 3833–3847. [CrossRef]
60. Ching, S.S.; Lee, P.C.; Lim, C.H.; Wong, A.S.Y.; Ng, A.Y.; Lin, J.; Lee, J. Study on weight loss outcomes after bariatric surgery to determine a metric least influenced by preoperative BMI. *Int. J. Obes.* **2023**, *47*, 993–999. [CrossRef]
61. Yarigholi, F.; Bahardoust, M.; Mosavari, H.; Tehrani, F.M.; Gholizadeh, H.; Shahmiri, S.S.; Rezvani, H.; Oshidari, B.; Garakani, K.; Eghbali, F. Predictors of Weight Regain and Insufficient Weight Loss According to Different Definitions After Sleeve Gastrectomy: A Retrospective Analytical Study. *Obes. Surg.* **2022**, *32*, 4040–4046. [CrossRef]
62. Saiki, A.; Yamaguchi, T.; Tanaka, S.; Sasaki, A.; Naitoh, T.; Seto, Y.; Matsubara, H.; Yokote, K.; Okazumi, S.; Ugi, S.; et al. Background characteristics and postoperative outcomes of insufficient weight loss after laparoscopic sleeve gastrectomy in Japanese patients. *Ann. Gastroenterol. Surg.* **2019**, *3*, 638–647. [CrossRef] [PubMed]
63. Van de Laar, A.W.; Nienhuijs, S.W.; Apers, J.A.; van Rijswijk, A.S.; de Zoete, J.P.; Gadiot, R.P. The Dutch bariatric weight loss chart: A multicenter tool to assess weight outcome up to 7 years after sleeve gastrectomy and laparoscopic Roux-en-Y gastric bypass. *Surg. Obes. Relat. Dis.* **2019**, *15*, 200–210. [CrossRef] [PubMed]
64. Sanchez-Cordero, S.; Garcia Ruiz de Gordejuela, A.; Vilallonga, R.; Gonzalez, O.; Ciscar, A.; Ciudin, A.; Zabalegui, A.; Armengol, M. Analysis of the Variability in Different Criteria to Define the Success of Bariatric Surgery: Retrospective Study 5-Year Follow-Up after Sleeve Gastrectomy and Roux-en-Y Gastric Bypass. *J. Clin. Med.* **2022**, *12*, 187. [CrossRef] [PubMed]
65. Li, Z.; Chen, G.; Wang, L.; Wuyun, Q.; Sang, Q.; Wang, J.; Tian, C.; Shang, M.; Wang, Z.; Du, D.; et al. Analysis of Correlation between Age and Satisfied Total Weight Loss Percentage Outcome at 1 Year after Bariatric Surgery using the Restricted Cubic Spline Function: A Retrospective Study in China. *Obes. Surg.* **2023**, *33*, 3133–3140. [CrossRef] [PubMed]
66. Kapała, J.; Maroszczuk, T.; Lewandowska, J.; Lech, P.; Dowgiałło-Gornowicz, N. Weight Regain in the Second Year after Sleeve Gastrectomy Could Be a Predictor of Long-Term Outcomes? *Medicina* **2023**, *59*, 766. [CrossRef] [PubMed]
67. Tu, Y.; Pan, Y.; Han, J.; Pan, J.; Zhang, P.; Jia, W.; Bao, Y.; Yu, H. A total weight loss of 25% shows better predictivity in evaluating the efficiency of bariatric surgery. *Int. J. Obes.* **2021**, *45*, 396–403. [CrossRef] [PubMed]

68. Holmes, C.J.; Racette, S.B. The Utility of Body Composition Assessment in Nutrition and Clinical Practice: An Overview of Current Methodology. *Nutrients* **2021**, *13*, 2493. [CrossRef]
69. Salmón-Gómez, L.; Catalán, V.; Frühbeck, G.; Gómez-Ambrosi, J. Relevance of body composition in phenotyping the obesities. *Rev. Endocr. Metab. Disord.* **2023**, *24*, 809–823. [CrossRef]
70. Bray, G.A. Beyond BMI. *Nutrients* **2023**, *15*, 2254. [CrossRef]
71. Von Berens, Å.; Obling, S.R.; Nydahl, M.; Koochek, A.; Lissner, L.; Skoog, I.; Frändin, K.; Skoglund, E.; Rothenberg, E.; Cederholm, T. Sarcopenic obesity and associations with mortality in older women and men—A prospective observational study. *BMC Geriatr.* **2020**, *20*, 199. [CrossRef]
72. Simó-Servat, A.; Ibarra, M.; Libran, M.; Quirós, C.; Puértolas, N.; Alonso, N.; Perea, V.; Simó, R.; Barahona, M.J. Usefulness of Ultrasound in Assessing the Impact of Bariatric Surgery on Body Composition: A Pilot Study. *Obes. Surg.* **2023**, *33*, 1211–1217. [CrossRef]

nutrients

MDPI

Article

Effect of Moderate-Intense Training and Detraining on Glucose Metabolism, Lipid Profile, and Liver Enzymes in Male Wistar Rats: A Preclinical Randomized Study

Hira Shakoor [1], Jaleel Kizhakkayil [1], Mariyam Khalid [2], Amar Mahgoub [3] and Carine Platat [1,*]

[1] Department of Nutrition and Health, College of Medicine and Health Sciences, United Arab Emirates University, Al Ain P.O. Box 15551, United Arab Emirates; 201890012@uaeu.ac.ae (H.S.)
[2] Department of Pharmacology, College of Medicine and Health Sciences, Khalifa University, Abu Dhabi P.O. Box 127788, United Arab Emirates
[3] Department of Pharmacology and Therapeutics, College of Medicine and Health Sciences, United Arab Emirates University, Al Ain P.O. Box 15551, United Arab Emirates
[*] Correspondence: platatcarine@uaeu.ac.ae

Abstract: Exercise training positively regulates glucose metabolism. This study investigated the impact of training and detraining on glucose metabolism, lipid profiles, and liver enzymes. Twenty-six rats completed an initial 4-week moderate-intense training (T0–T4). Then, the animals were randomly assigned to two groups at the end of week 4: AT4: detraining for 8 weeks; AT8: training for 8 weeks and 4-week detraining. Six animals were sacrificed at T0 and T4, four animals/group at T8, and three/group at T12. The study continued for 12 weeks, and all parameters were assessed at T0, T4, T8, and T12. IPGTT significantly improved after 4 weeks of training ($p < 0.01$) and was further reduced in AT8 at T8. In AT8, 8-week training significantly reduced total cholesterol at T4 and T12 vs. T0 ($p < 0.05$), LDL at T4, T8, and T12 vs. T0 ($p < 0.01$), ALP at T8, T12 vs. T0 ($p < 0.01$), and increased HDL at T8 and ALT at T8 and T12 vs. T0 ($p < 0.05$). Triglycerides and hexokinase activity increased significantly at T4 and T8 ($p < 0.05$) and then decreased at T12 in AT8. Pyruvate and glycogen increased at T12 in AT8 vs. AT4. Eight-week training improved LPL and ATGL expressions. Training positively modulated insulin, glucose metabolism, and lipid profiles, but detraining reduced the benefits associated with the initial training.

Keywords: endurance training; physical inactivity; glucose; metabolism; insulin; glycolysis; type 2 diabetes

1. Introduction

Industrialization and digitalization in modern societies affect our way of living, working, and eating. This resulted in decreased practice of physical activity. According to the World Health Organization (WHO), 23% of adults and 81% of adolescents (11–17 years) are insufficiently active in the world [1]. Since our genome has been selected for the body to function optimally under daily physical exertion conditions, a lack of physical activity inevitably induces major physiological and metabolic disturbances, including altered glucose metabolism and lipid profile, and insulin resistance, potentially leading to type 2 diabetes [2,3].

Physical activity is a bodily movement that induces energy expenditure above the basal energy level. It is recommended that adults practice at least 150 min of moderate-intensity aerobic physical activity every week [4]. Physical activity is also associated with several health benefits. Independent of its direct effect on energy expenditure, physical activity modulates body composition, lipid profiles, glucose homeostasis, and insulin sensitivity [5]. Evidence shows that regular physical training reduces blood glucose levels, HbA1c, and insulin resistance, similar to insulin treatment [6]. In addition, regular physical training can positively modulate hepatic lipid metabolism and blood lipid profiles by increasing high-density lipoprotein (HDL) and decreasing triglyceride (TG) and low-density lipoprotein (LDL) levels [7,8]. Moreover, physical training significantly increases the levels of liver enzymes (aspartate transaminase (AST) and alanine aminotransferase (ALT)) [9,10].

The mechanism through which regular physical training regulates glucose metabolism involves the modulation of glycolytic enzymes such as phosphofructokinase (PFK) and hexokinase (HK). Evidence has shown that high-intensity exercise training increases phosphofructokinase (PFK) activity [11–13], whereas endurance training decreases PFK activity in humans [14,15]. In addition, endurance training results in a transient increase in hexokinase II (HKII) transcription and mRNA levels and lipoprotein lipase (LPL) in human skeletal muscle [16,17]. Moderate-intensity training in mice for 6 weeks significantly increased glycogen storage in the muscle ($p < 0.05$), but no significant difference was observed in pyruvate [18]. Another recent study showed that repetition of long-term training in elderly men could decrease maximal fat oxidation and significantly upregulate HKII, glucose transporter type-4 (GLUT-4), and adipose triglyceride lipase (ATGL) expression, which in turn increases the capacity of glucose transport and muscle lipolysis of endogenous fat [19].

In contrast, stopping physical training results in partial or total loss of these physiological and metabolic adaptations, known as detraining [20,21]. Animal and human studies have reported that detraining is characterized by decreased glucose tolerance and insulin action [22,23]. This was observed in trained rats after only one week of training cessation [22]. Evidence in humans has shown that training cessation negatively affects insulin sensitivity and blood lipid profiles [24,25]. Some studies have been conducted on bed rest, and this model has been used to investigate how physical inactivity leads to the progression of chronic disease in healthy individuals. It has been reported that bed rest reduces insulin sensitivity and increases insulin resistance [26–30]. Additionally, evidence has shown that bed rest for 10–14 days enhances glucose intolerance and hyperinsulinemia following an oral glucose tolerance test (OGTT) [27,28,31]. Further, a study in male runners reported reduced HDL levels and post-heparin lipoprotein lipase activity with no change in total cholesterol, triglycerides, and LDL after 14–22 days of no physical activity [32]. Additionally, both continuous and interval training for 12 weeks followed by 4 weeks without training significantly reduced liver enzymes (ALT, AST, and alkaline phosphatase (ALP) in rats, compared to weeks 6 and 12 [33]. A study performed by Simoneau et al. did not report any impact on PFK after training cessation [13]. However, the impact of moderate-intensity training and detraining on glycolytic pathways still needs further exploration.

Indeed, training cessation has a negative impact on the body and leads to the progression of chronic diseases, including type 2 diabetes. Most adaptations gained during endurance training can be lost after detraining. Transitioning to sedentary behavior or physical inactivity would disrupt glucose metabolism. This is justified by Wendorf and Goldfine, who stated that human tribal people (Pima Indians) [34] and animals (spiny mice and the Egyptian sand rats) do not have type 2 diabetes when they are in their native state; however, when exposed to a sedentary environment with a constant food supply, they develop type 2 diabetes [35]. This shows that the human body must be involved in regular physical activity to function properly and prevent disease.

The lifestyle of our ancestors was challenging and, thus, physically demanding. Being physically active was mandatory for hunting, searching for food, and protecting against predators [36,37]. The body's functions have adapted to this daily metabolic stress. Due to advancements in technology, humans have evolved in an environment that demands less physical activity. This behavior likely outpaced the genome's ability to adapt, leading to a disconnect between physiological and metabolic functions and environmental factors [38]. The fact is that human genetic makeup has remained relatively identical since the appearance of the ancestral Homo sapiens 40,000 years ago [39]. This underscores the concept that our genome has not been optimized for a lifestyle characterized by inactivity and sedentarity, enforcing the idea. This mismatch resulted in the development of multiple chronic metabolic disorders, such as insulin resistance, leading to diseases like diabetes and cardiovascular disease [38]. To gain deeper insights into the development of these chronic metabolic disorders, it is critical to closely examine the transition towards inactivity. This scrutiny aims to uncover novel avenues for preventative and therapeutic interventions. Compelling evidence has demonstrated different physiological and metabolic functions between active and inactive states, accentuating the importance of comprehending the mechanisms of this transition [40–42]. As such, it becomes increasingly vital to delve into the intricacies of this shift. By comparing individuals who stopped being physically active with those who are regularly trained, this objective can be achieved. This comparison will help to pinpoint the most effective method of reintroducing physical activity to individuals who lead sedentary lives but are genetically programmed for a physically active life. Building on such a design, the current study seeks to investigate the changes in metabolic processes that occur as the body transitions from an active lifestyle to a state of physical inactivity. Additionally, this study also investigated the impact of physical training and detraining on insulin, glucose tolerance, lipid profiles, liver enzymes, and the glycolytic pathway.

2. Materials and Methods

2.1. Ethical Approval and Animal Care

The ethical approval for the animal study was obtained from the Animal Research Ethics Committee of the College of Medicine and Health Sciences at UAE University (ERA_2021_7238). The use and care of all animals in the experiment were according to the safe practice for animals in research guidelines as stipulated by the National Institutes of Health, USA.

Rats were maintained in an air-conditioned room (22 ± 2 °C) with a 12 h light/12 h dark cycle and 50% humidity. All animals received the same standard feed containing 24% protein, 5% fiber, and 8% ash.

2.2. Sample Size Calculation

The sample size was determined according to the estimation obtained from Mead's Resource Equation [43]. From this equation, two to three animals are required per group. Therefore, the final required sample size was equal to 26 (=6 + 6 + 7 + 7).

2.3. Training and Experimental Protocol

Twenty-six adult male Wistar rats (4–6 weeks old) were used in this study and bred in-house at the Animal Research Facility at the College of Medicine and Health Sciences at UAE University. The total duration of the study was 12 weeks.

At baseline (T0), six rats were sacrificed by decapitation. The remaining 20 rats underwent a 4-week exercise training program on a treadmill (6 Lanes; Columbus Instruments Treadmill Simplex II, Columbus, OH, USA). Each day during the first week, the protocol added 1 m/min to familiarize rats with the treadmill training. For the training protocol for 4 weeks, the treadmill speed was set to 5 m/min on the first day for 5 min per day. At the beginning of the third week, the treadmill speed reached 25 m/min. The 20-min duration was increased every week until it reached 60 min. After that, the speed and duration of running were kept constant. The treadmill was set at a 0% slope. Rats who stopped occasionally during running were gently prodded to help them continue running, and if required only, slight electrical stimuli (0.2 mA) were given.

After 4 weeks of training (T4) and 48 h after the last exercise session, to avoid any acute effect of exercise, 6 rats were sacrificed. The other remaining 14 animals were randomly divided into two groups: (1) training cessation till week 12 (group AT4); (2) aerobic training for 4 additional weeks, on the treadmill at 25 m/min for 1 h per day, 5 days per week, followed by 4 weeks with no training (Group AT8). Four animals per group were sacrificed at T8, and all remaining animals (n = 6) were sacrificed at T12 (Figure 1).

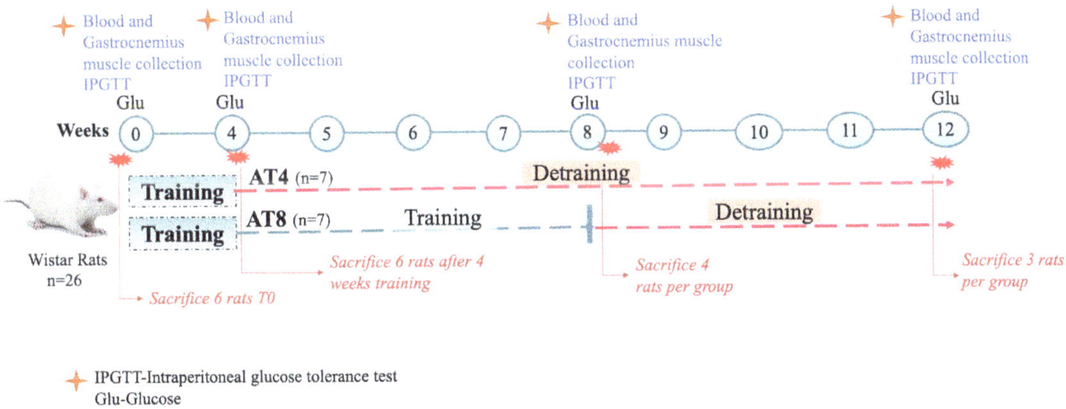

Figure 1. Study protocol. Aerobic training of 4 weeks (AT4), aerobic training of 8 weeks (AT8).

2.4. Blood Collection

Blood was collected immediately after each sacrifice at different times (T0, T4, T8, and T12). Blood samples were drawn into a dry and sterile Vacutainer for a serum with a gel clot activator. Blood samples were centrifuged at 1500× *g* for 20 min, and serum was collected and stored at −80 °C until analyzed.

2.5. Feed Intake, Body Weight, and Blood Glucose

During the 12-week study period, feed intake and body weight were measured at T0, T4, T8, and T12.

2.6. Intraperitoneal Glucose Tolerance Test (IPGTT)

The intraperitoneal glucose tolerance test (IPGTT) was performed at baseline (T0), 4 weeks (T4), 8 weeks (T8), and 12 weeks (T12). Animals were fasting for 10 h, and each conscious rat was intraperitoneally injected (2 g/kg body weight). For glucose solution preparation, 30 g was dissolved in 40 mL of distilled H_2O. Fasting (0 min) and stimulated blood glucose levels were measured 30, 60, 120, and 180 min after glucose administration. Blood was collected from the tail. The glucose area under the curve (AUC) was calculated based on individual animals' fasting blood glucose levels over time using GraphPad Prism 9.0 (GraphPad, San Diego, CA, USA).

2.7. Lipid Profile, Glucose, and Liver Enzyme

Glucose, total cholesterol, low-density lipoprotein (LDL), high-density lipoprotein (HDL), triglycerides, aspartate transaminase (AST), alanine transaminase (ALT), and alkaline phosphatase (ALP) were measured in serum using enzymatic colorimetric methods on Roche/Hitachi Cobas C systems (Integra 400 Plus, Mannheim, Germany).

2.8. Serum Insulin

Insulin was assessed using a commercially available ELISA kit, Merck Millipore (Cat# EZRMI-13K), and analysis was performed based on the manufacturer's instructions.

2.9. Enzymatic Activity

Following the manufacturer's instructions, gastrocnemius muscle tissues were homogenized in an ice-cooled assay buffer and centrifuged at 13,000× *g* at 4 °C for 15 min. Phosphofructokinase (PFK) and hexokinase (HK) enzyme activity was measured immediately in the supernatant using a commercially available PFK activity assay kit (ab155898, Abcam, Cambridge, UK) and HK activity assay kit (ab136957, Abcam, Cambridge, UK).

2.10. Muscle Glycogen and Pyruvate

A small portion of the gastrocnemius muscle (10 mg) was homogenized in 200 µL of ice-cold water (ddH_2O) using a pestle on ice. Homogenates were then boiled for 10 min at 100 °C to inactivate enzymes in the sample and centrifuged for 10 min at 13,000× *g* at 4 °C. Glycogen was determined in the supernatant using a glycogen assay kit (ab65620, Abcam, Cambridge, UK).

The gastrocnemius muscle (10 mg) was homogenized in 500 µL of a pyruvate assay buffer using a pestle kept on ice and centrifuged for 15 min at 13,000× *g* at 4 °C. Pyruvate was determined in the supernatant using a pyruvate assay kit (ab65342, Abcam, Cambridge, UK).

2.11. Lactate

In AT4, blood lactate concentration was measured at T4 and T12. In AT8, lactate was measured at T4, T8, and T12 by a Lactate Plus handheld blood lactate meter (Nova Biomedical, Waltham, MA, USA). One drop of blood was collected via tail vein puncture onto a disposable strip for lactate analysis. Before measurements in the resting condition, all rats were physically restrained for 30 min in small plastic containers to ensure that all rats were as physically inactive as possible. Lactate was measured at rest and after every 5 min while rats ran on a treadmill at 25 m/min speed for 25 min.

2.12. Immunoblot Analysis

The lipoprotein lipase (LPL), adipose triglyceride lipase (ATGL), and fatty acid transport protein 4 (FATP4) expressions were evaluated in skeletal muscle homogenates. Total protein was isolated from the gastrocnemius muscle using a RIPA lysis buffer (Sigma Aldrich, St. Louis, MO, USA) containing a 1% protease phosphatase inhibitor cocktail (Sigma Aldrich, St. Louis, MO, USA) using a homogenizer. The total protein in the supernatant was determined by the BCA Protein Assay Kit (Sigma Aldrich, St. Louis, MO, USA). Then, it was diluted, the supernatant was diluted in a 6× RIPA buffer and heated for 5 min at 90 °C.

For electrophoresis, 35 µg of protein from each sample was loaded per well and separated by SDS–PAGE. The protein was transferred onto a nitrocellulose membrane by wet transfer using a Bio-Rad Electro-transfer apparatus. Membranes were blocked with 5% skimmed milk in tris-buffered saline with 0.1% Tween-20 (TBS-T) at room temperature for 1 h. Then, membranes were incubated overnight with primary antibodies, including FATP4 and LPL antibodies (Abcam, Cambridge, UK), ATGL antibody (Cell Signaling Technology, Danvers, MA, USA), and GAPDH (ABclonal, Woburn, MA, USA). The appropriate horseradish peroxidase-conjugated secondary antibodies (Jackson Immune Research, Cambridge House, UK) were used to blot for 1 h after being washed three times with TBS-T. The band densities were detected using an enhanced chemiluminescence detection kit (Bio-Rad, Hercules, CA, USA). The band densities were quantified by the image analyzer Quantity One System (Bio-Rad, Hercules, CA, USA).

2.13. Statistical Analysis

Statistical analysis was performed using the SPSS software (v.28). A paired *t*-test was performed to analyze the intraperitoneal glucose tolerance test (IPGTT) at T0 and T4. An independent *t*-test was conducted to analyze the difference between groups at T8 and T12. To assess the normality assumptions of the data, Shapiro–Wilk's test was applied, and it was found that five variables (cholesterol, ALP, AST, ALT, and pyruvate) violated the normality assumptions. The non-parametric Kruskal–Wallis test was employed for these variables, and subsequent multiple comparisons were performed using Dunn's test. For non-parametric tests, data are expressed as median. A mixed model (two-way analysis of variance (ANOVA) with a Sidak Post Hoc test pairwise comparisons was performed to compare groups and time points. All experiments were carried out in duplicates. Data are expressed as means ± standard deviation (S.D.). In all analyses, $p \leq 0.05$ was considered statistically significant (* $p \leq 0.05$, ** $p \leq 0.01$).

3. Results

3.1. Body Weight

The mean weight at baseline (T0) was similar in AT4 (170.03 ± 20.80 g) and AT8 (173.77 ± 27.71 g) ($p < 0.05$) (Table 1). After 4 weeks of training, the weight significantly increased to 258.05 ± 17.34 and 258.25 ± 13.63 in AT4 and AT8, respectively ($p < 10^{-4}$). In both AT4 and AT8, the body weight further significantly increased at T8 (324.30 ± 36.34 g and 330.16 ± 22.26 g, respectively) and T12 (351.40 ± 46.86 g and 356.57 ± 8.86 g, respectively) compared to T0 and T4 ($p \leq 0.01$). However, in AT8, the body weight was greater than the AT4 group at both T8 ($p = 0.689$) and T12 ($p = 0.961$) but did not reach statistically significant.

Table 1. Weekly body weight, feed intake, and blood glucose level (Mean ± S.D.).

		T0	T4	T8	T12
Body Weight	AT4	170.03 ± 20.80	258.05 ± 17.34 a	324.30 ± 36.34 ab	351.40 ± 46.86 ab
	AT8	173.77 ± 27.71	258.25 ± 13.63 a	330.16 ± 22.26 ab	356.57 ± 8.86 ab
Feed Intake	AT4	24.35 ± 3.18	25.86 ± 4.47	23.73 ± 2.30	21.41 ± 1.33
	AT8	24.35 ± 3.18	25.86 ± 4.47	23.39 ± 4.43	23.33 ± 1.85

Aerobic training of 4 weeks (AT4), aerobic training of 8 weeks (AT8). Body weight and feed intake was measured in grams (g). a Statistically significant difference with T0. b Statistically significant difference with T4.

3.2. Feed Intake

Up to T4, the two groups of animals were not physically separated into different cages. The average daily feed intake of the rats at baseline was 24.35 ± 3.18 g, slightly increasing to 25.86 ± 4.47 g at T4. In AT4, feed intake decreased to 23.73 ± 2.30 g in T8 after exercise cessation, then 21.41 ± 1.33 g at T12. In AT8, the feed intake was lower at T8 (23.39 ± 4.43 g) and remained the same at T12. None of the differences were significant (Table 1).

3.3. Intraperitoneal Glucose Tolerance Test (IPGTT)

The total area under the curve (AUC) of IPGTT decreased significantly by 32% from 12,742 ± 1113 at T0 to 8580 ± 1132 at T4 as a result of 4 weeks of training ($p < 0.001$) (Figure 2A). In AT4, after 4 weeks without physical activity (T8), the AUC increased to 8873 ± 327 and even more at T12 (11,865 ± 2095). Inversely, the glucose AUC continued decreasing in AT8, at T8 (7971 ± 331), after 4 more weeks of training, and at T12 (7020 ± 371), after 4-week detraining (Figure 2B). At T12, even after 4 weeks of detraining, the glucose peak significantly decreased in AT8 ($p = 0.046$) at 60 min compared to AT4 (Figure 2C).

3.4. Serum Glucose

Serum glucose level was not significantly different between T0 and T4 (8.23 ± 0.78 mmol/L and 8.21 ± 0.61 mmol/L, respectively). In both groups, serum glucose levels did not change significantly over time. In addition, no change was observed in glucose levels between AT4 and AT8 groups neither at T8 nor at T12 (Figure 3).

3.5. Serum Insulin

After 4 weeks of moderate-intense training, the serum insulin level decreased from 7.66 ± 0.26 ng/mL to 6.93 ±1.44 ng/mL (Figure 4). In AT4, the serum insulin level increased to 7.67 ± 1.07 ng/mL after 4 weeks of detraining at T8, then decreased again at T12, but it was not significant. In AT8, the insulin level (7.03 ± 0.88 ng/mL) at T8 remained similar to T4. However, after 4 weeks of detraining, at T12, the insulin level was lowered (5.99 ± 0.94 ng/mL). Compared to AT4, the serum insulin level was lower in the AT8 group at T8 and T12, but this did not reach statistical significance.

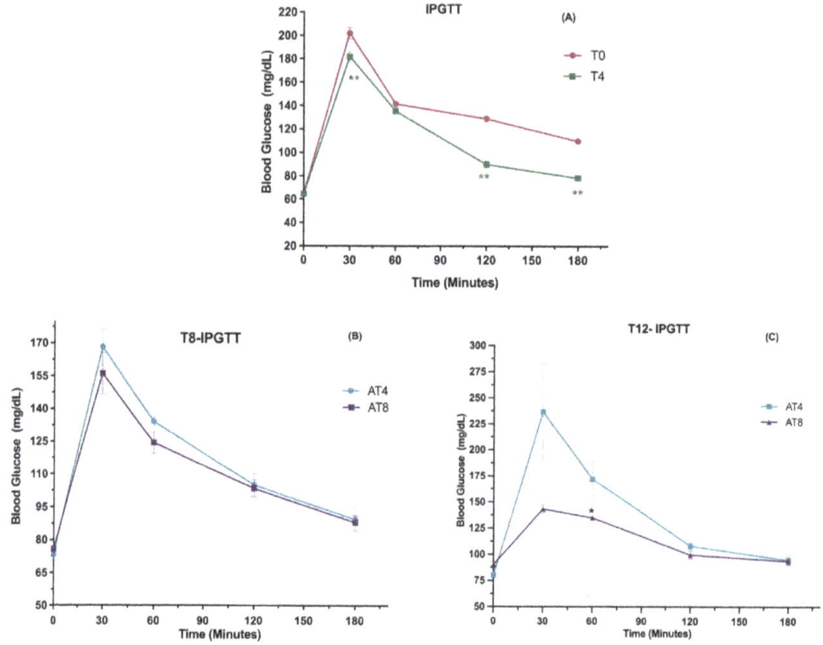

Figure 2. Intraperitoneal glucose tolerance test (IPGTT). (**A**) A paired *t*-test was performed to analyze the IPGTT at time points T0 and T4. (**B**) An independent *t*-test was performed to analyze the difference between AT4 and AT8 at T8. (**C**) An independent *t*-test was performed to analyze the difference between AT4 and AT8 at T12. Data are shown as Mean ± S.D. Statistical significance was set at $p \leq 0.05$. Statistically significant * ($p \leq 0.05$) and ** ($p \leq 0.01$).

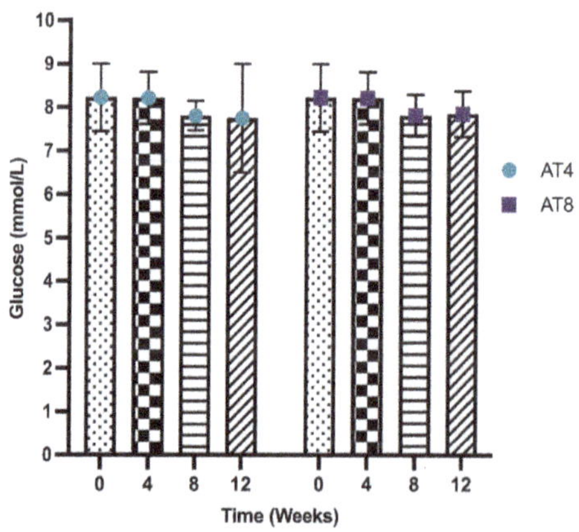

Figure 3. Serum glucose level. Data are shown as Mean ± S.D. of duplicate experiments. ANOVA with multiple comparisons was performed, and statistical significance was set at $p \leq 0.05$.

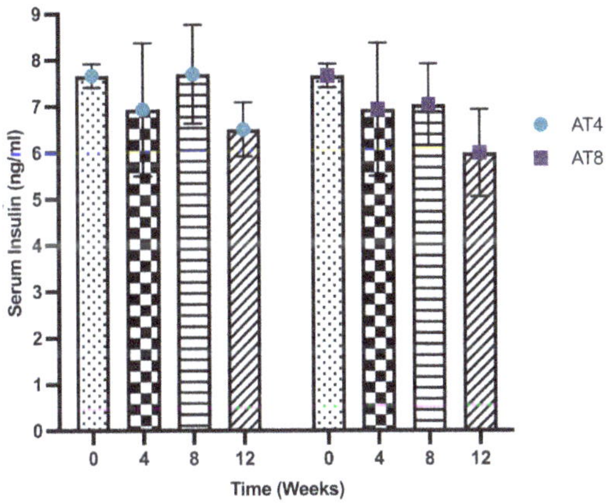

Figure 4. Serum insulin level. Data are shown as Mean ± S.D. of duplicate experiments. ANOVA with multiple comparisons was performed, and statistical significance was set at $p \leq 0.05$.

3.6. Serum Lipid Profiles

3.6.1. Serum Total Cholesterol Concentration

The serum total cholesterol concentration reduced significantly from 1.33 mmol/L, 95% CI at baseline, to 0.89 mmol/L, 95% CI after 4 weeks of training ($p < 10^{-4)}$). In AT4, the cholesterol level significantly increased at T8 (1.20 mmol/L, 95% CI) after 4 weeks of detraining compared to T4 ($p = 0.023$), and no further significant change was observed at T12, while in AT8, even after 4 weeks of detraining, the serum cholesterol level at T12 (1.04 mmol, 95% CI) remained significantly lower than the level at T0 ($p = 0.004$). Cholesterol levels remained lower in the AT8 group at T8 and T12 compared to AT4, but there was no significant difference among the groups (Figure 5).

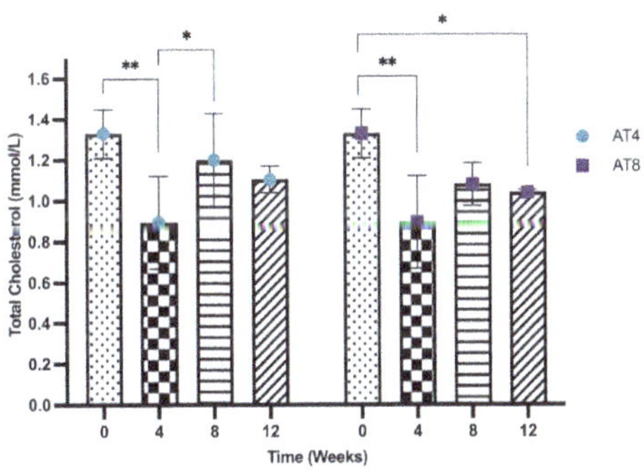

Figure 5. Serum cholesterol concentration. Data are shown as Median, 95% CI of duplicate experiments. A Kruskal–Wallis test with multiple comparisons of Dunn's test was performed, and statistical significance was set at $p \leq 0.05$. Statistically significant difference among time points * ($p \leq 0.05$) and ** ($p \leq 0.01$).

3.6.2. Serum Triglycerides Concentration

The serum triglyceride concentration significantly increased from 0.71 ± 0.14 mmol/L at baseline to 1.07 ± 0.35 mmol/L after 4 weeks of training ($p = 0.009$). In AT4, after training cessation, the triglyceride level started to decrease to reach 0.99 ± 0.13 mmol/L at T8, then 0.73 ± 0.17 mmol/L at T12, which is significantly lower than the value at T4 value but still similar to the baseline level. In contrast, in AT8, triglyceride levels increased significantly to 1.10 ± 0.12 mmol/L ($p = 0.021$) at T8 compared to baseline, and a slight reduction after training cessation of 0.96 ± 0.02 mmol/L was observed at T12. Moreover, at T12, in AT4, the serum triglycerides level was significantly lower than AT8 ($p = 0.011$) (Figure 6).

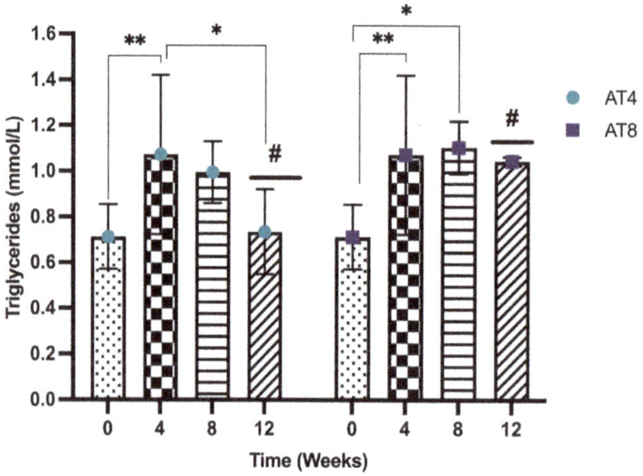

Figure 6. Serum triglycerides concentration. Data are shown as Mean ± S.D. of duplicate experiments. ANOVA with multiple comparisons was performed, and statistical significance was set at $p \leq 0.05$. Statistically significant difference among time points * ($p \leq 0.05$) and ** ($p \leq 0.01$). Statistically significant difference among groups # ($p \leq 0.05$).

3.6.3. Serum Low-Density Lipoprotein (LDL) and High-Density Lipoprotein (HDL) Concentration

The serum low-density lipoprotein (LDL) level decreased significantly ($p < 10^{-4}$) from 0.30 ± 0.04 mmol/L at baseline to 0.16 ± 0.04 mmol/L after 4 weeks of training (Figure 7A). An increasing LDL trend was observed in AT4 after detraining. However, LDL level at both T8 and T12 remains significantly lower than baseline ($p < 0.05$). A similar trend was observed in AT8; after detraining at T12, the serum LDL level increased.

The serum high-density lipoprotein (HDL) level was maintained at T4 (0.72 ± 0.08 mmol/L) compared to baseline (0.74 ± 0.16 mmol/L). In AT4, no change was observed at T8. Only a slight decrease was noted at T12, but it remained insignificant (Figure 7B). Interestingly, in AT8, 8 weeks of training (T8) significantly increased the HDL level to 0.88 ± 0.11 mmol/L ($p = 0.009$), while after 4 weeks of detraining (T12), the HDL level decreased significantly to 0.68 ± 0.01 mmol/L ($p = 0.013$). No significant difference was observed between the two groups.

3.7. Serum Liver Enzymes

The serum alkaline phosphatase (ALP) level decreased after 4 weeks of training from 200.7 U/L, 95% CI at T0 to 159.35 U/L, 95% CI at T4, but it is not significant. In AT4, after training cessation, the ALP level decreased drastically to a lower level of 110.5 U/L (95% CI, $p < 10^{-4}$) at T8 compared to T0. Then, it decreases to 98.15 U/L, 95% CI at T12, which is significantly lower than the baseline and T4 values ($p = 0.01$). The ALP level significantly ($p \leq 0.02$) decreased in AT8 to 116.75 U/L, 95% CI at T8 compared to T0 and T4. Then, in AT8, there was a decreasing trend in the ALP level after training cessation (104.1 U/L, 95% CI) at T12; the value is significantly ($p = 0.002$) lower than the baseline value. No significant difference was observed between AT4 and AT8 (Figure 8A).

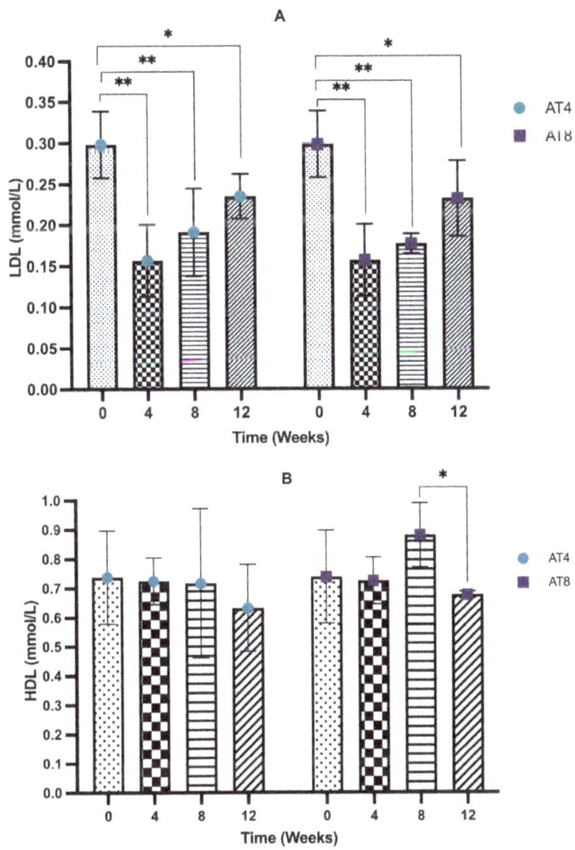

Figure 7. Serum low-density lipoprotein (LDL) and high-density lipoprotein (HDL) concentration. (**A**) LDL Comparison between time points and between groups. (**B**) HDL comparison between groups for each time point and between groups. ANOVA with multiple comparisons was performed, and statistical significance was set at $p < 0.05$. Statistically significant difference among time points * ($p \leq 0.05$) and ** ($p \leq 0.01$).

The serum alanine phosphatase (ALT) level was not altered significantly after 4 weeks of training. In AT4, 4 weeks of detraining elevated the ALT level (67.85 U/L, 95% CI) at T8. A similar trend was observed in AT8; after 4 weeks of detraining, the ALT level increased to 68.1 U/L, 95% CI, $p = 0.001$ at T12. AT4 and AT8 significantly differed at T8 ($p = 0.042$) (Figure 8B).

The serum aspartate aminotransferase (AST) level decreased from 134.65 U/L, 95% CI at baseline 119.95 U/L, and 95% CI at T4, but it was not significant. In AT4, the AST level abruptly increased to 185.8 U/L, 95% CI at T8 after training cessation, then decreased to 153.3 U/L, 95% CI at T12. In AT8, the AST level was maintained at T8 (130.15 U/L, 95% CI) and then increased at T12 (157.5 U/L, 95% CI) after training cessation. No significant difference was seen between the AT4 and AT8 (Figure 8C).

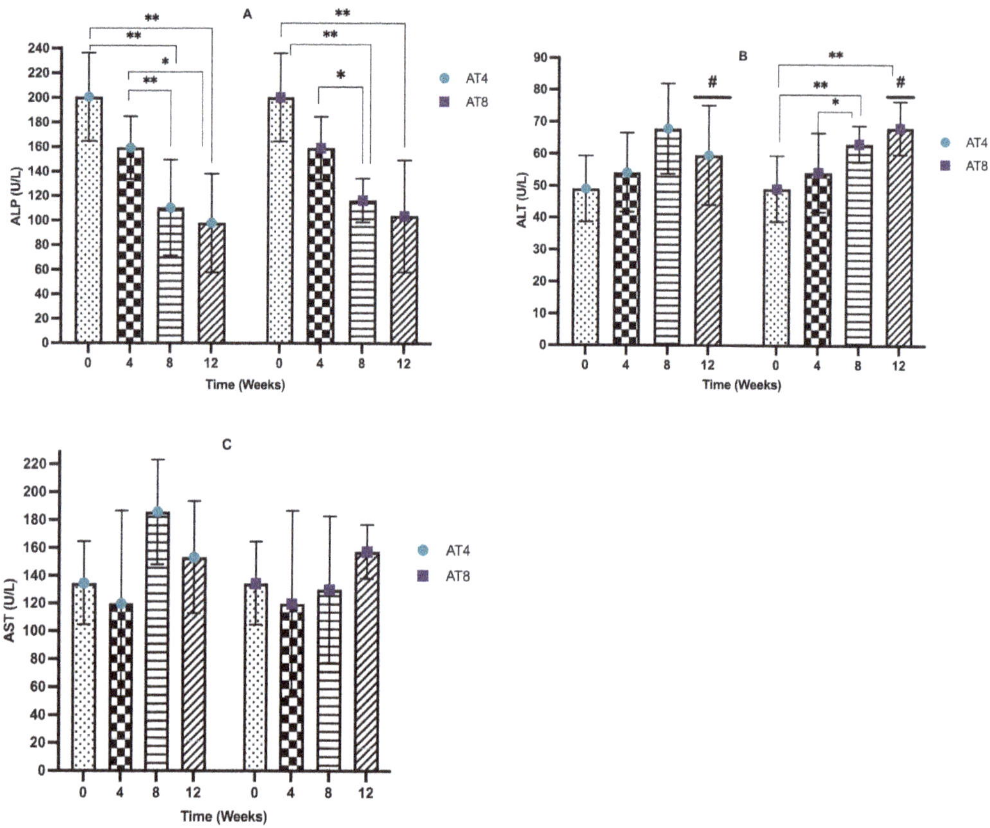

Figure 8. Serum liver enzymes. (**A**) Alkaline phosphatase (ALP) level comparison between time points and between groups. (**B**) Serum alanine transaminase (ALT) comparison between time points and between groups. (**C**) Aspartate aminotransferase (AST) comparison between time points and between groups. Data are shown as Median, 95% CI of duplicate experiments. A Kruskal–Wallis test with multiple comparisons of Dunn's test was performed, and statistical significance was set at $p \leq 0.05$. Statistically significant difference among time points * ($p \leq 0.05$) and ** ($p \leq 0.01$). Statistically significant difference among groups # ($p \leq 0.05$).

3.8. Phosphofructokinase (PFK)

Phosphofructokinases (PFK) were assessed in the gastrocnemius muscle of rats. The PFK level was 4.69 ± 0.17 mU/mL at baseline and 4.77 ± 0.27 mU/mL at T4. The PFK level was maintained in AT4 and AT8 at all time points. No significant change was observed between different time points or between groups (Figure 9).

3.9. Hexokinase (HK)

Hexokinase (HK) activity was assessed in the gastrocnemius muscle of rats, and it increased significantly after 4 weeks of training from 7.87 ± 2.09 mU/mL at T0 and 10.87 ± 1.89 mU/mL at T4 ($p \leq 0.05$). However, in AT4, after 4 weeks of detraining, HK decreased at T8 (4.25 ± 1.54 mU/mL) and was significantly lower than baseline and T4 values ($p < 10^{-4}$). No further change was observed at T12 compared to T8. In AT8, the HK continued to increase with 8 weeks of training (12.34 ± 4.54 mU/mL compared to baseline, $p = 0.004$). Then, it decreased drastically to 5.31 ± 0.39 mU/mL at T12 after 4 weeks of detraining ($p < 10^{-4}$). At T8, there was a significant ($p < 10^{-4}$) difference observed among AT4 (4 weeks of detraining) and AT8 (continuous training for 8 weeks) (Figure 10).

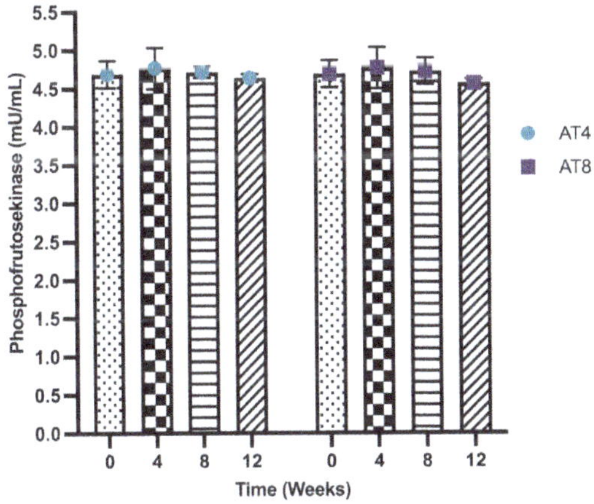

Figure 9. Phosphofructokinase (PFK) level in gastrocnemius muscle. Data are shown as Mean ± S.D. of duplicate experiments. ANOVA with multiple comparisons was performed, and statistical significance was set at $p \leq 0.05$.

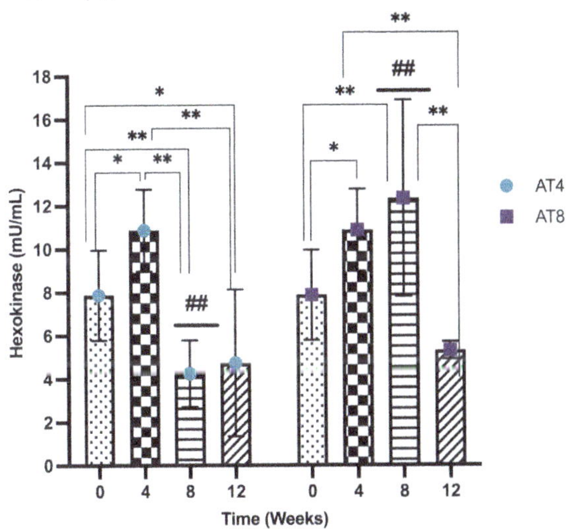

Figure 10. Hexokinase (HK) level in gastrocnemius muscle. Data are shown as Mean ± S.D. of duplicate experiments. ANOVA with multiple comparisons was performed, and statistical significance was set at $p \leq 0.05$. Statistically significant difference among time points * ($p \leq 0.05$) and ** ($p \leq 0.01$). Statistically significant difference among groups ## ($p \leq 0.01$).

3.10. Pyruvate

Pyruvate was assessed in the gastrocnemius muscle of rats, and it increased significantly after 4 weeks of training from 0.01 nmol/uL, 95%CI at baseline and 0.02 nmol/uL, 95% CI at T4 ($p = 0.002$). In AT4, the pyruvate level was then maintained at a similar level at T8 and T12 after training cessation. In AT8, the pyruvate level was maintained at T8 ($p = 0.02$) but increased significantly to 0.08 nmol/uL, 95% CI, $p < 10^{-4}$ at T12 after 4 weeks of training cessation compared to baseline, T4 and T8 ($p \leq 0.01$). A significant difference between AT4 and AT8 was observed at T12 ($p = 0.042$) (Figure 11).

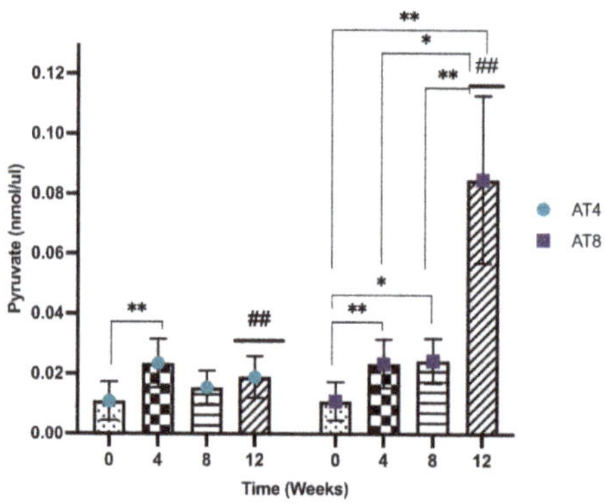

Figure 11. Pyruvate level in gastrocnemius muscle. Data are shown as the Median of duplicate experiments. Kruskal–Willis test with multiple comparisons Dunn's test was performed, and statistical significance was set at $p \leq 0.05$. Statistically significant difference among time points * ($p \leq 0.05$) and ** ($p \leq 0.01$). Statistically significant difference among groups ## ($p \leq 0.01$).

3.11. Glycogen

Glycogen increased significantly after 4 weeks of training from baseline (0.04 ± 0.00 ug/uL) to T4 (0.06 ± 0.01 ug/uL) ($p < 10^{-4}$). Then, the glycogen concentration decreased significantly in both groups (AT4 and AT8) at T8 ($p \leq 0.01$). In AT4, no further decrease was observed at T12, but the level remained lower than T4 ($p = 0.002$). In AT8, the glycogen level tended to increase at T12 after 4 weeks of training cessation and was higher than the baseline level ($p = 0.004$). At T12, the glycogen level was higher in AT8 compared to AT4 ($p = 0.16$) (Figure 12).

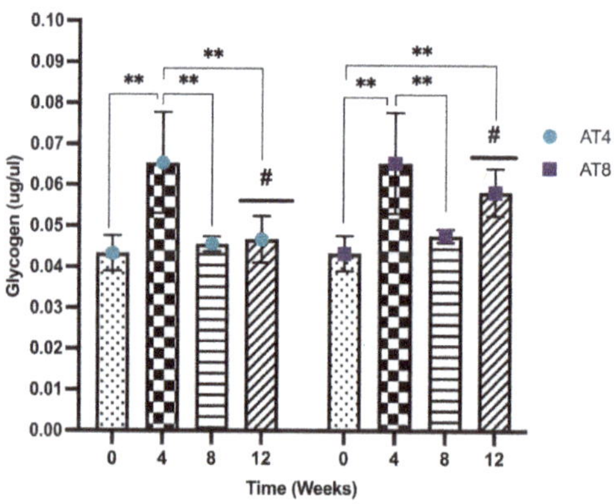

Figure 12. Glycogen level in gastrocnemius muscle. Data are shown as Mean ± S.D. of duplicate experiments. ANOVA with multiple comparisons was performed, and statistical significance was set at $p \leq 0.05$. Statistically significant difference among time points ** ($p \leq 0.01$). Statistically significant difference among groups # ($p \leq 0.05$).

3.12. Lactate

The lactate level was measured in running rats at various time points (0 min, 5 min, 10 min, 15 min, and 25 min) at a velocity of 25 m/min (Figure 13A). In AT4, overall values were lower at T12 compared to T4 after 8 weeks of detraining, but the results were not statistically significant. In AT8, lactate values were lower at T8 than T4, while at T12, values were higher, especially after 15 min of running at 25 m/min. There is a significant difference in the AT8 group at 5 min and 20 min between T8 and T4 ($p \leq 0.05$) (Figure 13B).

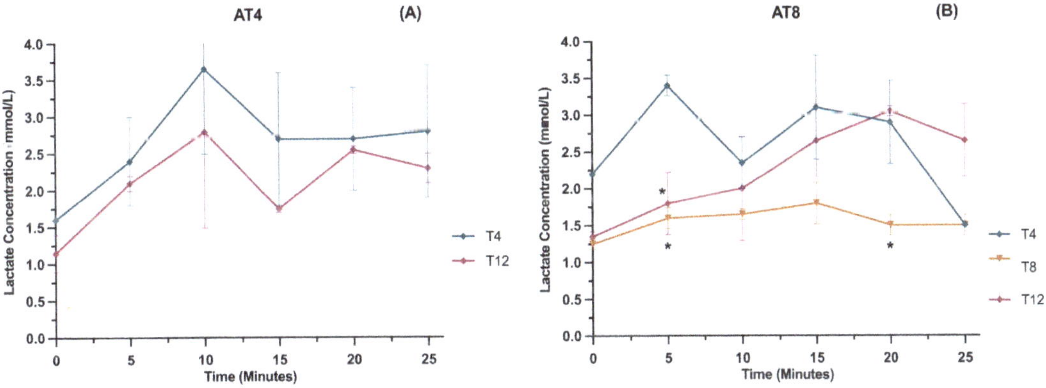

Figure 13. Blood lactate level in the AT8 group. (**A**) Lactate concentration in the AT4 group and (**B**) lactate concentration in the AT4 group. Data are shown as Mean ± S.D. of duplicate experiments. ANOVA with multiple comparisons was performed, and statistical significance was set at $p \leq 0.05$. Statistically significant difference among time points * ($p \leq 0.05$).

3.13. Protein Expressions

The level of protein expression of FATP4, ATGL, and LPL was assessed by Western blotting in the rat's gastrocnemius muscle (Figure 14A). Training slightly reduced the FATP4 protein expression, but the change was not statistically significant (Figure 14B). However, 4 weeks of detraining in AT4 slightly decreased FATP4 expression, but after 8 weeks, it increased by 11% ± 3.19. In AT8, 4 weeks of detraining at T12, increased FATP4 expression by 18% ± 2.77.

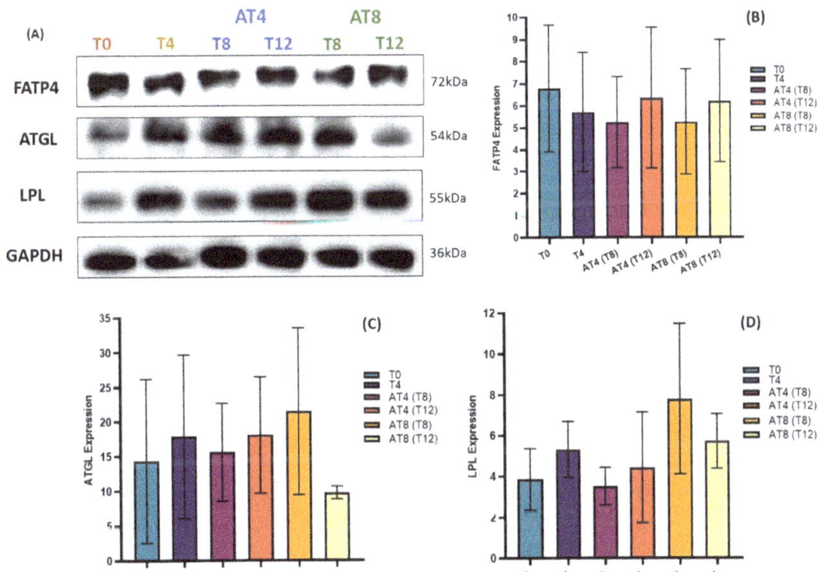

Figure 14. Effect of training and detraining on protein expression. (**A**) Immunoblot analysis, (**B**) level of FATP4, expression (**C**) level of ATGL expression, and (**D**) level of LPL expression. Data are shown as Mean ± S.D. of duplicate experiments. ANOVA with multiple comparisons was performed, and statistical significance was set at $p \leq 0.05$.

There was an increase in ATGL by 24% ± 7.07 at T4 compared to baseline. In AT4, after 4 weeks of detraining, AGTL decreased by 12% ± 7.07 at T8, but at T12, the expression level remained similar to T4. In AT8, ATGL increased by 37% ± 12.02 at T8 with 8 weeks of training but then decreased by 54% ± 0.92 at T12 (Figure 14C).

There was an increase in LPL by 37% ± 0.91 at T4 compared to T0. In AT4, after 4 weeks of detraining, LPL expression decreased by 33% ± 0.91 at T8 and 16% ± 2.69 at T12 compared to T4. In AT8, LPL increased by 121% ± 3.68 at T8 with 8 weeks training, then decreased by 26% ± 1.32 at T12 after detraining (Figure 14D).

4. Discussion

Physical activity is the naturally programmed status of the body. The present study reported the metabolic and biochemical adaptations to regular endurance training and the alteration in the metabolic process and glucose homeostasis when the body switched from training to detraining. In addition, the dose effect of moderately intense aerobic training and detraining from short duration (4 weeks) to long duration (8 weeks) was considered. Regular moderate-intense aerobic training positively regulates blood glucose, insulin levels, glucose tolerance, lipid profile, and glycolytic enzymes, but training cessation disrupts glucose homeostasis.

Increased physical activity is a clinically proven first-line strategy to improve glucose metabolism. The current study reported the beneficial effect of moderate-intensity aerobic training on glucose tolerance lost during the detraining period. The AUC of IPGTT was 11% greater in AT4 after training cessation compared to the AT8 group at T8. When the detraining continued for 8 weeks (T12) in the AT4 group, the AUC of IPGTT increased by 34% compared to T8. Previous findings reported that healthy individuals who underwent bed rest for 1–3 weeks showed abnormal intravenous glucose tolerance tests [44]. On the other hand, the AT8 group who continued exercise training for 8 weeks had improved glucose tolerance compared to AT4. Our results followed the findings of Abdolmaleki and Heidarianpour, which showed training positively improved glucose tolerance and reduced IPGTT-glucose peak [45], but after 4 weeks of detraining, the positive effects vanished. This supports a continuous training program throughout life to maintain glucose homeostasis.

This study revealed that detraining for 4 weeks after 4 weeks of training increased the insulin level at T8 in AT4. When the training continued for a longer duration (8 weeks), an insulin level at T12 did not elevate. Suggesting there might be a cumulative effect of 8 weeks of moderate-intense aerobic training that prevents insulin increase after detraining. Omidi and Yousefi (2019) reported that fasting glucose and insulin significantly improved after 8 weeks of aerobic training [46]. On the other hand, exercise intervention reduced the fasting glucose but increased insulin concentration ($p < 0.05$) [47].

Interestingly, in the present study, the serum cholesterol level significantly decreased after 4 weeks of training ($p < 10^{-4}$), which is consistent with previous results of Fahri et al. and Kraus et al. [48,49]. However, in AT4, after 4 weeks of detraining at T8, the cholesterol level increased by 36% compared to T4 ($p < 0.25$). Whereas in AT8, it was still significantly lower than baseline after 8 weeks of training and even after 4 weeks of detraining, showing that 8 weeks of training can limit the effects of detraining better than only 4 weeks of training. On the other hand, serum triglyceride levels decreased after detraining in AT4 (at T8 and T12, and AT8 at T12). However, the continuous training for 8 weeks has shown a significant increase in serum triglyceride levels compared to T0. This increase might be because of the increased energy requirement during exercise and the utilization of triglycerides as fuel. This is consistent with previous findings by Banz et al., who revealed that aerobic exercise training for 10 weeks increased triglycerides [50]. Contrarily, not all studies have found a significant alteration in lipid parameters after exercise training [51,52]. The present study reported a slight reduction in serum triglyceride levels after 4 weeks of detraining and even greater after 8 weeks.

HDL is the most sensitive parameter to aerobic exercise compared to LDL and triglycerides. It is well-known that changes in HDL levels are more obvious in rats than other lipid parameters. It might be related to the greater sensitivity of HDL to training but also to the abundance of HDL in rats compared to the other lipid components [53]. The current study reported that serum HDL levels only increased after 8 weeks of training, indicating a dose effect of training. Nevertheless, after 4 weeks of training cessation at T12, the HDL level decreased by 23% compared to T8 ($p < 0.05$). Similarly, a reduction in HDL after 8 weeks of detraining (T12) was observed in AT4. Similar to our findings, LeMura et al. demonstrated that sixteen weeks of aerobic training significantly elevated blood HDL in young women ($p < 0.05$), but these alterations vanish after 6 weeks of detraining [54], while in our study, a significant reduction in serum HDL level can be seen after 4 weeks of detraining. In another study, HDL levels decreased after a brief interval of detraining [32], which is in accordance with our results. Moreover, in the current study, trained animals had lower LDL level, which was maintained when exercise training continued for 8 weeks. However, the favorable adaptation to a lower LDL level was lost following detraining. It was found that 4 weeks of detraining increased LDL level, but a greater increase was observed after 8 weeks. Notably, the LDL level increased after detraining but remained lower than the baseline concentration. This is consistent with the previous finding of Rogerio et al., who showed that detraining for 4 weeks after 8 weeks of training increased LDL concentration [55].

The liver is an important organ that helps to regulate glycemia under metabolic alteration during exercise by controlling gluconeogenesis and blood glucose production [56]. Our results showed a reduction in serum ALP levels after 4 weeks of training and even after detraining. Similarly, a previous study reported a 6.1% reduction in the ALP enzyme after 2 weeks of aerobic exercise in overweight and obese men [57]. Additionally, 8 weeks of training significantly increased serum ALT levels ($p = 0.004$) and to a greater extent after 4 weeks of detraining at T12 ($p = 0.001$) compared to baseline. Similarly, the ALT level increased abruptly after 4 weeks of detraining in AT4. This increase in ALT after training cessation might be associated with an increased risk of insulin resistance. Hanley et al. indicated that the increased serum ALT activity predicts the development of insulin resistance and type 2 diabetes in human populations, but without any apparent sign of liver injury [58]. The current training program failed to evoke a significant alteration in serum AST levels, which is in accordance with the previous study. A study on professional sportsmen found no significant difference in AST levels after the training intervention [59]. However, the AST level increased at T8 in AT4 and AT8 at T12 after 4 weeks of detraining. Previously, it was noted that an increase in AST activity is associated with insulin resistance, metabolic syndrome, and type 2 diabetes [60]. Given that detraining has a negative association with AST levels.

Hexokinase is an important glycolysis enzyme involved in skeletal muscle glucose metabolism. Acute stimulation of skeletal muscle, either by insulin or by contraction through exercise, increased hexokinase activity in human and rodent skeletal muscle [61–63]. Similarly, our result showed that 4 weeks of training increased hexokinase activity by 38% vs. baseline, and 8 weeks of training further increased by 13% vs. T4. Indeed, exercise training has a positive impact on hexokinase levels, but when the body switches to inactivity, all these positive adaptations could be lost. We observed that detraining for 4 weeks in AT4 at T8 reduced hexokinase by 60%, while in AT8 at T12, it reduced by 56%. It was reported that the decreased hexokinase II expression during physical inactivity could trigger an alteration similar to type 2 diabetes, such as altered insulin response and muscle glucose transport [64].

Additionally, glycogen is the polysaccharide storage form of glucose in skeletal muscle. The present study found that initially, glycogen content increased after 4 weeks of training at T4 compared to T0, but glycogen content decreased in the AT4 group after detraining at T8 and T12. Previously, training-induced reduction in muscle glycogen was reported as a key driver to the post-training improvement in insulin sensitivity [65,66]. Interestingly, the glycogen content declined when training continued for 8 weeks in the AT8 group, possibly due to greater skeletal muscle training adaptation. Low glycogen availability during training could shift to other substrates' metabolism during and after exercise training [67,68]. However, after training cessation at T12 in the AT8 group, there was again a rise in glycogen content by 24% compared to AT4. Post-training skeletal muscle glycogen repletion might be influenced by hexokinase activity in the skeletal muscle, consistent with previous findings [69]. Evidence has shown that training significantly elevated the hexokinase II protein by 70%. In addition, an increase in muscle glycogen was not apparent after 1 day of training, but it increased by 40% after 4 days of training compared to pretraining [70].

Phosphofructokinase (PFK) is considered a rate-limiting enzyme when glucose enters glycolysis pathways and is allosterically activated by ADP, AMP, and Pi. The present study did not observe any significant change in PFK in either group during the training and detraining period. Our results are similar to the previous findings of Henriksson and Reitman, which demonstrated that training for 7–8 weeks did not cause alteration in phosphofructokinase activity in human skeletal muscle [71]. Unlike hexokinase, PFK was maintained during the training and detraining, suggesting that glucose may not have entered glycolysis pathways. This leads to the body's utilization of other energy sources like fats (triglycerides). For instance, fat is an important substrate for muscle contraction at rest and during exercise [72,73].

We observed an increase in serum triglyceride levels after training. Circulating triglycerides in the bloodstream could be broken down by an enzyme named lipoprotein lipase (LPL). These triglycerides are embedded in very low-density lipoproteins (VLDL) and chylomicrons traveling through the bloodstream [74]. LPL is also known to regulate lipoprotein and may reduce LDL [75]. LPL protein expression declined in AT4 after training cessation, which aligns with a previous study on rats that demonstrated that inactivity from 11 h to 11 days reduced LPL activity by 80%, indicating that physical inactivity may reduce muscle fat uptake [76]. In addition, adipose triglyceride lipase (ATGL) catalyzes adipose triglyceride and mobilizes lipids for energy production. ATGL also controls lipid homeostasis in other tissues [77]. We observed that 8 weeks of training increased protein expression of LPL by 6-fold and ATGL by 20-fold in the muscle, which is in line with former studies illustrating that regular endurance training results in greater muscle ATGL and LPL contents [78–80]. The increase in ATGL protein expression could maintain the low metabolic concentration of muscle fatty acids, thus improving insulin sensitivity [81]. The reduction in the expression of LPL and AGTL after detraining may reduce the catabolism of LDL; therefore, the LDL level increased during the detraining period. However, no significant change was found in fatty acid transporter FATP4 expression.

Training for 4 weeks slightly increased PFK and pyruvate, but further elevation was not observed with 8 weeks of training. Indeed, PFK is the rate-limiting enzyme in the glycolytic pathway; no change in PFK leads to the fact that the body has utilized other substrates to fulfill the energy requirement during exercise. Further, 4-week training increased glycogen content, which might be influenced by an increased hexokinase activity. However, when training continued for 8 weeks, the glycogen content decreased, while there was an increase in triglycerides level and protein expression of LPL and ATGL, suggesting that there might be a shift towards utilizing other substrate metabolisms when training continues for 8 weeks. The body might have started utilizing fat as fuel rather than carbohydrates at this stage. Additionally, training-induced elevated LPL expression may contribute to increased triglyceride-rich lipoprotein catabolism, thus reducing LDL levels. Thus, alterations in substrate use may contribute to the beneficial effect of regular exercise training to reduce the risk of obesity, insulin resistance, and type 2 diabetes.

Contrarily, we observed that training cessation after 4 weeks of training results in a loss of adaptations. For instance, training cessation reduced glucose tolerance, hexokinase activity, glycogen content, and protein expression (LPL and ATGL). Training cessation reduced LPL expression, which could reduce the catabolism of triglyceride and LDL. While detraining increased serum insulin, total cholesterol, LDL, and liver enzymes (ALT and AST) levels. All of these alterations have a negative impact on the metabolic function of the body and might be an indicator for the development of impaired glucose tolerance, insulin resistance, obesity, and eventually type 2 diabetes.

Notably, the increasing prevalence of type 2 diabetes and insulin resistance is not due to environmental disruption of genes, which is a common misconception. In fact, physical inactivity is an abnormal event for a genome programmed for physical activity. Therefore, insufficient physical activity fails to regulate normal biochemical and molecular events in maintaining glucose metabolism. Considering that the human body is designed to be physically active, the transition from a physically active lifestyle to an inactive lifestyle may have induced some metabolic changes, which is supported by the results of this study. Our study offers new insights by considering physically trained animals as controls for analyzing the downstream pathways involved in glucose metabolism. The current findings may have significant implications for preventing and treating diabetes, which is responsible for 6.7 million deaths (one in every five seconds), and the healthcare cost was about USD 966 billion in 2021 [82]. Therefore, it is necessary to promote regular physical activity, an innate behavior adopted by the human genome. Further research must be conducted to explore the alterations in metabolic pathways when the body switches from physical training to detraining. It is also required to identify the alteration in "active" genes that result in disease development when exposed to sedentary conditions.

There are some limitations in this study. Although a treadmill test was performed on each animal to assess their physical fitness through lactate release to individualize their training, it was challenging to apply specific training adapted to each animal. This is partially due to the equipment, which had six lanes but only a one-speed controller for all lanes. Another limitation is that only two detraining durations were selected. It is important to analyze different detraining durations to identify at exactly which time point the body starts losing the metabolic adaptations induced by exercise training.

5. Conclusions

This study identified the impact of training and detraining on metabolic adaptation, glucose metabolism, and the dose effect of training and detraining. Regular physical activity has improved glucose, insulin, lipid profile, liver enzymes, and glucose metabolism. A significant improvement was seen in the AUC for IPGTT, and the positive effect on glucose metabolism was lost during the detraining period. Further, no significant change was seen in HDL level after 4 weeks of training, but there was a significant elevation in HDL level at T8, indicating a dose effect of training. Training elicits a significant reduction in serum total cholesterol, LDL level, and ALP ($p < 0.05$) and an increased ALT level. Training increased hexokinase activity, but no change was seen in PFK. However, detraining increased glycogen recovery and pyruvate content after 8 weeks of training. Further, 8 weeks of training increased triglyceride levels, and enzymes (LPL, ATGL) were observed; the body lost this adaptation after 4 weeks of detraining. Further, detraining after 4 weeks of training immediately caused a loss of adaptations, thus resulting in the reduction of AUC of the glucose tolerance, hexokinase activity, glycogen content, and increased insulin level, total cholesterol, LDL level, and liver enzymes (ALT and AST). Conclusively, 4 weeks of daily physical training has shown beneficial effects in regulating glucose metabolism, with greater benefits associated with a longer training duration. Four weeks of detraining only were enough to start losing these positive adaptations. These results highlight the deleterious effects of physical inactivity and the importance of daily and constant endurance activity at moderate intensity to prevent the development of metabolic abnormalities likely to lead to complications such as type 2 diabetes.

Author Contributions: Conceptualization, C.P. and H.S.; methodology, C.P. and H.S.; software, H.S.; validation, C.P. and H.S.; formal analysis, C.P. and H.S.; investigation, H.S.; resources, C.P. and J.K.; data curation, H.S.; writing—original draft preparation, H.S.; writing—review and editing, C.P. and H.S.; visualization, J.K., M.K. and A.M.; animal work, H.S., J.K., M.K. and A.M.; supervision, C.P.; project administration, C.P.; funding acquisition, C.P. All authors have read and agreed to the published version of the manuscript.

Funding: This work was supported by the Ph.D. research fund (2021), fund code 31M522, from the United Arab Emirates University.

Institutional Review Board Statement: The animal study protocol was approved by the Animal Research Ethics Committee of the College of Medicine and Health Sciences at United Arab Emirates University (ERA_2021_7238, approved on 15 March 2021).

Data Availability Statement: The datasets generated and analyzed during the current study are available from the corresponding authors upon reasonable request.

Acknowledgments: All authors would like to acknowledge the College of Graduate Studies and Office of Associate Provost for Research, United Arab Emirates University, for their ongoing support.

Conflicts of Interest: The authors declare no conflict of interest.

Abbreviations

Intraperitoneal glucose tolerance test (IPGTT), pyruvate, glycogen, protein expression of lipoprotein lipase (LPL), adipose triglycerides lipase (ATGL), and fatty acid transport protein 4 (FATP4).

References

1. World Health Organization (WHO). Physical Inactivity. 2021. Available online: https://www.who.int/data/gho/indicator-metadata-registry/imr-details/3416 (accessed on 21 June 2023).
2. Helmrich, S.; Ragland, D.; Paffenbarger, R. Prevention of non—Insulin-dependent diabetes mellitus with physical activity. *Med. Sci. Sports Exerc.* **1994**, *26*, 824–830. [CrossRef] [PubMed]
3. Lee, I.M. Physical activity and cancer prevention—Data from epidemiologic studies. *Med. Sci. Sports Exerc.* **2003**, *35*, 1823–1827. [CrossRef] [PubMed]
4. World Health Organization. *Physical Activity*. 2020. Available online: https://www.who.int/health-topics/physical-activity#tab=tab_1 (accessed on 14 May 2023).
5. Richter, E.A.; Hargreaves, M. Exercise, GLUT4, and skeletal muscle glucose uptake. *Physiol. Rev.* **2013**, *93*, 993–1017. [CrossRef] [PubMed]
6. Shakoor, H.; Apostolopoulos, V.; Feehan, J.; Ali, H.I.; Ismail, L.C.; Al Dhaheri, A.S.O.S.; Stojanovska, L. Effect of Calorie Restriction and Exercise on Type 2 Diabetes. *Prilozi (Makedon. Akad. Nauk. Umet. Odd. Med. Nauki.)* **2021**, *42*, 109–126. [CrossRef]
7. Baba, C.S.; Alexander, G.; Kalyani, B.; Pandey, R.; Rastogi, S.; Pandey, A.; Choudhuri, G. Effect of exercise and dietary modification on serum aminotransferase levels in patients with nonalcoholic steatohepatitis. *J. Gastroenterol. Hepatol.* **2006**, *21*, 191–198. [CrossRef]
8. Guo, R.; Liong, E.C.; So, K.F.; Fung, M.-L.; Tipoe, G.L. Beneficial mechanisms of aerobic exercise on hepatic lipid metabolism in non-alcoholic fatty liver disease. *Hepatobiliary Pancreat. Dis. Int.* **2015**, *14*, 139–144. [CrossRef]
9. Georgakouli, K.; Manthou, E.; Fatouros, I.G.; Deli, C.K.; Spandidos, D.A.; Tsatsakis, A.M.; Kouretas, D.; Koutedakis, Y.; Theodorakis, Y.; Jamurtas, A.Z. Effects of acute exercise on liver function and blood redox status in heavy drinkers. *Exp. Ther. Med.* **2015**, *10*, 2015–2022. [CrossRef]
10. Smart, N.A.; King, N.; McFarlane, J.R.; Graham, P.L.; Dieberg, G. Effect of exercise training on liver function in adults who are overweight or exhibit fatty liver disease: A systematic review and meta-analysis. *Br. J. Sports Med.* **2018**, *52*, 834–843. [CrossRef]
11. Costill, D.L.; Coyle, E.F.; Fink, W.F.; Lesmes, G.R.; Witzmann, F.A. Adaptations in skeletal muscle following strength training. *J. Appl. Physiol.* **1979**, *46*, 96–99. [CrossRef]
12. Roberts, A.D.; Billeter, R.; Howald, H. Anaerobic muscle enzyme changes after interval training. *Int. J. Sports Med.* **1982**, *3*, 18–21. [CrossRef]
13. Simoneau, J.A.; Lortie, G.; Boulay, M.R.; Marcotte, M.; Thibault, M.C.; Bouchard, C. Effects of two high-intensity intermittent training programs interspaced by detraining on human skeletal muscle and performance. *Eur. J. Appl. Physiol. Occup. Physiol.* **1987**, *56*, 516–521. [CrossRef] [PubMed]
14. Evertsen, F.; Medbo, J.I.; Jebens, E.; Gjovaag, T.F. Effect of training on the activity of five muscle enzymes studied on elite cross-country skiers. *Acta Physiol. Scand.* **1999**, *167*, 247–258. [CrossRef] [PubMed]
15. Vestergaard, H.; Andersen, P.H.; Lund, S.; Schmitz, O.; Junker, S.; Pedersen, O. Pre-and posttranslational upregulation of muscle-specific glycogen synthase in athletes. *Am. J. Physiol.-Endocrinol. Metab.* **1994**, *266*, E92–E101. [CrossRef] [PubMed]
16. Pilegaard, H.; Keller, C.; Steensberg, A.; Wulff Helge, J.; Klarlund Pedersen, B.; Saltin, B.; Neufer, P.D. Influence of pre-exercise muscle glycogen content on exercise-induced transcriptional regulation of metabolic genes. *J. Physiol.* **2002**, *541*, 261–271. [CrossRef]
17. Pilegaard, H.; Ordway, G.A.; Saltin, B.; Neufer, P.D. Transcriptional regulation of gene expression in human skeletal muscle during recovery from exercise. *Am. J. Physiol.-Endocrinol. Metab.* **2000**, *279*, E806–E814. [CrossRef] [PubMed]

18. Fuller, S.; Simon, J.; Huang, T.Y.; Batdorf, H.; Scott, M.; Waskom, C.; Essajee, N.; Burke, S.; Collier, J.; Noland, R. Moderate Intensity Endurance Exercise Training Increases Muscle Glycogen Content but Does Not Alter Substrate Oxidation in C57BL6 Mice. *FASEB J.* **2018**, *32*, 855.30. [CrossRef]
19. Morville, T.; Rosenkilde, M.; Munch-Andersen, T.; Andersen, P.R.; Groenbæk, K.K.; Helbo, S.; Kristensen, M.; Hansen, A.V.; Mattsson, N.; Rasmusen, H.K. Repeated prolonged exercise decreases maximal fat oxidation in older men. *Med. Sci. Sports Exerc.* **2017**, *49*, 308–316. [CrossRef]
20. Mujika, I.; Padilla, S. Detraining: Loss of training-induced physiological and performance adaptations. Part I. *Sports Med.* **2000**, *30*, 79–87. [CrossRef]
21. Mujika, I.; Padilla, S. Detraining: Loss of training-induced physiological and performance adaptations. Part II. *Sports Med.* **2000**, *30*, 145–154. [CrossRef]
22. Neufer, P.D.; Shinebarger, M.H.; Dohm, G.L. Effect of training and detraining on skeletal muscle glucose transporter (GLUT4) content in rats. *Can. J. Physiol. Pharmacol.* **1992**, *70*, 1286–1290. [CrossRef]
23. King, D.S.; Dalsky, G.P.; Clutter, W.E.; Young, D.A.; Staten, M.A.; Cryer, P.E.; Holloszy, J.O. Effects of exercise and lack of exercise on insulin sensitivity and responsiveness. *J. Appl. Physiol.* **1988**, *64*, 1942–1946. [CrossRef] [PubMed]
24. Petibois, C.; Cassaigne, A.; Gin, H.; Déléris, G. Lipid profile disorders induced by long-term cessation of physical activity in previously highly endurance-trained subjects. *J. Clin. Endocrinol. Metab.* **2004**, *89*, 3377–3384. [CrossRef] [PubMed]
25. Ratel, S.; Gryson, C.; Rance, M.; Penando, S.; Bonhomme, C.; Le Ruyet, P.; Duclos, M.; Boirie, Y.; Walrand, S. Detraining-induced alterations in metabolic and fitness markers after a multicomponent exercise-training program in older men. *Appl. Physiol. Nutr. Metab.* **2012**, *37*, 72–79. [CrossRef] [PubMed]
26. Blanc, S.P.; Normand, S.; Pachiaudi, C.; Fortrat, J.-O.; Laville, M.; Gharib, C. Fuel homeostasis during physical inactivity induced by bed rest. *J. Clin. Endocrinol. Metab.* **2000**, *85*, 2223–2233. [CrossRef]
27. Dolkas, C.; Greenleaf, J. Insulin and glucose responses during bed rest with isotonic and isometric exercise. *J. Appl. Physiol.* **1977**, *43*, 1033–1038. [CrossRef]
28. Lipman, R.L.; Schnure, J.J.; Bradley, E.M.; Lecocq, F.R. Impairment of peripheral glucose utilization in normal subjects by prolonged bed rest. *J. Lab. Clin. Med.* **1970**, *76*, 221–230.
29. Mikines, K.J.; Richter, E.A.; Dela, F.; Galbo, H. Seven days of bed rest decrease insulin action on glucose uptake in leg and whole body. *J. Appl. Physiol.* **1991**, *70*, 1245–1254. [CrossRef]
30. Stuart, C.A.; Shangraw, R.E.; Prince, M.J.; Peters, E.J.; Wolfe, R.R. Bed-rest-induced insulin resistance occurs primarily in muscle. *Metabolism* **1988**, *37*, 802–806. [CrossRef]
31. Lipman, R.L.; Raskin, P.; Love, T.; Triebwasser, J.; Lecocq, F.R.; Schnure, J.J. Glucose intolerance during decreased physical activity in man. *Diabetes* **1972**, *21*, 101–107. [CrossRef]
32. Mankowitz, K.; Seipa, R.; Semenkovich, C.F.; Daugherty, A.; Schonfeld, G. Short-term interruption of training affects both fasting and post-prandial lipoproteins. *Atherosclerosis* **1992**, *95*, 181–189. [CrossRef]
33. Barzegarzadeh, H.; Dabidi, R.V. Effects of a 12-Week aerobic Training Course Followed by a 4-Week Detraining Period on Alanine Aminotransferase, Aspartate Aminotransferase, Alkaline Phosphatase and Blood Lipids Level Changes in Menopausal Rats. *J. Rafsanjan Univ. Med. Sci.* **2012**, *11*, 207–218.
34. Ravussin, E. Energy metabolism in obesity: Studies in the Pima Indians. *Diabetes Care* **1993**, *16*, 232–238. [CrossRef] [PubMed]
35. Wendorf, M.; Goldfine, I.D. Archaeology of NIDDM: Excavation of the "thrifty" genotype. *Diabetes* **1991**, *40*, 161–165. [CrossRef]
36. O'Kane, M.; Parrotti, H.M.; Pinkney, J.; Welbourn, R.; Hughes, C.A.; Mok, J.; Walker, N.; Thomas, D.; Devin, J.; Coulman, K.D. British Obesity and Metabolic Surgery Society Guidelines on perioperative and postoperative biochemical monitoring and micronutrient replacement for patients undergoing bariatric surgery—2020 update. *Obes. Rev.* **2020**, *21*, e13087. [CrossRef] [PubMed]
37. O'Keefe, J.H.; Vogel, R.; Lavie, C.J.; Cordain, L. Exercise like a hunter-gatherer: A prescription for organic physical fitness. *Prog. Cardiovasc. Dis.* **2011**, *53*, 471–479. [CrossRef]
38. Center for disease control and prevention (CDC). *Physical Activity and Health: A Report of the Surgeon General*; US Department of Health and Human Services: Washington, DC, USA, 1996. Available online: https://www.cdc.gov/nccdphp/sgr/index.htm (accessed on 2 May 2023).
39. Eaton, S.B.; Konner, M. Paleolithic nutrition: A consideration of its nature and current implications. *N. Engl. J. Med.* **1985**, *312*, 283–289. [CrossRef]
40. Gastebois, C.; Chanon, S.; Rome, S.; Durand, C.; Pelascini, E.; Jalabert, A.; Euthine, V.; Pialoux, V.; Blanc, S.; Simon, C. Transition from physical activity to inactivity increases skeletal muscle miR-148b content and triggers insulin resistance. *Physiol. Rep.* **2016**, *4*, e12902. [CrossRef]
41. Laye, M.J.; Rector, R.S.; Borengasser, S.J.; Naples, S.P.; Uptergrove, G.M.; Ibdah, J.A.; Booth, F.W.; Thyfault, J.P. Cessation of daily wheel running differentially alters fat oxidation capacity in liver, muscle, and adipose tissue. *J. Appl. Physiol.* **2009**, *106*, 161–168. [CrossRef]
42. Bergouignan, A.; Momken, I.; Lefai, E.; Antoun, E.; Schoeller, D.A.; Platat, C.; Chery, I.; Zahariev, A.; Vidal, H.; Gabert, L. Activity energy expenditure is a major determinant of dietary fat oxidation and trafficking, but the deleterious effect of detraining is more marked than the beneficial effect of training at current recommendations. *Am. J. Clin. Nutr.* **2013**, *98*, 648–658. [CrossRef]

43. Arifin, W.N.; Zahiruddin, W.M. Sample size calculation in animal studies using resource equation approach. *Malays. J. Med. Sci. MJMS* **2017**, *24*, 101.
44. Lutwak, L.; Whedon, G.D. The effect of physical conditioning on glucose tolerance. *Clin. Res.* **1959**, *7*, 143–144.
45. Abdolmaleki, F.; Heidarianpour, A. The response of serum Glypican-4 levels and its potential regulatory mechanism to endurance training and chamomile flowers' hydroethanolic extract in streptozotocin–nicotinamide-induced diabetic rats. *Acta Diabetol.* **2018**, *55*, 935–942. [CrossRef] [PubMed]
46. Omidi, M.; Yousefi, M. The effect of 8 weeks of aerobic exercise and 4 weeks detraining on serum fast blood sugar, insulin and glycosylated hemoglobin in. *J. Pract. Stud. Biosci. Sport* **2019**, *7*, 55–64.
47. Eizadi, M.; Bagheri, G.; Kasparast, J.M.; Zahedmanesh, F.; Afsharmand, Z. Effects of training on body composition, blood lipids, and glucose homeostasis assessed by the homeostasis model assessment. *Sci. Sports* **2013**, *28*, 75–80. [CrossRef]
48. Kraus, W.E.; Houmard, J.A.; Duscha, B.D.; Knetzger, K.J.; Wharton, M.B.; McCartney, J.S.; Bales, C.W.; Henes, S.; Samsa, G.P.; Otvos, J.D. Effects of the amount and intensity of exercise on plasma lipoproteins. *N. Engl. J. Med.* **2002**, *347*, 1483–1492. [CrossRef]
49. Akçakoyun, F. Changes in serum lipid profile following moderate exercise. *Afr. J. Pharm. Pharmacol.* **2010**, *4*, 829–833.
50. Banz, W.J.; Maher, M.A.; Thompson, W.G.; Bassett, D.R.; Moore, W.; Ashraf, M.; Keefer, D.J.; Zemel, M.B. Effects of resistance versus aerobic training on coronary artery disease risk factors. *Exp. Biol. Med.* **2003**, *228*, 434–440. [CrossRef] [PubMed]
51. Kelley, G.A.; Kelley, K.S. Effects of aerobic exercise on lipids and lipoproteins in adults with type 2 diabetes: A meta-analysis of randomized-controlled trials. *Public Health* **2007**, *121*, 643–655. [CrossRef] [PubMed]
52. Mirghani, S.J.; Yousefi, M.S. The effect of interval recovery periods during HIIT on liver enzymes and lipid profile in overweight women. *Sci. Sports* **2015**, *30*, 147–154. [CrossRef]
53. Wang, Y.; Xu, D. Effects of aerobic exercise on lipids and lipoproteins. *Lipids Health Dis.* **2017**, *16*, 132. [CrossRef] [PubMed]
54. LeMura, L.M.; von Duvillard, S.P.; Andreacci, J.; Klebez, J.M.; Chelland, S.A.; Russo, J. Lipid and lipoprotein profiles, cardiovascular fitness, body composition, and diet during and after resistance, aerobic and combination training in young women. *Eur. J. Appl. Physiol.* **2000**, *82*, 451–458. [CrossRef] [PubMed]
55. Sertie, R.A.L.; Andreotti, S.; Proença, A.R.G.; Campana, A.B.; Lima-Salgado, T.M.; Batista, M.L., Jr.; Seelaender, M.C.L.; Curi, R.; Oliveira, A.C.; Lima, F.B. Cessation of physical exercise changes metabolism and modifies the adipocyte cellularity of the periepididymal white adipose tissue in rats. *J. Appl. Physiol.* **2013**, *115*, 394–402. [CrossRef]
56. Gonzalez, J.T.; Fuchs, C.J.; Betts, J.A.; Van Loon, L.J.C. Liver glycogen metabolism during and after prolonged endurance-type exercise. *Am. J. Physiol.-Endocrinol. Metab.* **2016**, *311*, E543–E553. [CrossRef]
57. Zhao, X.-G.; Huang, H.-M.; Du, C.-Y. Effect of a combination of aerobic exercise and dietary modification on liver function in overweight and obese men. *J. Mens Health* **2021**, *17*, 176–182.
58. Hanley, A.J.; Wagenknecht, L.E.; Festa, A.; D'Agostino Jr, R.B.; Haffner, S.M. Alanine aminotransferase and directly measured insulin sensitivity in a multiethnic cohort: The Insulin Resistance Atherosclerosis Study. *Diabetes care* **2007**, *30*, 1819–1827. [CrossRef] [PubMed]
59. Hazar, S.; Hazar, M.; Korkmaz, Ş.; Bayil, S.; Gürkan, A.C. The effect of graded maximal aerobic exercise on some metabolic hormones, muscle damage and some metabolic end products in sportsmen. *Sci. Res. Essays* **2011**, *6*, 1337–1343.
60. Cho, N.H.; Jang, H.C.; Choi, S.H.; Kim, H.R.; Lee, H.K.; Chan, J.C.; Lim, S. Abnormal liver function test predicts type 2 diabetes: A community-based prospective study. *Diabetes Care* **2007**, *30*, 2566–2568. [CrossRef]
61. O'Doherty, R.M.; Bracy, D.P.; Osawa, H.; Wasserman, D.H.; Granner, D.K. Rat skeletal muscle hexokinase II mRNA and activity are increased by a single bout of acute exercise. *Am. J. Physiol.-Endocrinol. Metab.* **1994**, *266*, E171–E178. [CrossRef]
62. Koval, J.A.; DeFronzo, R.A.; O'Doherty, R.M.; Printz, R.; Ardehali, H.; Granner, D.K.; Mandarino, L.J. Regulation of hexokinase II activity and expression in human muscle by moderate exercise. *Am. J. Physiol.-Endocrinol. Metab.* **1998**, *274*, E304–E308. [CrossRef] [PubMed]
63. Biensø, R.S.; Olesen, J.; Gliemann, L.; Schmidt, J.F.; Matzen, M.S.; Wojtaszewski, J.F.P.; Hellsten, Y.; Pilegaard, H. Effects of exercise training on regulation of skeletal muscle glucose metabolism in elderly men. *J. Gerontol. Ser. A Biomed. Sci. Med. Sci.* **2015**, *70*, 866–872. [CrossRef]
64. Biensø, R.S.; Ringholm, S.; Kiilerich, K.; Aachmann-Andersen, N.-J.; Krogh-Madsen, R.; Guerra, B.; Plomgaard, P.; Van Hall, G.; Treebak, J.T.; Saltin, B. GLUT4 and glycogen synthase are key players in bed rest–induced insulin resistance. *Diabetes* **2012**, *61*, 1090–1099. [CrossRef] [PubMed]
65. Fell, R.D.; Terblanche, S.E.; Ivy, J.L.; Young, J.C.; Holloszy, J.O. Effect of muscle glycogen content on glucose uptake following exercise. *J. Appl. Physiol.* **1982**, *52*, 434–437. [CrossRef] [PubMed]
66. Bogardus, C.; Thuillez, P.; Ravussin, E.; Vasquez, B.; Narimiga, M.; Azhar, S. Effect of muscle glycogen depletion on in vivo insulin action in man. *J. Clin. Investig.* **1983**, *72*, 1605–1610. [CrossRef]
67. Blomstrand, E.; Saltin, B. Effect of muscle glycogen on glucose, lactate and amino acid metabolism during exercise and recovery in human subjects. *J. Physiol.* **1999**, *514*, 293. [CrossRef] [PubMed]
68. Weltan, S.M.; Bosch, A.N.; Dennis, S.C.; Noakes, T.D. Preexercise muscle glycogen content affects metabolism during exercise despite maintenance of hyperglycemia. *Am. J. Physiol.-Endocrinol. Metab.* **1998**, *274*, E83–E88. [CrossRef] [PubMed]

69. Takahashi, Y.; Sarkar, J.; Yamada, J.; Matsunaga, Y.; Nonaka, Y.; Banjo, M.; Sakaguchi, R.; Shinya, T.; Hatta, H. Enhanced skeletal muscle glycogen repletion after endurance exercise is associated with higher plasma insulin and skeletal muscle hexokinase 2 protein levels in mice: Comparison of level running and downhill running model. *J. Physiol. Biochem.* **2021**, *77*, 469–480. [CrossRef]
70. Ryan, B.J.; Schleh, M.W.; Ahn, C.; Ludzki, A.C.; Gillen, J.B.; Varshney, P.; Van Pelt, D.W.; Pitchford, L.M.; Chenevert, T.L.; Gioscia-Ryan, R.A. Moderate-intensity exercise and high-intensity interval training affect insulin sensitivity similarly in obese adults. *J. Clin. Endocrinol. Metab.* **2020**, *105*, e2941–e2959. [CrossRef]
71. Henriksson, J.; Reitman, J.S. Quantitative measures of enzyme activities in type I and type II muscle fibres of man after training. *Acta Physiol. Scand.* **1976**, *97*, 392–397. [CrossRef] [PubMed]
72. Ranallo, R.F.; Rhodes, E.C. Lipid metabolism during exercise. *Sports Med.* **1998**, *26*, 29–42. [CrossRef]
73. Zierler, K.L. Fatty acids as substrates for heart and skeletal muscle. *Circ. Res.* **1976**, *38*, 459–463. [CrossRef] [PubMed]
74. Pirahanchi, Y.; Anoruo, M.; Sharma, S. *Biochemistry, Lipoprotein Lipase*; StatPearls: Orlando, FL, USA, 2021.
75. Mohammad, P.; Esfandiar, K.Z.; Abbas, S.; Ahoora, R. Effects of moderate-intensity continuous training and high-intensity interval training on serum levels of resistin, chemerin and liver enzymes in streptozotocin-nicotinamide induced type-2 diabetic rats. *J. Diabetes Metab. Disord.* **2019**, *18*, 379–387. [CrossRef] [PubMed]
76. Bey, L.; Hamilton, M.T. Suppression of skeletal muscle lipoprotein lipase activity during physical inactivity: A molecular reason to maintain daily low-intensity activity. *J. Physiol.* **2003**, *551*, 673–682. [CrossRef] [PubMed]
77. Trites, M.J.; Clugston, R.D. The role of adipose triglyceride lipase in lipid and glucose homeostasis: Lessons from transgenic mice. *Lipids Health Dis.* **2019**, *18*, 204. [CrossRef]
78. Alsted, T.J.; Nybo, L.; Schweiger, M.; Fledelius, C.; Jacobsen, P.; Zimmermann, R.; Zechner, R.; Kiens, B. Adipose triglyceride lipase in human skeletal muscle is upregulated by exercise training. *Am. J. Physiol.-Endocrinol. Metab.* **2009**, *296*, E445–E453. [CrossRef] [PubMed]
79. Kiens, B.; Lithell, H.; Mikines, K.J.; Richter, E.A. Effects of insulin and exercise on muscle lipoprotein lipase activity in man and its relation to insulin action. *J. Clin. Investig.* **1989**, *84*, 1124–1129. [CrossRef]
80. Seip, R.L.; Angelopoulos, T.J.; Semenkovich, C.F. Exercise induces human lipoprotein lipase gene expression in skeletal muscle but not adipose tissue. *Am. J. Physiol.-Endocrinol. Metab.* **1995**, *268*, E229–E236. [CrossRef] [PubMed]
81. Turnbull, P.C.; Longo, A.B.; Ramos, S.V.; Roy, B.D.; Ward, W.E.; Peters, S.J. Increases in skeletal muscle ATGL and its inhibitor G0S2 following 8 weeks of endurance training in metabolically different rat skeletal muscles. *Am. J. Physiol.-Regul. Integr. Comp. Physiol.* **2016**, *310*, R125–R133. [CrossRef]
82. International Diabetes Federation (IDF). *IDF Diabetes Atlas 2021*, 10th ed.; International Diabetes Federation (IDF): Brussels, Belgium, 2021. Available online: https://idf.org/about-diabetes/diabetes-facts-figures/ (accessed on 11 June 2023).

nutrients

MDPI

Article

Modified Mediterranean-Ketogenic Diet and Carboxytherapy as Personalized Therapeutic Strategies in Lipedema: A Pilot Study

Laura Di Renzo [1,†], Paola Gualtieri [1,*,†], Samanta Zomparelli [2], Gemma Lou De Santis [3], Silvia Seraceno [2], Claudia Zuena [2], Giulia Frank [2,3], Rossella Cianci [4], Domenico Centofanti [5] and Antonino De Lorenzo [1]

1 Section of Clinical Nutrition and Nutrigenomics, Department of Biomedicine and Prevention, University of Rome Tor Vergata, Via Montpellier 1, 00133 Rome, Italy
2 School of Specialization in Food Science, University of Tor Vergata, Via Montpellier 1, 00133 Rome, Italy
3 PhD School of Applied Medical-Surgical Sciences, University of Rome Tor Vergata, Via Montpellier 1, 00133 Rome, Italy
4 Department of Translational Medicine and Surgery, Fondazione Policlinico Universitario A. Gemelli, IRCCS, 00168 Rome, Italy
5 Società Italiana di Medicina Estetica, 00195 Rome, Italy
* Correspondence: paola.gultieri@uniroma2.it
† These authors contributed equally to this work.

Abstract: In recent years, the use of the ketogenic diet as a proper nutritional treatment for lipedema has been hypothesized in the literature. This is the first clinical study evaluating the ketogenic diet and carboxytherapy in lipedema patients. In the present study, it was decided to use a modified Mediterranean ketogenic diet (MMKD) in combination with carboxytherapy. Since lipedema is characterized by microangiopathy, local hypoxia, and increased subcutaneous adipose tissue (SAT) deposition, carboxytherapy could improve painful symptoms and skin tone. A total of 22 subjects were included in the data analysis, divided into three groups; 8 patients underwent MMKD combined with carboxytherapy sessions (KDCB group), 8 underwent MMKD nutritional treatment alone (KD group), and 6 patients underwent only carboxytherapy sessions (CB group), for a total of 10 weeks of treatment for all three groups. It was observed that the ketogenic diet effectively induced weight and fat mass loss, including in the limbs, areas considered unresponsive to diet therapy in lipedema patients. However, the best results were obtained from the combination of the ketogenic diet and carboxytherapy, which showed improvements in both body composition and skin texture and a reduction in pain, along with an improvement in sleep quality. It would be helpful to conduct a clinical trial on a larger scale and over a more extended period to observe the results in the long term as well.

Keywords: nutrition; ketogenic diet; carboxytherapy; SAT diseases; lipedema; body composition

1. Introduction

Lipedema is an autosomal dominant inheritance, progressive, multifactorial, and disabling disease, characterized by an accumulation of pathological subcutaneous adipose tissue (SAT) in the superfascial area, microangiopathy, chronic tissue inflammation, and pain. Symptoms usually occur at puberty, pregnancy, or menopause, assuming the role of estrogens in the pathophysiological process. The diagnosis is clinical, the adipose tissue develops descending symmetrically and bilaterally, and the lower limbs are the most affected sites. It is classified into five types based on the distribution of the lipo-edematous adipose tissue and into four stages based on the severity of the disease [1]. The first clinical study on diet therapy in lipedema was published by our research group, and showed an improvement in overall body composition and in specifically affected areas (upper and lower limbs) with consumption of a low-carb diet and high-antioxidant-content foods, inspired by the Mediterranean diet [2]. In recent years, there has been a sharp increase in studies on the use of the ketogenic diet for various diseases, such as obesity, diabetes mellitus type II, Alzheimer's disease, multiple sclerosis, and cancer [3,4]. It is characterized by an intake of carbohydrates <30 g/day, shifting from a glucose cellular metabolism to a lipid metabolism, thus inducing the oxidation of fats and ketosis (defined as a blood concentration of beta-hydroxybutyrate >0.5 mmol/L) [5,6]. In January 2021, a review was published encouraging the ketogenic diet in patients suffering from lipedema as the most effective therapy. Hypothesized mechanisms involved are a reduction in insulin and, therefore, in the lipogenesis and lipo-hypertrophy promoted by hyperinsulinemia; increased sense of satiety, both due to the intake of a greater quantity of lipids and by improving the cerebral sensitivity to leptin (which in subjects with an increase in adipose tissue can be reduced) [7]; modulation of inflammation; reduction in oxidative stress, carried out by beta-hydroxy-butyrate [8]; reduction in sensitivity to mechanical, thermal, and/or neuropathic pain after several weeks of ketosis [9]. Masino and Ruskin hypothesized that the restriction of carbohydrates reduces the neurons' excitability, suppressing pain perception, reducing inflammation, and increasing the levels of adenosine, a natural analgesic [3]. Moreover, a decrease in appearance-related discomfort and depression following a reduction in weight and body fat, particularly in the most affected areas, was highlighted [10]. Additionally, several studies have shown that adopting a ketogenic regimen reduces depression, and improves attention, mood, and social interactions [11]. Recently, Cannataro et al. published a case report of a lipedema patient following a ketogenic diet as a nutritional intervention for two years, achieving significant weight loss, reducing pain, and, therefore, improving quality of life. However, to our knowledge, there are no clinical studies regarding the ketogenic diet in a group of lipedema patients.

Also, we wanted to evaluate the efficacy of carboxytherapy for a reduction in subcutaneous fat and a reduction in painful symptoms. Its use for therapeutic purposes dates back to the 1930s, when it was used as thermal therapy (baths in carbonated water) for treating patients with obliterating peripheral arterial disease [12]. The goal of carboxytherapy is to improve or restore circulatory function when damaged. This procedure is characterized by the administration of carbon dioxide (CO2) in the gaseous state by a subcutaneous or intradermal route through tiny needles (30 G) [13]. In addition, carboxytherapy stimulates microcirculation and increases the local blood flow, with a concomitant positive effect on fibroblastic activity and a lipolytic effect with an improvement in skin elasticity and skin irregularities caused by fat accumulation [14]. Since lipedema is characterized by microangiopathy, local hypoxia, and increased SAT deposition, carboxytherapy could improve painful symptoms and skin tone. Therefore, the primary outcome of this pilot study is to identify potential therapeutic strategies in a group of lipedema patients evaluating the efficacy of a personalized modified Mediterranean ketogenic diet (MMKD), with or without carboxytherapy, for a limited period on body composition parameters. The secondary outcome is to evaluate the effects of the treatments above on the state of health, pain perception, and quality of life.

2. Materials and Methods

2.1. Subjects and Study Design

Between May 2022 and May 2023, a pilot study was conducted at the Section of Clinical Nutrition and Nutrigenomics, University of Rome Tor Vergata, and 34 patients diagnosed with lipedema were enrolled. Inclusion criteria were diagnosis of lipedema, female sex, and consent to the protocol. Exclusion criteria were age <18 or >65 years; diagnosis of lymphedema; stage 4 lipedema; drug or alcohol abuse; psychotic disorders; acute or chronic renal failure; liver failure; neoplastic disease under treatment; pregnancy and lactation; menopause for more than 2 years; hepatitis B and C; HIV/AIDS; and COVID-19. Four patients declined to participate. Therefore, 30 patients were randomly divided into three groups; 11 patients underwent MMKD combined with carboxytherapy sessions (KDCB group), 12 underwent MMKD nutritional treatment alone (KD group), and 7 patients underwent only carboxytherapy sessions (CB group), for a total of 10 weeks of treatment for all three groups. From the KDCB group, 3 patients withdrew; from the KD group, 4 patients withdrew; from the CD group, 1 patient withdrew (major surgery, pregnancy, bereavement, COVID-19, relocation for work reasons). In the end, 22 patients completed the study, 8 in the KDCB group, 8 in the KD group, and 6 in the CB group (Figure 1).

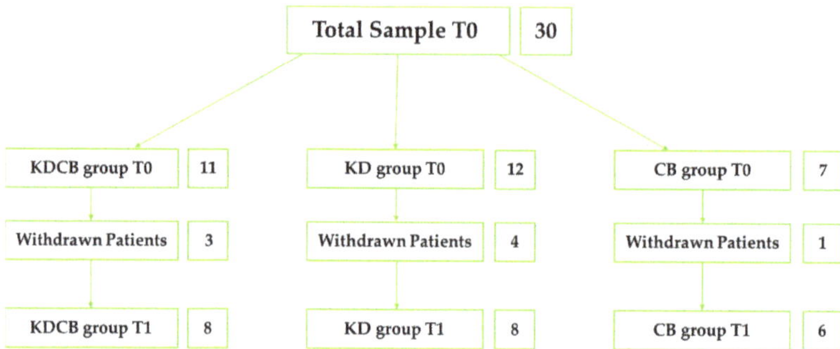

Figure 1. Flowchart.

A complete medical and nutritional evaluation was performed at baseline (T0) and after ten weeks (T1). All patients were interviewed via telephone every two weeks with a nutritional recall of the previous 24 h to monitor compliance with the dietary treatment and were questioned about any complications or side effects. Carboxytherapy sessions were performed once a week for the ten weeks of treatment by the same operator (S.S.).

All enrolled patients signed an informed consent form according to the principles of the Declaration of Helsinki. This trial is registered with ClinicalTrial.gov NCT01890070. Approval was obtained from the Ethics Committee of the Calabria Region Central Area Section (register protocol no. 146 17/05/2018).

2.2. Dietary Assessment and Intervention

At T0 and T1, a trained nutritionist assessed the subjects' eating habits through a thorough food history. A 24 h recall and a food frequency questionnaire were conducted to identify the amount of intake and weekly frequency of different foods [15].

All subjects received the MMKD with a 20% calorie restriction of daily energy requirements. Daily protein intake was calculated as 2 g/kg of total lean mass (LM), according to Colica et al. [16]. The diet indicated for each day of the week the foods to be consumed, divided into five meals daily. The mean calorie distribution of the meals was as follows: 15%—breakfast, 10%—morning snack, 35%—lunch, 10%—afternoon snack, and 30%—dinner. The daily macronutrient intake of the diet was divided as follows: <10% of total kcal/day of carbohydrates (<30 g day), 15 g of fiber, 20–25% of total kcal/day of protein (of which 20% was of vegetable origin), and 70% of total kcal/day of lipids (of which 48% was of polyunsaturated fatty acids (PUFA) and monounsaturated fatty acids (MUFA)). The bromatological composition of the diet was obtained using Dietosystem® dietary analysis software (version 12.00.13, DS Medica SRL, Milan, Italy).

The main characteristics of the MMKD are as follows: seasonal vegetables; foods rich in mono- and polyunsaturated fats, such as olive oil, nuts, avocado, oily fish, and fresh cheeses with reduced saturated fat content; lean meat of organic origin; and use of herbs and spices to reduce the amount of added salt. Processed and preserved foods such as frozen ready meals, cured meats, canned products and sausages, simple carbohydrates and sugars, sugary alcoholic and soft drinks, and fresh fruits (except for red fruits) were excluded.

The Mediterranean adequacy index (MAI) was calculated using the ratio of caloric intake (% kcal/day) from typical Mediterranean carbohydrates and foods (such as fruits, vegetables, bread, pasta, extra virgin olive oil, fish, and wine) to nontypical foods (such as milk and dairy products, meat, eggs, sweets, sugar, and alcoholic beverages). MAI values are considered acceptable when the value is >5 and 100% adequate if >15 [17].

2.3. Carboxytherapy

The method consists of the supply of CO2 through highly sophisticated electronic machinery (CarbomedCO2, Physioled, Taumed, Rome, Italy), which allows supplying of pure gas, free from contaminants, with specific preset parameters of dose, flow, speed, and temperature. The CO2 passes through a disposable sterile tube at the end of which a 30-gauge 13 mm needle or 4 mm microlance is inserted. The dose and speed depend on the treatment site and the clinical indication. The injection can be superficial, intradermal, or subcutaneous. The rate that CO2 takes to cross the tissue varies according to the characteristics of the tissue of the subject being treated [18]. In our study, CO2 was delivered subcutaneously via a 30-gauge needle angled at 45° to the tissue to be treated at a temperature of 43 °C. Up to 500 mL per side per session can be administered. A total of 2400 mL per session was delivered, with an average flow of 80 mL/min. The protocol included ten sessions, one time a week. Carboxytherapy was performed on the lower limbs bilaterally in the following areas: trochanteric, midthigh anterior, inner thigh, posterior thigh, and popliteal.

CO2 determines increased local blood flow rate; increased arteriolar and metarteriolar sphygmicity (short-term effect); stimulation of true and false neoangiogenesis, with an increase in microcirculation (long-term effect); extero-receptor activation, linked to hyperdistension of subcutaneous tissues, with the production of bradykinin, increase in cyclic adenosine monophosphate (cAMP), and activation of intra-adipocyte lipase; and Bohr effect amplification, with the more significant release of oxygen (O2) at the tissue level [19]. Possible adverse effects are local pain associated with crepitus or burning sensation and possible bruising. Serious adverse events are rare and were not detected during our protocol. It cannot cause embolism, and it is not toxic [20].

2.4. Anthropometrics, Body Composition, and Basal Metabolism

After a 12 h overnight fast, an anthropometric assessment was performed for each patient. Body weight and height were measured with a scale and stadiometer (Invernizzi, Rome, Italy) while the subject was standing wearing underwear. Data were collected to the nearest 0.1 kg and 0.1 cm, respectively. Body mass index (BMI) was calculated as body weight (kg)/height (m^2) and classified according to the World Health Organization (WHO) [21]. Hip and waist circumferences were measured with a flexible, non-stretchable metric tape.

Body composition was assessed according to the standard method [22]. Patients were asked to remove all clothing (except underwear), shoes, and any metal objects. Whole and segmental fat mass (FM) (kg) were assessed using dual X-ray absorptiometry (DXA) (Primus, X-ray densitometer; software version 1.2.2, Osteosys Co., Ltd., Guro-gu, Seoul, Republic of Korea). The effective radiation dose for this procedure is about 0.01 mSv. The intra- and intersubject coefficient of variation (CV% = 100 SD/mean) ranged from 1 to 5%. The coefficients for this instrument for five participants undergoing six scans over 9 months were 2.2% for FM and 1.1% for fat-free mass (FFM) and LM. Total FM (% FM) was calculated as total body FM (total FM) divided by the total mass of all tissues, including total body bone (TBBone), as follows: % FM = [total FM/(total FM + total LM + TBBone)] × 100.

Based on % FM, subjects are classified as normal weight (NW) for % FM < 30, and obese for % FM $\geq$ 30. Android and gynoid distribution were confirmed when gynoid and android total fat tissue (%) were >30 [23,24].

The appendicular skeletal muscle mass index (ASMMI) was calculated as follows:

(LM legs + LM arms)/height (m^2). The intermuscular adipose tissue (IMAT) was calculated according to Colica et al. [16] with the following formulas: Log (IMAT) = −2.21 + (0.12 × fat) + (−0.0013 × fat^2) for women.

Basal metabolic rate (BMR) was calculated using the De Lorenzo formula [25]:

$$BMR = [(3941 \times VO2) + (1106 \times VCO2)] \times 1.44$$

$$VO2 = LM\ kg\ (DXA) \times 5.3\ (f)$$

$$VCO2 = VO2 \times 0.85$$

2.5. EUROQOL-5 Dimension (EQ-5D)

This test was constructed to become a generic measure of quality of life, and to be short, easy to use, and self-administered. It was validated through collaboration with researchers from Northern Europe (Finland, the Netherlands, UK, Sweden), who have worked on the European Quality of Life project since 1990. It is a standardized instrument that can be used for different purposes; in this case, it was used to assess the possible changes in health status at other times (T0 and T1) and to contribute to the standardized assessment of the verification of the effectiveness of the dietary treatment used in patients with lipedema.

The second section of the EQ-5D includes an assessment using visual analog scale (VAS) graphically represented by a graded scale ranging from 0 (the worst possible health status) to 100 (the best possible health status) on which the respondent indicates the level of perceived health status. In this case, the EQ-5D evaluates the comparison of the change in the numbers obtained between the first part and the second part at T0 and T1, particularly in assessing any improvements regarding not only general health status but also pain, discomfort, and the psychological aspect related to depression and anxiety [26].

The EQ-5D is reported in Appendix A.

2.6. Fibromyalgia Tests

2.6.1. Fibromyalgia Assessment Status (FAS)

Examinations of patients with lipedema showed that the areas of increased pain and soreness overlapped with those of fibromyalgia, even though this condition does not characterize lipedema. Therefore, to assess the effect of diet and carboxytherapy on pain and asthenia, it was decided that the FAS would be used. This simple self-administered test assesses asthenia, pain, and sleep disturbances based on the 16 non-joint sites listed on the self-assessment pain scale (SAPS) in a single measure (range: 0 to 10) [27].

The FAS is reported in Appendix A.

2.6.2. Fibromyalgia Severity Scale (FSS)

This is an instrument used to assess symptoms and signs related to pain in fibromyalgia pathology. It consists of the diffuse pain index, which refers to the distribution of the pain symptom in the last week at the time of observation; generalized pain index, which details the body regions affected by pain; and symptom severity index, which considers symptoms such as asthenia, nonrestorative sleep, and cognitive problems, reported in the last week, and symptoms such as migraine, abdominal pain or cramps, and depression, reported in the last six months [27].

The FSS is reported in Appendix A.

2.6.3. Revised Fibromyalgia Impact Questionnaire (FIQR)

The FIQR is an updated version of the fibromyalgia impact questionnaire (FIQ). It consists of twenty-one numerical rating scales from 0 to 10 (where 10 is "worst") that explore the three main domains of function, widespread impact, and symptoms. The revised version expanded the original scale by adding new questions about sensitivity, balance, memory, and environmental sensitivity. All questions refer to the previous seven days. The final score (range 0–100, with higher values indicating greater severity of illness) is calculated as follows: the algebraic sum of the 9-item function domain (range 0–90) is divided by three; the algebraic sum of the 2-item general impact domain (range 0–20) remains unchanged; and the algebraic sum of the 10-item symptom domain (range 0–100) is divided by two. These three partial scores are then added together [28].

The FIQR is reported in Appendix A.

2.7. Difficulties in Emotional Regulation Scale (DERS)

The DERS is a self-reported measure that aims to assess emotion dysregulation. It is widely used in treatment and research settings for adults with emotional disorders (e.g., bipolar, anxiety, depression, obsessive-compulsive disorder, trauma, and stress-related disorders), so it is useful for investigating the possible presence of psychological disorders in patients with lipedema.

The model on which DERS is based proposes six emotion regulation factors, translated into six subscales: (a) lack of awareness and understanding of emotions ("I am mindful of my feelings", with reverse scoring); (b) lack of acceptance of emotions ("I have difficulty making sense of my feelings"); (c) difficulty controlling impulses ("When I am angry, I get out of control"); (d) difficulty engaging in goal-oriented cognitions and behaviors when distressed (goals; "When I'm angry, I have a hard time getting the job done"); (e) unwillingness to accept specific emotional responses ("When I'm angry, I get angry at myself for feeling that way"); and (f) lack of access to strategies for feeling better when distressed ("When I'm angry, I think there's nothing I can do to feel better"). Developed initially as a 36-question measure, a short 18-question form was created that retains the original six subscales. The measure is scored so that higher scores reflect more significant impairment or dysregulation [29–31].

The DERS is reported in Appendix A.

2.8. Yale Food Addiction Scale 2.0 (YFAS 2.0)

Lipedema patients may present with eating disorders. Therefore, a validated diagnostic tool for food addiction (FA), the YFAS, was used to identify individuals with addictive eating behaviors. The original YFAS (25 questions) was based on the Diagnostic and Statistical Manual of Mental Disorders (DSM) IV for substance dependence, including the consumption of highly palatable foods (e.g., pizza, ice cream, and chocolate). Later, the scale was replaced with the YFAS 2.0 (35 questions) in response to the revised criteria for substance-related disorders and addictions in the DSM-5. YFAS 2.0 introduced the following diagnostic criteria: use despite interpersonal or social consequences and, in physically dangerous situations, craving. A severity classification was also introduced.

The YFAS version 2.0 is a thirty-five-question questionnaire with an eight-point response scale. It measures the eleven criteria of substance-related disorders and addictions to food and eating. For the potential "diagnosis" of food addiction, at least two of the eleven addiction and substance use disorder criteria must be met, and significant impairment must be present. The YFAS also measures eating behavior impairment.

Both versions have two scoring options: a symptom count (YFAS range = 0–7, YFAS 2.0 range = 0–11), a diagnostic score that predicts the achievement of a symptom threshold (YFAS $\geq$ 3, YFAS 2.0 $\geq$ 2), and the presence of clinically significant impairment or distress (self-perceived). With respect to the first version, the YFAS 2.0 differentiates the severity level of FA based on symptom count (mild 2–3, moderate 4–5, severe $\geq$ 6), paralleling the DSM-5 severity [32,33].

The YFAS 2.0 is reported in Appendix A.

2.9. Statistical Analysis

The data collected before statistical evaluations were analyzed for the presence of outliers, and the Shapiro–Wilk test was performed to evaluate variable distribution. The data presented are expressed as mean and standard deviation, to evaluate differences between the times. Related sample t-tests or Wilcoxon signed rank tests were used to assess the differences in the variables examined at the follow-up. Results were significant for p-value < 0.05. Statistical analysis was performed using IBM SPSS Statistics V25.0 (SPSS, Chicago, IL, USA).

3. Results

3.1. Dietary Components

At T0 and T1, the results of dietary component analysis (macro- and micronutrients and nutritional indices) were calculated using food frequency. The average dietary components of the patients' eating habits at T0 and the average dietary components of KD at T1 were compared (Table 1). Significant differences are shown for the following parameters: decreased carbohydrates (%) ($p = 0.001$), reduced sugars (%) ($p = 0.001$), decreased fiber (g) ($p = 0.011$), and increased animal proteins (%) ($p = 0.001$). In addition, statistically significant results were obtained for increased MUFA and PUFA content ($p = 0.001$). Statistically significant increases in vitamin D (μcg) ($p = 0.001$) and vitamin E (mg) ($p = 0.001$) content were also observed, while vitamin C (mg) was significantly reduced ($p = 0.07$). A significant increase in the MAI when comparing the dietary patterns followed at T0 and T1 ($p = 0.001$) was observed.

Table 1. Average dietary components of the patients' eating habits at T0 and average dietary components of the KD at T1.

	Media T0	Media T1	*p*-Value
Energy (Kcal)	1551.69 [329.96]	1512.5 [140.73]	0.617
Proteins (% Kcal)	22.88 [7.12]	22.81 [0.7]	0.969
Vegetable proteins (% Kcal)	22.52 [10.17]	20.08 [2.12]	0.373
Animal proteins (% Kcal)	65.96 [9.93]	77.95 [2.07]	<0.001 *
Carbohydrates (% Kcal)	28.9 [11.85]	5.95 [0.67]	<0.001 *
Sugars (% Kcal)	22.68 [13.79]	3.5 [0.26]	<0.001 *
Fiber (g)	18.32 [5.97]	14.17 [0.9]	0.011 *
Lipids (% Kcal)	47.84 [10.36]	71.23 [0.93]	<0.001 *
SFA (% Kcal)	14.92% [9.93%]	15.70% [0.82%]	0.759
PUFA (% Kcal)	5.10% [1.93%]	8.55% [0.51%]	<0.001 *
MUFA (% Kcal)	22.80% [4.96%]	40.60% [0.70%]	<0.001 *
Vit C (mg)	154.41 [72.32]	101.34 [10.21]	0.007 *
Vit D (μcg)	2.42 [1.89]	4.91 [0.68]	<0.001 *
Vit E (mg)	14.94 [5.75]	22.87 [1.81]	<0.001 *
MAI	0.87 [0.65]	2.63 [0.75]	<0.001 *

SFA, saturated fatty acid; PUFA, polyunsaturated fatty acid; MUFA, monounsaturated fatty acid; Vit, vitamin; MAI, Mediterranean adequacy index; KDCB, ketogenic diet and carboxytherapy group; KD, ketogenic diet group. Standard deviation in square brackets. Statistical significance was attributed as * $p < 0.05$.

3.2. Sample Description, Anthropometrics, and Body Composition

After screening through the inclusion criteria, 30 subjects, all female, were included in the data analysis (Table 2).

According to BMI and % FM, 13.8% of patients were found to be normal weight, 20.7% normal weight obese, and 65.5% obese. According to the distribution of FM, 44.8% had a gynoid distribution, 55.2% had a mixed-type distribution, and none had an android distribution. An ANOVA test was performed to analyze the BMI and % FM differences between the three groups at T0. No differences were highlighted (respectively $p = 0.63$ and $p = 0.83$).

Table 2. Description of total sample at T0.

Sample T0	
Total (n)	30
Sex (M/F)	30 (F)
Age (years)	46 [7.4]
Height (cm)	160.65 [6.2]
Weight (kg)	73.8 [17]
BMI (kg/m^2)	28.6 [6.5]

Standard deviation in square brackets.

The percentage of different stages of lipedema identified in the sample was as follows: 20% of patients were stage 1, 60% were stage 2, 20% were stage 3, and none were stage 4.

Then, the sample was divided into three groups: 11 patients treated with the ketogenic diet and carboxytherapy (KDCB group), 12 with the ketogenic diet only (KD group), and 7 with carboxytherapy only (CB group).

After 10 weeks of treatment, a significant decrease in most of the parameters analyzed was shown (Table 3). Weight and BMI were significantly reduced in both the KDCB ($p = 0.009$, $p = 0.008$) and the KD groups ($p = 0.003$, $p = 0.008$). These parameters were not significantly different in the CB group. In relation to circumferences, only the hip was significantly different in both the KDCB and KD groups ($p = 0.02$, $p = 0.0001$), while waist circumference was significantly reduced only in the KD group ($p = 0.03$). No difference in the CB group was detected.

Table 3. Comparison of anthropometrics at T0 and at T1 in the 3 treatment groups.

	KDCB T0	KDCB T1	*p*-Value	KD T0	KD T1	*p*-Value	CB T0	CB T1	*p*-Value
Weight (Kg)	72.64 [21.17]	69.29 [21.5]	0.009 *	74.26 [11.53]	70.73 [11.55]	0.003 *	76.78 [24.88]	76.07 [24.78]	0.168
BMI (Kg/m^2)	28.33 [7.3]	27.02 [7.51]	0.008 *	27.18 [4.66]	25.88 [4.39]	0.006 *	30.68 [10.93]	30.4 [10.92]	0.211
Waist Circumference (cm)	80.5 [16.06]	77.38 [15.26]	0.069	82.25 [10.94]	79.19 [10.52]	0.03 *	83.37 [17.03]	83.02 [16.57]	0.527
Hip Circumference (cm)	107.41 [13.4]	104.94 [13.04]	0.02 *	109.66 [7.87]	105.19 [8.54]	0.0001 *	112.32 [20.8]	113.55 [19.93]	0.239

KDCB, ketogenic diet and carboxytherapy group; KD, ketogenic diet group; CB, carboxytherapy group; T0, baseline; T1, after 10 weeks. Standard deviation in square brackets. Statistical significance was attributed as * $p < 0.05$.

Regarding DXA parameters, in the KDCB group, total FM (expressed in grams and percentage) was significantly reduced ($p = 0.005$, $p = 0.012$), as was leg FM, in grams and percentage ($p = 0.001$, $p = 0.02$). The same results were obtained in the KD group for total FM g and % ($p = 0.019$ and $p = 0.044$), while FM in legs was significantly reduced only in g ($p = 0.015$). Differently, in the CB group, no significant results related to these parameters were found. In addition, significant decreases in the percentage of android and gynoid FM and IMAT were shown in both the KDCB group ($p = 0.0011$, $p = 0.003$, $p = 0.026$) and the KD group ($p = 0.029$, $p = 0.03$, $p = 0.007$). In contrast, in the CB group, none of these parameters changed significantly (Table 4).

Table 4. Comparison of body composition parameters at T0 and T1 in the 3 treatment groups.

DXA Parameters	KDCB T0	KDCB T1	*p*-Value	KD T0	KD T1	*p*-Value	CB T0	CB T1	*p*-Value
Total fat tissue (%)	36.39 [9.21]	34.38 [9.6]	0.012 *	38.03 [7.69]	36.35 [9.83]	0.044 *	38.78 [9.52]	37.42 [10.43]	0.153
Total fat tissue (g)	26,825.88 [15,049.11]	24,619.63 [15,214.81]	0.005 *	29,135.88 [9149.12]	26,489.17 [11,013.63]	0.019 *	32,070.5 [18,361.24]	29,948.5 [17,215.04]	0.064
Total leg fat tissue (%)	42.44 [8.45]	40.49 [8.93]	0.020 *	46.08 [6.02]	44.97 [8.03]	0.075	45.63 [6.37]	45.27 [5.98]	0.598
Total leg fat tissue (g)	13,008.63 [5692.33]	11,702.88 [5722.94]	0.001 *	14,616.63 [4120.1]	13,264.5 [4021.63]	0.015 *	14,243.5 [6219.5]	14,108.33 [6473.1]	0.673
Total arm fat tissue (g)	2177.25 [682.81]	2266 [955.18]	0.676	2336.38 [884.28]	2167.5 [959.96]	0.664	2557.67 [1551.81]	2674.67 [1820.62]	0.564
Android total fat tissue (%)	37.63 [12.71]	33.75 [13.56]	0.0011 *	41.44 [10.09]	35.47 [17.34]	0.029 *	41.67 [11.91]	40.97 [12.45]	0.666
Gynoid total fat tissue (%)	43.95 [7.54]	40.91 [7.91]	0.003 *	46.66 [5.92]	43.27 [8.63]	0.030 *	47.55 [6.4]	46.48 [6.55]	0.314
Total lean mass (g)	41,295.75 [10,954.4]	40,645.25 [10,826.55]	0.243	43,512.38 [4267.88]	41,546 [5058.08]	0.139	43,379 [7137.34]	42,949.67 [6532.6]	0.530
Total leg lean mass (g)	15,772.88 [3054.57]	15,197.63 [3291.54]	0.114	15,725 [2284.37]	14,888.33 [1940.51]	0.397	15,160.55 [3177.59]	15,301.67 [3907.32]	0.815
Total arm lean mass (g)	3488.5 [596.14]	3833.5 [398.06]	0.121	3509 [723.16]	3634.17 [333.77]	0.426	3580 [700.9]	3921.17 [831.92]	0.346
IMAT	0.94 [0.45]	0.83 [0.45]	0.026 *	1.17 [0.43]	1.05 [0.48]	0.007 *	1.16 [0.61]	1.1 [0.62]	0.111
ASMMI	7.54 [0.87]	7.45 [1.08]	0.585	7.03 [0.8]	6.63 [0.41]	0.384	7.42 [1.5]	7.62 [1.7]	0.538

KDCB, ketogenic diet and carboxytherapy group; KD, ketogenic diet group; CB, carboxytherapy group; IMAT, intramuscular adipose tissue; ASMMI, appendicular skeletal muscle mass index; T0, baseline; T1, after 10 weeks. Standard deviation in square brackets. Statistical significance was attributed as * $p < 0.05$.

The total LM obtained from DXA analysis was also found to be statistically unaffected in all three groups. Also, the ASMMI was statistically unaffected in all three groups. Evaluation of LM in legs for the KDCB, KD, and CB groups confirmed the unaltered statistical trend associated with total LM.

In all three groups, for the other DXA parameters, after ten weeks no statistical differences were observed.

In the KDCB and CB groups, an improvement in skin texture in the legs was observed, as shown in the pictures (Figure 2a–c).

3.3. *Quality of Life, Fibromyalgia, and Psychometric Tests*

Different tests on quality of life and pain were administered to the three groups at baseline and follow-up. A statistically significant improvement was found in the KDCB group at the level of the FAS, which investigates asthenia, pain, and sleep disturbance ($p = 0.049$), and of the FIQR, which explores the three main domains of symptoms, function, and general impact ($p = 0.032$), indicating significant improvements in sleep quality and quality of life and a reduction in pain after 10 weeks of treatment.

(a) Skin texture pre- and post-carboxytherapy in one patient of the KDCB group

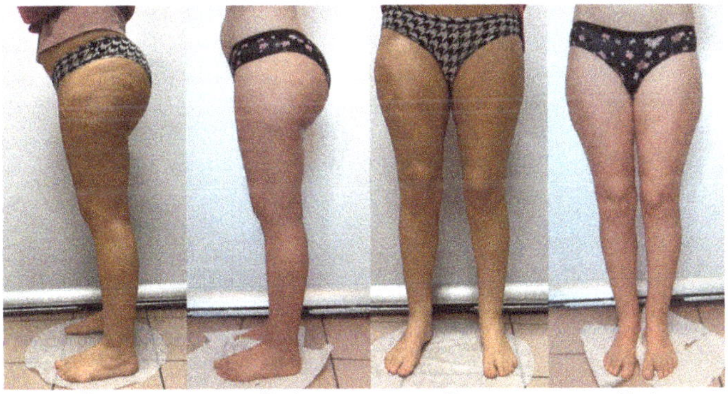

(b) Skin texture pre- and post-carboxytherapy in one patient of the CB group

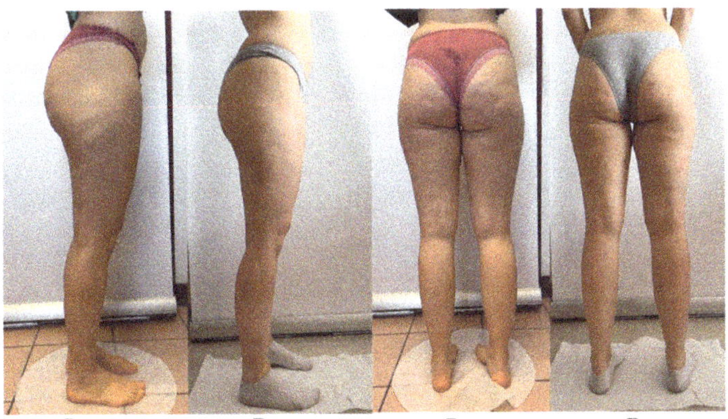

(c) Skin texture pre- and post-carboxytherapy in one patient of the CB group

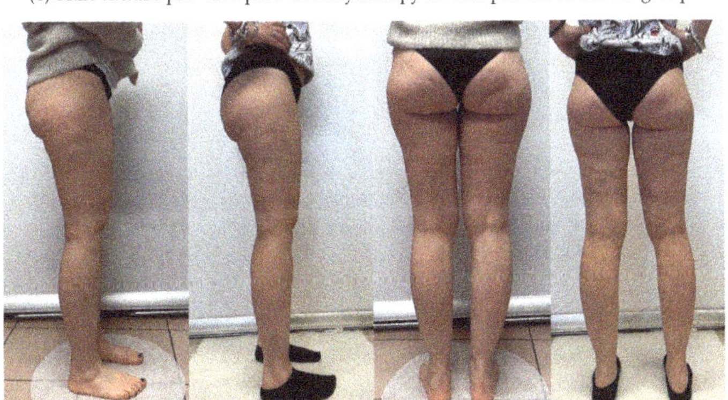

Figure 2. Skin texture pre- and post-carboxytherapy.

No other significant changes were found in the other test scores and in the other groups (Table 5).

Table 5. Comparison of test parameters in the three groups.

	KDCB T0	KDCB T1	*p*-Value	KD T0	KD T1	*p*-Value	CB T0	CB T1	*p*-Value
EuroQ_tot	45.14 [11.98]	35 [16.41]	0.141	63.63 [38.65]	75.71 [31.42]	0.729	46.83 [33.2]	56.67 [27.51]	0.067
FAS	12.51 [5.88]	8.63 [6.06]	0.049 *	16.88 [6.71]	16.44 [6.32]	0.860	10.9 [7.25]	15.2 [2.11]	0.155
FIQR_tot	41.43 [24.52]	31.33 [21.42]	0.032 *	66.5 [42.14]	64.52 [40.32]	0.730	51.06 [36.26]	66.39 [23.59]	0.138
FSS	12.29 [8.42]	9.63 [7.82]	0.119	16.38 [8.6]	16 [5.86]	0.643	12.17 [9.41]	15.83 [8.13]	0.175
DERS tot	81.14 [22.45]	76.63 [24.77]	0.408	84.38 [29.13]	79.71 [25.34]	0.250	70.67 [16.27]	67.83 [13.36]	0.586
YFAS level of FA	0.86 [1.46]	0.38 [1.06]	0.356	0.5 [1.07]	1.14 [1.35]	0.280	0.17 [0.41]	0.67 [1.21]	0.363

EuroQ_tot, European Quality of Life total score; FAS, fibromyalgia assessment status; FIQR_tot, revised fibromyalgia impact questionnaire total score; FSS, fibromyalgia severity scale; DERS, difficulties in emotional regulation scale; YFAS, Yale food addiction scale; FA, food addiction; KDCB, ketogenic diet and carboxytherapy group; KD, ketogenic diet group; CB, carboxytherapy group; T0, baseline; T1, after ten weeks. Standard deviation in square brackets. Statistical significance was attributed as * $p < 0.05$.

4. Discussion

Conservative therapeutic strategies in lipedema aim to reduce symptoms and prevent complications and progression of the disease [34]. Thus, to improve the quality of life of patients with lipedema, it is essential to find a dietary strategy aimed at weight loss and FM reduction in the typical areas of lipedema, such as the lower limbs, but also aimed at reducing pain caused by the orthostatic edema and the expansion of inflamed subcutaneous tissue. There seems to be a widespread misconception that limb volume and symptoms of lipedema do not respond to weight loss [1,35]. In fact, this concept has recently been challenged as contrary to the clinical experience of other scholars [2]. Regardless of BMI, early nutritional therapy is recommended at the time of diagnosis to prevent the development of obesity and the progression of lipedema [36].

The nutritional treatment, in this case, is a diet inspired by the Mediterranean diet in terms of food choice but ketogenic given that it is low in carbohydrate intake, low in salt and simple sugars, includes no processed foods, and is high in antioxidant foods, such as foods with high concentrations of PUFA and MUFA (e.g., oily fish, nuts, and extra virgin olive oil). These nutrients play an essential role in the inflammatory process by promoting an anti-inflammatory effect [37]. In fact, the values of some vitamins typical of the Mediterranean diet involved in antioxidative processes, such as vitamin D and vitamin E, appear to be increased ($p = 0.001$). Moreover, our results showed an improvement in the MAI between the diet followed by the patients before our dietary intervention and the diet followed according to our MMKD pattern, although it did not reach the level of Mediterranean adequacy (the KD being devoid of complex carbohydrates, fruits, and legumes), as expected given the low amount of carbohydrates. This goes to underscore how the MMKD used was rich in antioxidant and health-beneficial foods [38,39]. However, the observed significant reduction in vitamin C could be related to the lack of foods such as fresh fruit.

In fact, it has already been seen that a low-calorie diet based on foods rich in anti-inflammatory and antioxidant nutrients could contribute to the well-being of patients with lipedema [2]. In our previous study, after four weeks of treatment, an unexpected significant loss of FM in the legs and arms was detected, resulting in the first effective nutritional treatment for lipedema. A second important result was the improvement in quality of life, with reductions in asthenia, pain, and anxiety.

In recent years, the use of the ketogenic diet as a valid nutritional treatment for lipedema has been hypothesized in the literature [40]. In fact, it has an interesting rational application in this disease, both for the reduction in insulinemia (and thus hyperinsulinemia-promoted adipogenesis) and for an anti-inflammatory effect [7]. However, at present, there is a lack of clinical trials in the literature on the evaluation of the efficacy of the ketogenic diet in patients with lipedema.

In the present study, it was decided to use an MMKD, for the reasons discussed above, in combination with carboxytherapy. Indeed, lipedema is characterized by microangiopathy and local hypoxia, so we hypothesized that carboxytherapy, through the restoration of microcirculation, could improve painful symptoms and skin tone. Brandi et al. studied the effect of CO2 therapy on skin laxity in the knee and thigh region, observing an improvement in skin texture, as also expected for lipedema [14]. In addition, Pianez et al. [41] evaluated the efficacy of carboxytherapy in reducing cellulite in the buttocks and thigh area, noting an improvement due to the remodeling of collagen fibers and an increase in their quantity. A local lipolytic effect was also observed.

However, data on carboxytherapy are quite divergent in the literature, and many authors do not mention the parameters used regarding volume, infusion rate, and application technique, thus making it difficult to suggest a more effective procedure.

In any case, to the best of our knowledge, this is the first clinical study evaluating the effect of carboxytherapy on women with lipedema. What was found in our study was a significant improvement in skin texture, as shown (Figure 2a–c).

In contrast to the previous literature [1,35,42,43], which indicates lipedema fat as resistant to weight loss, our results show statistically significant losses of body weight, waist and hip circumferences, and total FM (g, %), and a reduction in IMAT, but especially a loss of lower limb (g) and gynoid (%) FM in both the KDCB and KD groups ($p = 0.001$, $p = 0.015$ and $p = 0.003$, $p = 0.03$, respectively). These results confirm and strengthen the evidence on diet therapy from our previous study [2].

Furthermore, contrary to what was observed for very low-calorie ketogenic diets (VLCKD) [16], LM was maintained throughout the duration of the study. This was also confirmed by the sarcopenia index ASMMI, which did not change in all groups ($p = 0.585$, $p = 0.384$, $p = 0.538$).

The same results for FM were not found in the group that performed only carboxytherapy. In fact, the primary goal of carboxytherapy is to restore and improve skin microcirculation, not to reduce fat mass; any lipolysis is only a secondary effect [44,45]. Other results to note are the significant improvements in sleep quality, asthenia, and pain reduction in the KDCB group ($p = 0.049$, $p = 0.032$). These data could reflect a reduction in inflammatory phenomena induced by adipose tissue as a consequence of a customized MMKD rich in antioxidant nutrients [46], in combination with the synergistic effect of carboxytherapy, which would induce an improvement in microcirculation and thus pain.

Moreover, a relationship between vitamin D levels and the development of anxiety and depression was previously observed [47]. The increased vitamin D content compared with baseline may have contributed to improving symptoms (pain), quality of sleep, and daily life functions in general in our patients.

The main limitations of this study are the small number of participants and the short intervention period. It will be necessary to further investigate the efficacy of the proposed treatments on a larger sample and for longer periods of time. In addition, this study lacks a comparison with a sample of non-lipedema patients to compare the results obtained. Moreover, it might be useful to assess patients' oxidative and inflammatory status to check the antioxidative and anti-inflammatory power of nutrients administered through the diet.

5. Conclusions

To our knowledge, this is the first clinical study evaluating the ketogenic diet and carboxytherapy in lipedema patients.

It was observed that the ketogenic diet effectively induced weight and fat mass loss, including in the limbs, areas considered unresponsive to diet therapy in lipedema patients. The best results were obtained from the combination of the ketogenic diet and carboxytherapy, which showed both an improvement in body composition and a reduction in pain, along with an improvement in sleep quality.

This study confirms the need, according to the consensus of the various international guidelines, to maintain a multidisciplinary and integrated approach to lipedema, demonstrating that no isolated treatment, at present, can be completely effective.

Nutrition should have a primary role in the management of lipedema, as it could be, in the long term, an effective tool to reduce the low-grade inflammation that is almost always present in this condition. In parallel, it is necessary to continue studying this disease and its pathophysiology to have targeted therapeutic strategies.

Given the promising results of this pilot study, it would be useful to conduct a clinical trial over a more extended period and on a larger scale to observe the results in the long term as well.

Author Contributions: Conceptualization, L.D.R. and P.G.; methodology, L.D.R.; formal analysis, P.G.; investigation, S.Z., G.F., G.L.D.S., S.S., C.Z. and D.C.; data curation, P.G., S.Z. and G.L.D.S.; writing—original draft preparation, L.D.R., P.G., S.Z. and G.L.D.S.; writing—review and editing, L.D.R., P.G., G.L.D.S., S.Z., G.F., R.C., D.C. and A.D.L.; project administration, L.D.R.; supervision, A.D.L. All authors have read and agreed to the published version of the manuscript.

Funding: This research received no external funding.

Institutional Review Board Statement: This study was conducted in accordance with the Declaration of Helsinki, approved by the Institutional Review Calabria Region Center Area Section (register protocol no. 146 17/05/2018), and registered with ClinicalTrials.gov NCT01890070.

Informed Consent Statement: Informed consent was obtained from all subjects involved in the study.

Data Availability Statement: The data presented in this study are available on request from the corresponding author. The data are not publicly available due to privacy.

Acknowledgments: The authors thank all the lipedema patients who participated as volunteers in the study. The authors thank Petronilla Nocerino for planning the diet and the staff of the Section of Clinical Nutrition and Nutrigenomics, Department of Biomedicine and Prevention, University of Rome Tor Vergata, for supporting the study.

Conflicts of Interest: The authors declare no conflict of interest.

Appendix A

In Appendix A, the EQ-5D, FAS, FSS, FIQR, DERS, and YFAS 2.0 questionnaires are reported.

Euro-Qol 5D

Indicare quali delle seguenti affermazioni descrive meglio il suo stato di salute oggi, segnando con una crocetta (☒) una sola casella di ciascun gruppo

Capacità di movimento

Non ho difficoltà nel camminare ☐

Ho qualche difficoltà nel camminare ☐

Sono costretto/a a letto ☐

Cura della persona

Non ho difficoltà nel prendermi cura di me stesso ☐

Ho qualche difficoltà nel lavarmi o vestirmi ☐

Non sono in grado di lavarmi o vestirmi ☐

Attività abituali
(per es. lavoro, studio, lavori domestici, attività familiari o di svago)
Non ho difficoltà nello svolgimento delle attività abituali ☐
Ho qualche difficoltà nello svolgimento delle attività abituali ☐
Non sono in grado di svolgere le mie attività abituali ☐
Dolore, Fastidio o malessere
Non provo alcun dolore o fastidio ☐
Provo dolore o fastidio moderati ☐
Provo estremo dolore o fastidio ☐
Ansia o Depressione
Non sono ansioso o depresso ☐
Sono moderatamente ansioso o depresso ☐
Sono estremamente ansioso o depresso ☐

Per aiutarla ad esprimere il suo stato di salute attuale abbiamo disegnato una scala graduate (simile ad un termometro) sulla quale il migliore stato di salute immaginabile è contrassegnato dal numero 100 e il peggiore dallo 0.

Vorremmo che indicasse su questa scala quale è, secondo lei, il livello del suo stato di salute oggi, tracciando una linea dal riquadro sottostante fino al punto che corrisponde al suo stato di salute attuale.

Migliore stato di salute immaginabile

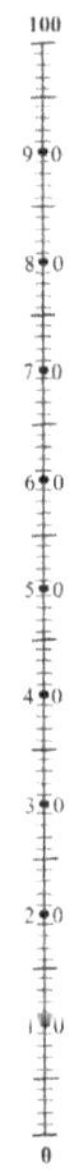

Peggiore stato di salute immaginabile

Fibromyalgia Assessment Status

(1) Quale numero da 0 a 10 descrive nel miglioro modo il livello di fatica che hai provato nella scorsa settimana?

	○	○	○	○	○	○	○	○	○	○	
Nessuna stanchezza	1	2	3	4	5	6	7	8	9	10	La peggior stanchezza

(2) Quanti problemi ha avuto per dormire nella scorsa settimana?

	○	○	○	○	○	○	○	○	○	○	
Nessun problema	1	2	3	4	5	6	7	8	9	10	Numerosi problemi

(3) Si prega di indicare sotto la sensazione di dolore da o a 4 che hai provato nella settimana passata per ciascuna parte del corpo inserendo una X nelle caselle. Si prega di essere sicuri di contrassegnare entrambi i lati destro e sinistro separatamente.

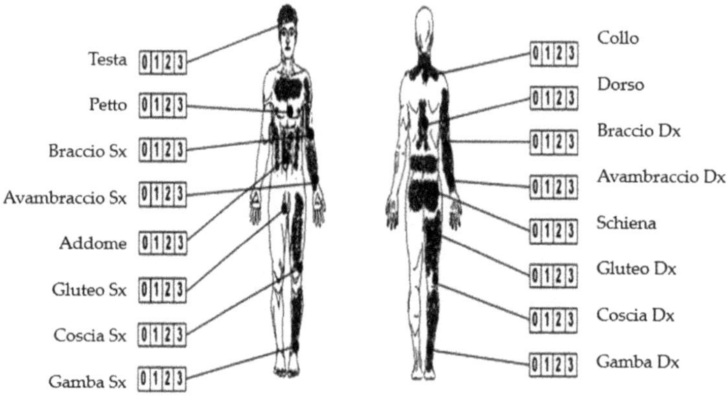

Fibromyalgia Severity Scale

Indice di dolore diffuso

Indicare le aree in cui il paziente ha riferito dolore **nell'ultima settimana**

Punteggio: ___su 19 aree

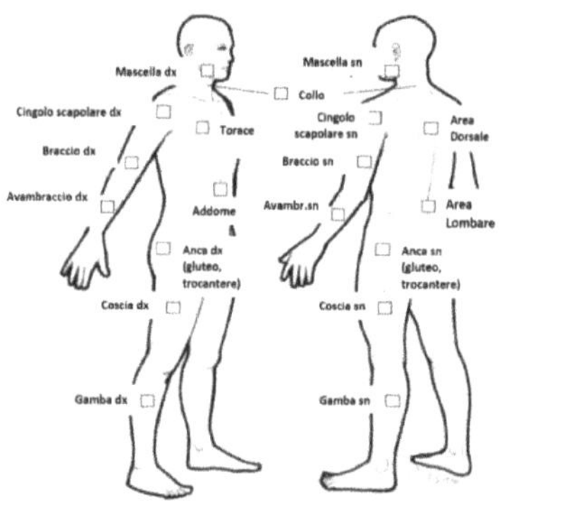

Dolore generalizzato

Indicare le regioni **Punteggio: ___ su 5 regioni**

Aree	Regione	Presenza
Cingolo scapolare	**Superiore** sinistra	
Braccio		
Avambraccio		
Cingolo scapolare	**Superiore** destra	
Braccio		
Avambraccio		
Anca (gluteo, trocantere)	**Inferiore** sinistra	
Coscia		
Gamba		
Anca (gluteo, trocantere)	**Inferiore** destra	
Coscia		
Gamba		
Collo	**Assiale**	
Area dorsale		
Area Lombare		

Indice di gravità dei sintomi

Punteggio: ____ su 12

Indicare il livello di gravità dei 3 sintomi (A,B,C) nell'ultima settimana

	Nessun problema 0	Problema lieve 1	Problema moderato 2	Problema grave 3
A. Astenia	☐	☐	☐	☐
B. Sonno non ristoratore	☐	☐	☐	☐
C. Problemi cognitivi (es. attenzione, memoria)	☐	☐	☐	☐

Indicare la presenza o la assenza dei 3 sintomi (D,E,F) negli ultimi 6 mesi

	Assente 0	Presente 1
D. Emicrania	☐	☐
E. Dolore o crampi addominali	☐	☐
F. Depressione	☐	☐

VERSIONE ITALIANA DEL REVISED FIBROMYALGIA IMPACT QUESTIONNAIRE (ITALIAN-FIQR)

Nome: ____________ Età: ____________

Cognome: ____________ Durata dei sintomi (anni): ____________

DOMINIO 1 – FUNZIONE FISICA

Per ognuna delle seguenti NOVE domande, segni la casella che meglio indica il grado di difficoltà da Lei avvertito, ***nel corso dell'ultima settimana,*** nel compiere ciascuna delle attività elencate, a causa della fibromialgia: *(scegliere un solo numero).*

1. SPAZZOLARE O PETTINARE I CAPELLI

Nessuna difficoltà ❑ 0 ❑ 1 ❑ 2 ❑ 3 ❑ 4 ❑ 5 ❑ 6 ❑ 7 ❑ 8 ❑ 9 ❑ 10 Estrema difficoltà

2. CAMMINARE ININTERROTTAMENTE PER 20 MINUTI

Nessuna difficoltà ❑ 0 ❑ 1 ❑ 2 ❑ 3 ❑ 4 ❑ 5 ❑ 6 ❑ 7 ❑ 8 ❑ 9 ❑ 10 Estrema difficoltà

3. PREPARARE I PASTI

Nessuna difficoltà ❑ 0 ❑ 1 ❑ 2 ❑ 3 ❑ 4 ❑ 5 ❑ 6 ❑ 7 ❑ 8 ❑ 9 ❑ 10 Estrema difficoltà

4. PASSARE L'ASPIRAPOLVERE E LAVARE I PAVIMENTI

Nessuna difficoltà ❑ 0 ❑ 1 ❑ 2 ❑ 3 ❑ 4 ❑ 5 ❑ 6 ❑ 7 ❑ 8 ❑ 9 ❑ 10 Estrema difficoltà

5. SOLLEVARE E PORTARE LE BORSE DELLA SPESA

Nessuna difficoltà ❑ 0 ❑ 1 ❑ 2 ❑ 3 ❑ 4 ❑ 5 ❑ 6 ❑ 7 ❑ 8 ❑ 9 ❑ 10 Estrema difficoltà

6. SALIRE UN PIANO DI SCALE

Nessuna difficoltà ❑ 0 ❑ 1 ❑ 2 ❑ 3 ❑ 4 ❑ 5 ❑ 6 ❑ 7 ❑ 8 ❑ 9 ❑ 10 Estrema difficoltà

7. CAMBIARE LE LENZUOLA DEL LETTO

Nessuna difficoltà ❑ 0 ❑ 1 ❑ 2 ❑ 3 ❑ 4 ❑ 5 ❑ 6 ❑ 7 ❑ 8 ❑ 9 ❑ 10 Estrema difficoltà

8. STARE SEDUTO SU UNA SEDIA PER ALMENO 45 MINUTI

Nessuna difficoltà ❑ 0 ❑ 1 ❑ 2 ❑ 3 ❑ 4 ❑ 5 ❑ 6 ❑ 7 ❑ 8 ❑ 9 ❑ 10 Estrema difficoltà

9. ANDARE A FARE LA SPESA

Nessuna difficoltà ❑ 0 ❑ 1 ❑ 2 ❑ 3 ❑ 4 ❑ 5 ❑ 6 ❑ 7 ❑ 8 ❑ 9 ❑ 10 Estrema difficoltà

DOMINIO 1 – SUBTOTALE: ________

DOMINIO 2 – STATO DI SALUTE GENERALE

Per ognuna delle seguenti DUE domande, segni la casella che meglio indica il grado di difficoltà da Lei avvertito, ***nel corso dell'ultima settimana,*** nel compiere ciascuna delle attività elencate, a causa della fibromialgia: *(scegliere un solo numero).*

10. LA FIBROMIALGIA MI HA IMPEDITO DI PORTARE A TERMINE I LAVORI/COMPITI DELLA SETTIMANA

Mai ❑ 0 ❑ 1 ❑ 2 ❑ 3 ❑ 4 ❑ 5 ❑ 6 ❑ 7 ❑ 8 ❑ 9 ❑ 10 Sempre

11. SONO STATO/A COMPLETAMENTE SOPRAFFATTO/A DAI SINTOMI DELLA FIBROMIALGIA

DOMINIO 3 – SINTOMI

Per ognuna delle seguenti DIECI domande, segni la casella che meglio indica il grado di severità del sintomo da Lei avvertito, ***nel corso dell'ultima settimana,*** a causa della fibromialgia: *(scegliere un solo numero).*

12. ASSEGNI UN PUNTEGGIO AL SUO LIVELLO DI DOLORE

Nessun dolore	❑ 0	❑ 1	❑ 2	❑ 3	❑ 4	❑ 5	❑ 6	❑ 7	❑ 8	❑ 9	❑ 10	Estremo dolore

13. ASSEGNI UN PUNTEGGIO AL SUO LIVELLO DI STANCHEZZA

Nessuna stanchezza	❑ 0	❑ 1	❑ 2	❑ 3	❑ 4	❑ 5	❑ 6	❑ 7	❑ 8	❑ 9	❑ 10	Estrema stanchezza

14. ASSEGNI UN PUNTEGGIO AL SUO LIVELLO DI RIGIDITA'

Nessuna rigidità	❑ 0	❑ 1	❑ 2	❑ 3	❑ 4	❑ 5	❑ 6	❑ 7	❑ 8	❑ 9	❑ 10	Estrema rigidità

15. ASSEGNI UN PUNTEGGIO ALLA QUALITA' DEL SUO SONNO

Ben riposato/a al risveglio	❑ 0	❑ 1	❑ 2	❑ 3	❑ 4	❑ 5	❑ 6	❑ 7	❑ 8	❑ 9	❑ 10	Estremamente stanco/a al risveglio

16. ASSEGNI UN PUNTEGGIO AL SUO GRADO DI DEPRESSIONE

Per nulla depresso/a	❑ 0	❑ 1	❑ 2	❑ 3	❑ 4	❑ 5	❑ 6	❑ 7	❑ 8	❑ 9	❑ 10	Estremamente depresso/a

17. ASSEGNI UN PUNTEGGIO AI SUOI PROBLEMI DI MEMORIA

Buona memoria	❑ 0	❑ 1	❑ 2	❑ 3	❑ 4	❑ 5	❑ 6	❑ 7	❑ 8	❑ 9	❑ 10	Scarsissima memoria

18. ASSEGNI UN PUNTEGGIO AL SUO GRADO DI ANSIA

Per nulla ansioso/a	❑ 0	❑ 1	❑ 2	❑ 3	❑ 4	❑ 5	❑ 6	❑ 7	❑ 8	❑ 9	❑ 10	Estremamente ansioso/a

19. ASSEGNI UN PUNTEGGIO AL SUO LIVELLO DI DOLORABILITA' (dolore percepito al tatto)

Nessuna dolorabilità	❑ 0	❑ 1	❑ 2	❑ 3	❑ 4	❑ 5	❑ 6	❑ 7	❑ 8	❑ 9	❑ 10	Estrema dolorabilità

20. ASSEGNI UN PUNTEGGIO AI SUOI DISTURBI DI EQUILIBRIO

Nessun problema di equilibrio	❑ 0	❑ 1	❑ 2	❑ 3	❑ 4	❑ 5	❑ 6	❑ 7	❑ 8	❑ 9	❑ 10	Scarsissimo equilibrio

21. ASSEGNI UN PUNTEGGIO AL LIVELLO DELLE SUA SENSIBILITA' AI RUMORI, ALLE LUCI, AGLI ODORI ED AL FREDDO

Nessuna sensibilità	❑ 0	❑ 1	❑ 2	❑ 3	❑ 4	❑ 5	❑ 6	❑ 7	❑ 8	❑ 9	❑ 10	Estrema sensibilità

DOMINIO 3 – SUBTOTALE: ________

PUNTEGGIO:

1. *Sommare i punteggi di ogni singolo item per i tre domini (funzione fisica, stato di salute generale e sintomi);*
2. *Dividere per 3 il punteggio relativo al dominio FUNZIONE FISICA, lasciare il punteggio inalterato per il dominio STATO GENERALE DI SALUTE e dividere per 2 il punteggio del dominio SINTOMI*
3. *Sommare i risultanti punteggi dei 3 domini per ottenere il totale*

PUNTEGGIO TOTALE FIQR ☐

DERS Istruzioni Utilizzando la seguente scala di valori, le chiediamo di segnare quanto spesso le seguenti affermazioni possono essere applicate alla sua esperienza, indicando il numero appropiato a fianco di ogni item. 1 Quasi mai (0–10%); 2 A volte (11–35%); 3 Circa la metà delle volte (36–65%); 4 Molte volte (66–90%); 5 Quasi sempre (91–100%).		Quasi sempre	Molte volte	Circa la metà delle volte	A volte	Quasi mai
1	Sono sereno riguardo a ciò che provo	1	2	3	4	5
2	Presto attenzione a come mi sento	1	2	3	4	5
3	Vivo le mie emozioni come travolgenti e fuori dal controllo	5	4	3	2	1
4	Non ho idea di come mi sento	5	4	3	2	1
5	Ho difficoltà a dare un senso a ciò che provo	5	4	3	2	1
6	Presto attenzione alle mie emozioni	1	2	3	4	5
7	So esattamente come mi sento	1	2	3	4	5
8	Mi interessa come mi sento	1	2	3	4	5
9	Sono confuso riguardo a ciò che provo	5	4	3	2	1
10	Quando sono turbato, riconosco le mie emozioni	1	2	3	4	5
11	Quando sono turbato, mi arrabbio con me stesso perché mi sento in quel modo	5	4	3	2	1
12	Quando sono turbato mi imbarazza sentirmi in quel modo	5	4	3	2	1
13	Quando sono turbato, ho delle difficoltà a completare il mio lavoro	5	4	3	2	1
14	Quando sono turbato, perdo il controllo	5	4	3	2	1
15	Quando sono turbato, credo che rimarrò in quello stato per molto tempo	5	4	3	2	1
16	Quando sono turbato, credo che finirò per sentirmi depresso	5	4	3	2	1
17	Quando sono turbato, credo che i miei sentimenti siano validi e importanti	1	2	3	4	5
18	Quando sono turbato, faccio fatica a focalizzarmi su altre cose	5	4	3	2	1
19	Quando sono turbato, mi sento senza controllo	5	4	3	2	1
20	Quando sono turbato, posso comunque finire le cose che devo fare	1	2	3	4	5
21	Quando sono turbato, mi vergogno con me stesso perché mi sento in quel modo	5	4	3	2	1
22	Quando sono turbato, so che alla fine posso trovare un modo per sentirmi meglio	1	2	3	4	5
23	Quando sono turbato, mi sento debole	5	4	3	2	1
24	Quando sono turbato, sento di poter avere ancora il controllo dei miei comportamenti	1	2	3	4	5
25	Quando sono turbato, mi sento in colpa perchè mi sento in quel modo	5	4	3	2	1
26	Quando sono turbato, ho delle difficoltà a concentrarmi	5	4	3	2	1
27	Quando sono turbato, ho delle difficoltà nel controllare i miei comportamenti	5	4	3	2	1
28	Quando sono turbato, credo che non ci sia niente che io possa fare per sentirmi meglio	5	4	3	2	1
29	Quando sono turbato, mi irrito con me stesso perché mi sento in quel modo	5	4	3	2	1
30	Quando sono turbato, inizio a sentirmi molto male con me stesso	5	4	3	2	1
31	Quando sono turbato, credo che crogiolarmi in questa emozione sia l'unica cosa che io possa fare	5	4	3	2	1
32	Quando sono turbato, perdo il controllo sui miei comportamenti	5	4	3	2	1
33	Quando sono turbato, faccio fatica a pensare a qualcosa di diverso	5	4	3	2	1
34	Quando sono turbato, mi prendo del tempo per riflettere su quello che sto provando veramente	1	2	3	4	5
35	Quando sono turbato, mi ci vuole molto tempo per sentirmi meglio	5	4	3	2	1
36	Quando sono turbato, le mie emozioni sono travolgenti	5	4	3	2	1

I-YFAS 2.0									
ISTRUZIONI									
Il questionario vuole indagare sulle sue abitudini alimentari nell'ultimo anno. Alcune persone hanno difficoltà a controllare l'assunzione di determinati cibi come: -Dolci quali gelati, cioccolato, ciambelle, biscotti, torte, caramelle -Amidi quali pane bianco, pasta e riso -Snack salati quali patatine, crackers ecc -Cibi grassi quali hamburger, pancetta, pizza, patatine fritte ecc -Bevande gassate quali coca cola, fanta ecc Nelle domande la dizione "certi cibi" si riferisce a qualsiasi tipo di cibo menzionato sopra o comunque a qualsiasi tipo di cibo che ritenga possa essere coinvolto.		Ogni Giorno	4–6 Volte a settimana	2–3 Volte a Settimana	1 Volta a settimana	2–3 Volte al Mese	1 Volta al Mese	Non Mensilemtente	Mai
1	Quando inizio a mangiare "certi cibi" finisco per mangiare molto più di quanto pianificato.	7	6	5	4	3	2	1	0
2	Continuo a mangiare "certi cibi" nonostante non sia più affamato.	7	6	5	4	3	2	1	0
3	Mangio fino a sentirmi male fisicamente.	7	6	5	4	3	2	1	0
4	Non mangiare "certi cibi" o ridurne certi altri è qualcosa che mi preoccupa.	7	6	5	4	3	2	1	0
5	Trascorro tanto tempo sentendomi pieno o affaticato per aver mangiato troppo.	7	6	5	4	3	2	1	0
6	Mi trovo costantemente a mangiare "certi cibi" durante tutto il giorno.	7	6	5	4	3	2	1	0
7	Trovo il modo di procurarmi "certi cibi" quando non sono disponibili. Per esempio, sarei disposto ad allungare il mio percorso di guida verso un negozio per comprarli, anche quando ho altre opzioni disponibili a casa.	7	6	5	4	3	2	1	0
8	Ho mangiato "certi cibi" così spesso o in quantità tale che ho smesso di fare altre cose importanti, come lavorare o passare il tempo con la mia famiglia o con gli amici.	7	6	5	4	3	2	1	0
9	Ho avuto problemi con la mia famiglia o con i miei amici per aver mangiato troppo.	7	6	5	4	3	2	1	0
10	Ho evitato la scuola, il lavoro o attività sociali per paura di mangiare in eccesso lì	7	6	5	4	3	2	1	0
11	Quando ho ridotto o smesso di mangiare "certi cibi" mi sono sentito irritabile, nervoso/a o triste.	7	6	5	4	3	2	1	0
12	Quando ho avuto sintomi fisici, per non aver mangiato "certi cibi", li ho mangiati per sentirmi meglio.	7	6	5	4	3	2	1	0
13	Quando ho avuto disturbi emotivi, per non aver mangiato "certi cibi", li ho mangiati per sentirmi meglio.	7	6	5	4	3	2	1	0
14	Quando ho ridotto o smesso di mangiare "certi cibi" ho avuto sintomi fisici. Per esempio ho avuto mal di testa o stanchezza.	7	6	5	4	3	2	1	0
15	Quando ho ridotto o smesso di mangiare "certi cibi" ho avuto gran voglia di mangiarli.	7	6	5	4	3	2	1	0
16	La mia condotta alimentare mi ha causato molto malessere.	7	6	5	4	3	2	1	0
17	Ho avuto problemi significativi nella mia vita a causa del cibo e della alimentazione. Questi problemi possono essere relazionati con la mia routine, il lavoro, la scuola, gli amici, la famiglia o la salute.	7	6	5	4	3	2	1	0
18	Mi sono sentito male per aver mangiato in eccesso, tanto da non fare altre cose importanti. Tra cui lavorare o passare il tempo con la famiglia e gli amici.	7	6	5	4	3	2	1	0
19	Mangiare in eccesso ha interferito nel adempimento dei miei doveri familiari o nel fare i servizi domestici.	7	6	5	4	3	2	1	0
20	Ho evitato il lavoro, la scuola o le attività perché in queste situazioni non potevo mangiare "certi cibi".	7	6	5	4	3	2	1	0
21	Ho evitato occasioni/incontri sociali perché la gente non avrebbe approvato quanto mangio.	7	6	5	4	3	2	1	0
22	Nonostante sapessi che la mia alimentazione avrebbe causato disturbi emotivi, ho continuato a mangiare "certi cibi".	7	6	5	4	3	2	1	0
23	Nonostante sapessi che la mia alimentazione mi avrebbe causato problemi fisici, ho continuato a mangiare "certi cibi"	7	6	5	4	3	2	1	0
24	Mangiare la stessa quantità di cibo non mi da più tanta soddisfazione come prima.	7	6	5	4	3	2	1	0
25	Realmente ho voluto ridurre o smettere di mangiare "certi cibi", però semplicemente non ci sono riuscito.	7	6	5	4	3	2	1	0
26	Avevo bisogno di mangiare ogni volta di più per raggiungere la sensazione che volevo raggiungere mangiando. Ciò includeva, ridurre le emozioni negative (come la tristezza) o aumentare le emozioni positive (come il piacere).	7	6	5	4	3	2	1	0
27	Non ho reso molto a lavoro o a scuola perché stavo mangiando troppo.	7	6	5	4	3	2	1	0
28	Ho continuato a mangiare "certi cibi", nonostante sapessi che era dannoso per la mia salute. Per esempio, ho continuato a mangiare dolci pur avendo il diabete, o cibi grassi, pur avendo malattie cardiovascolari.	7	6	5	4	3	2	1	0
29	Ho avuto impulsi tanto forti per mangiare "certi cibi" che non potevo pensare ad altro.	7	6	5	4	3	2	1	0
30	Ho avuto desideri tanto intensi per "certi cibi" che sentivo che avrei dovuto mangiarli nell'immediato.	7	6	5	4	3	2	1	0
31	Ho provato a ridurre o smettere di mangiare "certi cibi", però non ho avuto successo.	7	6	5	4	3	2	1	0
32	Ho provato a ridurre o smettere di mangiare "certi cibi" ed ho fallito.	7	6	5	4	3	2	1	0
33	Sono stato tanto distratto/a mangiando che ho rischiato di ferirmi (ad esempio guidando l'auto, attraversando la strada, maneggiando macchinari).	7	6	5	4	3	2	1	0
34	Sono stato tanto distratto/a pensando al cibo che ho rischiato di ferirmi (ad esempio guidando l'auto, attraversando la strada, maneggiando macchinari).	7	6	5	4	3	2	1	0
35	I miei amici o familiari sono stati molto preoccupati perché ho esagerato con il cibo.	7	6	5	4	3	2	1	0

References

1. Buck, D.W.; Herbst, K.L. Lipedema: A relatively common disease with extremely common misconceptions. *Plast. Reconstr. Surg-Glob. Open* **2016**, *4*, e1043. [CrossRef]
2. Di Renzo, L.; Cinelli, G.; Romano, L.; Zomparelli, S.; De Santis, G.L.; Nocerino, P.; Bigioni, G.; Arsini, L.; Cenname, G.; Pujia, A.; et al. Potential effects of a modified mediterranean diet on body composition in lipoedema. *Nutrients* **2021**, *13*, 358. [CrossRef] [PubMed]
3. Susan, P.; Masino, A.; Ruskin, D.N. Ketogenic Diets and Pain. *Bone* **2008**, *23*, 993–1001. [CrossRef]
4. Athinarayanan, S.J.; Adams, R.N.; Hallberg, S.J.; McKenzie, A.L.; Bhanpuri, N.H.; Campbell, W.W.; Volek, J.S.; Phinney, S.D.; McCarter, J.P. Long-term effects of a novel continuous remote care intervention including nutritional ketosis for the management of type 2 diabetes: A 2-year nonrandomized clinical trial. *Front. Endocrinol.* **2019**, *10*, 348. [CrossRef] [PubMed]
5. McKenzie, A.L.; Hallberg, S.J.; Creighton, B.C.; Volk, B.M.; Link, T.M.; Abner, M.K.; Glon, R.M.; McCarter, J.P.; Volek, J.S.; Phinney, S.D. A novel intervention including individualized nutritional recommendations reduces hemoglobin A1c level, medication use, and weight in type 2 diabetes. *JMIR Diabetes* **2017**, *2*, e5. [CrossRef]
6. Volek, J.S.; Fernandez, M.L.; Feinman, R.D.; Phinney, S.D. Dietary carbohydrate restriction induces a unique metabolic state positively affecting atherogenic dyslipidemia, fatty acid partitioning, and metabolic syndrome. *Prog. Lipid Res.* **2008**, *47*, 307–318. [CrossRef] [PubMed]
7. Keith, L.; Seo, C.; Rowsemitt, C.; Pfeffer, M.; Wahi, M.; Staggs, M.; Dudek, J.; Gower, B.; Carmody, M. Ketogenic diet as a potential intervention for lipedema. *Med. Hypotheses* **2021**, *146*, 110435. [CrossRef]
8. Puchalska, P.; Crawford, P.A. Multi-dimensional roles of ketone bodies. *Physiol. Behav.* **2019**, *176*, 139–148. [CrossRef]
9. Cooper, M.A.; Menta, B.W.; Perez-Sanchez, C.; Jack, M.M.; Khan, Z.W.; Ryals, J.M.; Winter, M.; Wright, D.E. A ketogenic diet reduces metabolic syndrome-induced allodynia and promotes peripheral nerve growth in mice. *Exp. Neurol.* **2018**, *306*, 149–157. [CrossRef]
10. Dudek, J.E.; Białaszek, W.; Ostaszewski, P.; Smidt, T. Depression and appearance-related distress in functioning with lipedema. *Psychol. Health Med.* **2018**, *23*, 846–853. [CrossRef]
11. Murphy, P.; Likhodii, S.; Nylen, K.; Burnham, W.M. The antidepressant properties of the ketogenic diet. *Biol. Psychiatry* **2004**, *56*, 981–983. [CrossRef]
12. Sadala, A.Y.; Machado, A.F.P.; Liebano, R.E. Effects of transcutaneous electrical nerve stimulation on pain intensity during application of carboxytherapy in patients with cellulite: A randomized placebo-controlled trial. *J. Cosmet. Dermatol.* **2018**, *17*, 1175–1181. [CrossRef]
13. Alam, M.; Sadhwani, D.; Geisler, A.; Aslam, I.; Makin, I.R.S.; Schlessinger, D.I.; Disphanurat, W.; Pongprutthipan, M.; Voravutinon, N.; Weil, A.; et al. Subcutaneous infiltration of carbon dioxide (carboxytherapy) for abdominal fat reduction: A randomized clinical trial. *J. Am. Acad. Dermatol.* **2018**, *79*, 320–326. [CrossRef] [PubMed]
14. Brandi, C.; D'Aniello, C.; Grimaldi, L.; Caiazzo, E.; Stanghellini, E. Carbon dioxide therapy: Effects on skin irregularity and its use as a complement to liposuction. *Aesthetic Plast. Surg.* **2004**, *28*, 222–225. [CrossRef] [PubMed]
15. Buscemi, S.; Rosafio, G.; Vasto, S.; Massenti, F.M.; Grosso, G.; Galvano, F.; Rini, N.; Barile, A.M.; Maniaci, V.; Cosentino, L.; et al. Validation of a food frequency questionnaire for use in Italian adults living in Sicily. *Int. J. Food Sci. Nutr.* **2015**, *66*, 426–438. [CrossRef]
16. Colica, C.; Merra, G.; Gasbarrini, A.; De Lorenzo, A.; Cioccoloni, G.; Gualtieri, P.; Perrone, M.A.; Bernardini, S.; Bernardo, V.; Di Renzo, L.; et al. Efficacy and safety of very-low-calorie ketogenic diet: A double blind randomized crossover study. *Eur. Rev. Med. Pharmacol. Sci.* **2017**, *21*, 2274–2289. [PubMed]
17. Alberti-Fidanza, A.; Fidanza, F. Mediterranean Adequacy Index of Italian diets. *Public Health Nutr.* **2004**, *7*, 937–941. [CrossRef]
18. Varlaro, F.P.; Manzo, V.; Mugnaini, G.; Bisacci, C. Carboxytherapy: Effects on microcirculation and its use in the treatment of severe lymphedema. *Acta Phlebol.* **2007**, *8*, 79–91.
19. Lee, G.S.K. Quality survey on efficacy of carboxytherapy for localized lipolysis. *J. Cosmet. Dermatol.* **2016**, *15*, 484–492. [CrossRef]
20. Hartmann, B.R.; Bassenge, E.; Pittler, M. Effect of carbon dioxide-enriched water and fresh water on the cutaneous microcirculation and oxygen tension in the skin of the foot. *Angiology* **1997**, *48*, 337–343. [CrossRef]
21. World Health Organization. Obesity. Available online: https://www.who.int/health-topics/obesity (accessed on 3 July 2023).
22. Di Renzo, L.; Bertoli, A.; Bigioni, M.; Gobbo, V.; Premrov, M.G.; Calabrese, V.; Di Daniele, N.; De Lorenzo, A. Body composition and -174G/C interleukin-6 promoter gene polymorphism: Association with progression of insulin resistance in normal weight obese syndrome. *Curr. Pharm. Des.* **2008**, *14*, 2699–2706. [CrossRef]
23. De Lorenzo, A.; Romano, L.; Di Renzo, L.; Di Lorenzo, N.; Cenname, G.; Gualtieri, P. Obesity: A preventable, treatable, but relapsing disease. *Nutrition* **2020**, *71*, 110615. [CrossRef]
24. Di Renzo, L.; Bigioni, M.; Bottini, F.G.; Del Gobbo, V.; Premrov, M.G.; Cianci, R.; De Lorenzo, A. Normal Weight Obese syndrome: Role of single nucleotide polymorphism of IL-1 5Ralpha and MTHFR 677C-->T genes in the relationship between body composition and resting metabolic rate. *Eur. Rev. Med. Pharmacol. Sci.* **2006**, *10*, 235–245.
25. De Lorenzo, A.; Di Renzo, L.; Morini, P.; de Miranda, R.C.; Romano, L.; Colica, C. New equations to estimate resting energy expenditure in obese adults from body composition. *Acta Diabetol.* **2018**, *55*, 59–66. [CrossRef] [PubMed]
26. Oliveira, J.S.; Hayes, A. Clinimetrics: The EuroQol-5 Dimension (EQ-5D). *J. Physiother.* **2020**, *66*, 133. [CrossRef] [PubMed]

27. Salaffi, F.; Di Carlo, M.; Bazzichi, L.; Atzeni, F.; Govoni, M.; Biasi, G.; Di Franco, M.; Mozzani, F.; Gremese, E.; Dagna, L.; et al. Definition of fibromyalgia severity: Findings from a cross-sectional survey of 2339 Italian patients. *Rheumatol* **2021**, *60*, 728–736. [CrossRef] [PubMed]
28. Lee, M. Clinimetrics: The Revised Fibromyalgia Impact Questionnaire. *J. Physiother.* **2021**, *67*, 220–221. [CrossRef]
29. Hallion, L.S.; Steinman, S.A.; Tolin, D.F.; Diefenbach, G.J. Psychometric properties of the difficulties in emotion regulation scale (DERS) and its short forms in adults with emotional disorders. *Front. Psychol.* **2018**, *9*, 539. [CrossRef]
30. Semborski, S.; Henwood, B.; Rhoades, H.; Mason, T.; Wenzel, S.; Rice, E. Construct, concurrent, and real-world predictive validity of the Difficulties in Emotion Regulation (DERS-18) among young adults with history of homelessness. *Psychol. Assess.* **2021**, *33*, 385–394. [CrossRef]
31. Bjureberg, J.; Ljótsson, B.; Tull, M.; Hedman-Lagerlöf, E.; Sahlin, H.; Lundh, L.-G.; Bjärehed, J.; DiLillo, D.; Messmanmoore, T.L.; Gumpert, C.H.; et al. In Emotion Regulation Scale: The DERS-16. *J. Psychopathol. Behav. Assess.* **2016**, *38*, 284–296. [CrossRef]
32. Koehler, A.; Aguirre, T.; Schulte, E.; Bowman, R.; Struwe, L. Secondary analysis of YFAS 2.0 symptom counts, impairment/distress, and food addiction severity in adults with overweight/obesity. *Eat. Weight. Disord.* **2021**, *26*, 2393–2399. [CrossRef] [PubMed]
33. Hauck, C.; Cook, B.; Ellrott, T. Food addiction, eating addiction and eating disorders. *Proc. Nutr. Soc.* **2020**, *79*, 103–112. [CrossRef]
34. Todd, M. Diagnosis and management of lipoedema in the community. *Br. J. Community Nurs.* **2016**, *21*, S6–S12. [CrossRef] [PubMed]
35. Herbst, K.L. Rare adipose disorders (RADs) masquerading as obesity. *Acta Pharmacol. Sin.* **2012**, *33*, 155–172. [CrossRef] [PubMed]
36. Ghods, M.; Georgiou, I.; Schmidt, J.; Kruppa, P. Disease progression and comorbidities in lipedema patients: A 10-year retrospective analysis. *Dermatol. Ther.* **2020**, *33*, e14534. [CrossRef]
37. De Lorenzo, A.; Bernardini, S.; Gualtieri, P.; Cabibbo, A.; Perrone, M.A.; Giambini, I.; Di Renzo, L. Mediterranean meal versus Western meal effects on postprandial ox-LDL, oxidative and inflammatory gene expression in healthy subjects: A randomized controlled trial for nutrigenomic approach in cardiometabolic risk. *Acta Diabetol.* **2017**, *54*, 141–149. [CrossRef]
38. Di Daniele, N.; Di Renzo, L.; Noce, A.; Iacopino, L.; Ferraro, P.M.; Rizzo, M.; Sarlo, F.; Domino, E.; De Lorenzo, A. Effects of Italian Mediterranean organic diet vs. low-protein diet in nephropathic patients according to MTHFR genotypes. *J. Nephrol.* **2014**, *27*, 529–536. [CrossRef]
39. Nagpal, R.; Neth, B.J.; Wang, S.; Craft, S.; Yadav, H. Modified Mediterranean-ketogenic diet modulates gut microbiome and short-chain fatty acids in association with Alzheimer's disease markers in subjects with mild cognitive impairment. *EBioMedicine* **2019**, *47*, 529–542. [CrossRef]
40. Cannataro, R.; Michelini, S.; Ricolfi, L.; Caroleo, M.C.; Gallelli, L.; De Sarro, G.; Onorato, A.; Cione, E. Management of Lipedema with Ketogenic Diet: 22-Month Follow-Up. *Life* **2021**, *11*, 1402. [CrossRef]
41. Pianez, L.R.; Custódio, F.S.; Guidi, R.M.; de Freitas, J.N.; Sant'Ana, E. Effectiveness of carboxytherapy in the treatment of cellulite in healthy women: A pilot study. *Clin. Cosmet. Investig. Dermatol.* **2016**, *9*, 183–190. [CrossRef]
42. La Torre, Y.S.D.; Wadeea, R.; Rosas, V.; Herbst, K.L. Lipedema: Friend and foe. *Horm. Mol. Biol. Clin. Investig.* **2018**, *33*, 20170076. [CrossRef] [PubMed]
43. Wold, L.E.; Hines, E.A.; Allen, E.V. Lipedema of the legs; a syndrome characterized by fat legs and edema. *Ann. Intern. Med.* **1951**, *34*, 1243–1250. [CrossRef] [PubMed]
44. Brandi, C.; Campana, M.; Russo, F.; Brafa, A.; Nisi, G.; Grimaldi, L.; D'aniello, C. Carbon dioxide: Maybe not the only one but an efficient and secure gas for treating local adiposities. *Aesthetic Plast. Surg.* **2012**, *36*, 218–219. [CrossRef]
45. Koutná, N. Carboxytherapy--a new non-invasive method in aesthetic medicine. *Cas. Lek. Cesk* **2006**, *145*, 841–843. [PubMed]
46. Di Renzo, L.; Di Pierro, D.; Bigioni, M.; Sodi, V.; Galvano, F.; Cianci, R.; La Fauci, L.; De Lorenzo, A. Is antioxidant plasma status in humans a consequence of the antioxidant food content influence? *Eur. Rev. Med. Pharmacol. Sci.* **2007**, *11*, 185–192.
47. Al-Wardat, M.; Alwardat, N.; De Santis, G.L.; Zomparelli, S.; Gualtieri, P.; Bigioni, G.; Romano, L.; Di Renzo, L. The association between serum vitamin D and mood disorders in a cohort of lipedema patients. *Horm. Mol. Biol. Clin. Investig.* **2021**, *42*, 351–355. [CrossRef]

nutrients

MDPI

Article

Adherence to a Mediterranean Diet, Body Composition and Energy Expenditure in Outpatients Adolescents Diagnosed with Anorexia Nervosa: A Pilot Study

Giulia Cinelli [1], Ileana Croci [1,*], Gemma Lou De Santis [2], Ilenia Chianello [3], Kiersten Pilar Miller [1], Paola Gualtieri [4], Laura Di Renzo [4], Antonino De Lorenzo [4], Alberto Eugenio Tozzi [1] and Valeria Zanna [3]

1 Predictive and Preventive Medicine Research Unit, Bambino Gesù Children's Hospital IRCCS, 00165 Rome, Italy; giulia.cinelli@opbg.net (G.C.); kiersten.millerpilar@opbg.net (K.P.M.); albertoeugenio.tozzi@opbg.net (A.E.T.)

2 PhD School of Applied Medical-Surgical Sciences, University of Rome Tor Vergata, 00133 Rome, Italy; gemmaloudesantis@gmail.com

3 Anorexia Nervosa and Eating Disorder Unit, Child and Adolescent Neuropsychiatry Unit, Bambino Gesù Children's Hospital, IRCCS, 00165 Rome, Italy; ilenia.chianello@opbg.net (I.C.); valeria.zanna@opbg.net (V.Z.)

4 Section of Clinical Nutrition and Nutrigenomics, Department of Biomedicine and Prevention, University of Rome Tor Vergata, 00133 Rome, Italy; paola.gualtieri@uniroma2.it (P.G.); laura.di.renzo@uniroma2.it (L.D.R.); delorenzo@uniroma2.it (A.D.L.)

* Correspondence: ileana.croci@opbg.net; Tel.: +39-06-68594814

Abstract: Weight restoration is the primary goal of treatment for patients with Anorexia Nervosa (AN). This observational pilot study aims to describe adherence to the Mediterranean Diet (MD) and the consequent process of weight and functional recovery in outpatient adolescents diagnosed with AN. Eight patients with a median age of 15.1 (14.0–17.1) years were seen at baseline and after six months. Anthropometrics, body composition, and resting energy expenditure (REE) were assessed. The KIDMED questionnaire, the 24 h recall, and a quantitative food frequency questionnaire were used to evaluate adherence to the MD. The median KIDMED score increased from 5.5 (T0) to 10 (T1), which was not significant. Intakes of grams of carbohydrates, lipids, mono-unsaturated fatty acids, and fiber increased ($p = 0.012$, $p = 0.036$, $p = 0.036$, $p = 0.025$). Weight significantly increased ($p = 0.012$) as well as lean body mass ($p = 0.036$), with a resulting improvement of the REE ($p = 0.012$). No association between anthropometrics and body composition and the KIDMED score was found. The MD could represent an optimal dietary pattern for weight gain and nutritional restoration in patients with AN, and it could lead to an improvement in body composition and resting energy expenditure.

Keywords: anorexia nervosa; Mediterranean diet; anthropometrics; body composition

1. Introduction

Anorexia Nervosa (AN) is an eating disorder with serious physical repercussions and the highest mortality and relapse rate among psychiatric illnesses [1]. The main characteristic of patients with AN is severe food restriction, with an energy intake lower than daily requirements, which leads to significant weight loss and a consequent reduction in both fat and lean body mass [2]. The primary goal of treatment for patients with AN is weight restoration through the refeeding intervention, which is necessary to reduce the risk of physical complications or death [3].

The incidence of AN is increasing among younger girls [1]. In adolescence, many patients do not require hospitalization, and, if necessary, after that, outpatient treatment continues with nutritional rehabilitation managed at home. Based on the clinical experience of the Neuropsychiatry Unit at Bambino Gesù Children's Hospital, adolescent patients who are not hospitalized may experience differences in the process of refeeding, especially in their food choices. Some patients may reintroduce processed foods, such as snacks or fruit juices, early and with high frequency. While their high-energy-density may help in weight gain, the excess of saturated fatty acids and sugar deviates from the National Guidelines on Healthy Eating recommendations [4].

Body composition is altered in patients with AN. Both fat mass and fat free mass are significantly lower compared to healthy subjects, and they are only partially restored after treatment [5]. Unbalanced nutritional rehabilitation may put patients at risk of metabolic alterations related to dysbiosis of the intestinal microbiome and visceral adiposity. Partial weight gain following a condition of severe physical wasting has, in fact, been associated with a characteristic fat deposition in the abdominal region [5–8]. This phenomenon may be related to the imbalanced insulin sensitivity detected in AN patients [9], but it has also been linked to potential pathological consequences on the patient's metabolism, such as insulin resistance [10].

The evaluation of body composition may be of importance to monitor the beneficial effects of a nutritional treatment and to understand both the nature and the course of AN [5]. Improvements in both fat and lean mass have, in fact, been highlighted as markers of menstrual recovery and restoration of health status in the medium and long term [11].

Nutritional rehabilitation should aim to restore health as well as to educate the individual and their family on healthy eating habits, which is essential to ensure the acquisition of the underlying principles needed for a healthy lifestyle. Nutritional education must include restructuring the lifestyle habits of the entire family in order to achieve therapeutic success and prevent complications or relapses in the rehabilitation process. These may include the phenomenon of transitioning from AN to Bulimia Nervosa (BN) and Binge Eating Disorder (BED), which is characterised by events of uncontrolled overeating [12].

The Mediterranean Diet (MD) is characterized by: (i) high intake of complex carbohydrates and fiber from grains, vegetables, and legumes, (ii) moderate consumption of fatty fish and extra-virgin olive oil, and (iii) low consumption of dairy products and meats (red and white) [13]. In the MD, the distribution and quality of macronutrients provide a high amount of monounsaturated fats, fiber, prebiotics, and antioxidants. Population studies on the MD have demonstrated a reduction in the risk of cardiovascular disease, the onset of tumor disease, and insulin resistance in relation to adherence [14–16]. An inverse association has been observed between the MD and waist circumference, and, thus, a lower distribution of fat mass at the abdominal level [17–19]. Leone et al. suggested that a better adherence to the MD may prevent the occurrence of AN and BN. The hypothesis is that of the overall dietary pattern, tryptophan, unsaturated fatty acids, vitamins, and antioxidant intake may protect against eating disorders [20] and probably against possible relapses.

To date, there are no studies investigating adherence to the MD or its short- or long-term effects in AN patients treated on an outpatient basis. The main aim of the following pilot study is to describe adherence to the MD in a small group of adolescents diagnosed with AN during the outpatient refeeding intervention. Secondly, the study aims to investigate the subsequent process of recovery in terms of weight, body composition, and energy metabolism.

2. Materials and Methods

2.1. Subjects and Study Design

This observational pilot study analysed data from patients who were admitted to the Neuropsychiatry Unit at Bambino Gesù Children's Hospital in the period between March 2019 and February 2020 who were diagnosed with anorexia nervosa. Male and female patients, aged 12 to 18 years old, with a primary diagnosis of an eating disorder based on DSM-5 criteria, were invited to take part in the study. Exclusion criteria were the presence of intellectual disabilities and a non-eating disorder primary diagnosis.

All the patients who agreed to participate were enrolled and sent to the Section of Clinical Nutrition and Nutrigenomics, Department of Biomedicine and Prevention of the University of Rome Tor Vergata for nutritional assessment, which included dietary assessment, anthropometrics, body composition, and indirect calorimetry. Visits were performed in the presence of at least one parent or a caregiver. A Mediterranean Diet was prescribed to all the patients, and the complete nutritional follow-up was performed after 3 and 6 months. Adherence to the dietary intervention was monitored every 2 weeks with face-to-face follow-ups or by telephone interviews when needed. All the patients received outpatient psychological treatment throughout the six-month intervention. The study was reviewed and approved by the Ethical Committees of the Bambino Gesù Children Hospital (protocol code 1555_OPBG_2018, 20 November 2018) and was conducted in accordance with the Declaration of Helsinki. All the patients and their parents signed a written informed consent to participate in the study.

2.2. Dietary Intervention

All the subjects who participated in the study were given a Mediterranean Diet to follow. The diet was designed to meet the macro- and micronutrient needs of each patient and was personalized according to their preferences. The energy intake was calculated in relation to the BW at T0 as 30–40 kcal/kg/day and increased according to the weight gain in a tailored way for each patient, according to the Italian Ministry Guidelines [21].

The MD was mainly plant based, including seasonal fruits and vegetables, legumes, and nuts. According to the national dietary reference intakes [22], the diet was composed of 45–60% carbohydrates (sugars less than 15%), 20–35% lipids (with less than 10% being saturated fats, 6–10% being polyunsaturated fatty acids, and 15% being monounsaturated fatty acids) and 15–20% proteins. In addition, the daily fiber intake was about 25 g per day.

The diet plan consisted of five meals per day and the distribution of calories across the meals was as follows: breakfast (15–20%), morning snack (5–10%), lunch (35%), afternoon snack (5–10%), and dinner (30%).

2.3. Dietary and MD Adherence Assessment

Eating habits were investigated by a trained nutritionist during an interview by using the standard 24 h recall methods and the Italian Version of the medium-length quantitative Food Frequency Questionnaire validated by Buscemi et al. [23]. The "Istituto Scotti Bassani" photo atlas was used to determine the portion sizes and the weight of food consumed [24]. The estimated intake of total daily energy and macronutrients was calculated by using Metadieta dietary software v.4.4 (METEDA S.r.l., Rome, Italy).

The adherence to the MD was assessed using the KIDMED questionnaire for individuals aged 2 to 24 [25]. The questionnaire was administered through an interview conducted by a trained nutritionist. It consisted of 16 questions, with a scoring range of 0 to 12 points. The questions mainly inquired about the frequency of consuming various food groups and their portions, without specifying the quantities in grams. A score of +1 is assigned for positive adherence to the MD, while a score of −1 indicates negative adherence. The sum of the scores was then categorized into three levels: >8 represents "high" adherence to the MD, 4–7 indicates a need for improvement in daily intake according to MD guidelines ("medium"), and ≤3 signifies a lack of conformity with the MD model ("low").

2.4. Anthropometrics

While standing in their underwear, body weight and height were measured using a scale and stadiometer (Invernizzi, Rome, Italy) with precision to the nearest 0.1 kg and 0.1 cm, respectively. Height was measured with the Frankfurt plane of the participant's head aligned by eye to be parallel to the ground. Body circumferences (waist, abdomen, hip, mid-arm, and mid-thigh) were measured on the non-dominant side using a flexible, non-extensible metric tape. The participant's body mass index (BMI) was calculated as body weight (in kg) divided by height (in meters) squared. BMI percentile (pBMI) showed how the child's weight compares to that of other children of the same age and sex, and was determined using the WHO Anthro software v.1.0.4 [26]. In case the software assigned a "Not-Applicable" value to pBMI, a value of 0.1 was used in the analysis by convention.

The International Obesity Task Force (IOTF) childhood BMI cut-offs for thinness, based on and linked to the corresponding adult BMI cut-offs, were used to classify BMI [27,28].

2.5. Body Composition

The Bioelectrical Impedance Analysis (BIA) (BIA101S, Akern/RJL Systems, Florence, Italy) was used to measure resistance (Rz) and reactance (Xc). A dedicated piece of software was used to process data and calculate the total body water (TBW, L), the extracellular body water (ECW, L), the body cell mass (BCM) and its index (calculated by dividing it by height (in meters) squared (BCMI)), and the phase angle (PA).

Dual-energy X-ray absorptiometry (DXA; I-DXA Lunar) was used to assess body composition. Standard quality control and calibration measures were performed before each session, and participants were required to remove any metal jewellery or accessories before the measurement. They were positioned in a supine position with their arms at their sides and their ankles fastened together with a Velcro belt to ensure that they remained in a standard position for approximately 20 min while the DXA scan recorded their results. The coefficient of variation (CV% = 100 × SD/mean) for intra and inter subjects ranged from 1% to 5%, with a coefficient of variation for bone measurements of less than 1%. The radiation dose for the procedure was 0.01 mSv. A dedicated software was used to process data from the body scan and produce measurements for limbs and trunk, including Fat Mass (FM) and Lean Body Mass (LBM). FM% was calculated as FM (in kg) divided by BW.

The Fat Mass Index (FMI) and the Lean Body Mass Index (LBMI) were calculated by dividing the FM and LBM in kilograms by the height in metres squared, respectively. FMI and LBMI were compared to the reference population curve for age and sex [29]. Percentiles between the 10th and the 75th were normal.

2.6. Indirect Calorimetry

To determine the resting energy expenditure (REE), indirect calorimetry was conducted using a Vyntus CPX Canopy (CareFusion, Höchberg, Germany) and the Sentry Suite™ software (CareFusion, Höchberg, Germany), according to the method described by De Lorenzo et al. [30]. The gas mixture comprised 12.0% O_2, 5.0% CO_2, and N_2, and the subjects were instructed to fast for 12 h before the measurement. The participants were asked to lie down on a laboratory bed in a supine position for 25–30 min in a room with an ambient temperature of 22 °C until a steady-state condition was achieved, at which point VO_2 and VCO_2 values were recorded. The Weir formula [31] was then used to calculate the REE.

2.7. Handgrip Strength

The mean handgrip strength of both hands was measured with a portable electronic dynamometer (DynEx, Akern, Florence, Italy). It was regulated for each subject to fit the hand and allow flexion at the metacarpophalangeal joints. The scale of the dynamometer indicated handgrip strength in kilograms (kg). Both non-dominant and dominant hands were measured. The testing protocol consisted of three maximal voluntary isometric contractions maintained for 5 s on both hands, with a rest period of at least 60 s. The mean values for each hand were calculated and considered during the analysis.

During the hand strength testing protocol, the subject sat upright against the back of a chair with feet flat on the floor, and the arm 13 position was standardized with the shoulder adducted and neutrally rotated, with the elbow flexed to 90°. The forearm and wrist were in a neutral position resting on the support surface; the hand was maintained in line with the forearm holding the instrument upright on its base on the short side. Specific verbal instructions were given to subjects before the evaluations, and the experiments were performed with verbal encouragement [32].

2.8. Statistical Analysis

Categorical variables were summarized as frequencies and percentages while continuous variables were presented as median and interquartile range (IQR).

The Wilcoxon Signed Rank and the McNemar tests were used to analyze differences between T0 and T1 for continuous and categorical variables, respectively. Spearman's correlation was applied to test the relationship between anthropometrics and body composition variables and KIDMED score. The Kruscal–Wallis test was used to analyse differences in anthropometrics and body composition variables among the three KIDMED level's groups.

Data analysis was performed with Stata 17 (Stata Corporation, College Station, TX, USA).

3. Results

3.1. Subjects

A total of 20 patients were enrolled in the study. Four of them did not give their consent, one was hospitalized before the first visit, and one was not seen for the first visit due to the COVID-19 restrictions. In the end, 14 patients were included in the study, of which only 9 were seen for the follow-up visit at 6 months due to the COVID-19 restrictions. One patient was excluded since she shifted to overeating and was an outlier for weight gain. In the end, eight patients were used for the present analysis. The median age was 15.1 (14.0–17.1) years. At T0, seven patients (87.5%) had secondary amenorrhea since 7.8 (6.2–11.4) months, while 1 (12.5%) was in prepuberty. Two (25%) were in treatment with psychiatric drugs. At T1, menses resumption was observed in four patients over seven (57.1%). The patient in prepuberty did not change her menstrual status at T1.

3.2. Dietary Components

The mean dietary components (macronutrients) of the baseline (T0) diet and the follow-up (T1) were calculated using the 24 h recall and the FFQ (Table 1). Only two patients (at T0) and one (at T1) took oral nutritional supplements (200 mL/day corresponding to 300 kcal).

Table 1. Dietary intakes before (T0) and after (T1) the nutritional rehabilitation (n = 8).

	T0	T1	p
Energy (Kcal)	1219.1 (587.9–1536.2)	1854.7 (1689.4–2051.6)	**0.025**
Carbohydrates (g)	154.7 (64.5–190.7)	220.2 (210.0–245.4)	**0.012**
Carbohydrates (%)	45.2 (37.4–48.5)	48.1 (44.1–49.1)	0.069
Sugars (g)	47.7 (22.8–62.0)	66.4 (52.8–69.6)	**0.012**
Sugars (%)	13.9 (13.4–16.0)	13.2 (12.0–15.4)	0.161
Proteins (g)	59.6 (35.6–84.8)	87.6 (79.4–95.6)	**0.036**
Proteins (%)	22.8 (21.8–23.8)	19.1 (17.6–20.0)	**0.025**
Animal/plant-based proteins *	2.4 (1.8–3.8)	2.0 (1.6–2.3)	0.124
Lipids (g)	37.6 (24.7–56.4)	70.6 (57.5–83.9)	**0.036**
Lipids (%)	33.5 (30.2–38.4)	32.5 (30.6–36.8)	1.000
Saturated fatty acids (g)	9.6 (6.7–11.8)	21.7 (15.5–25.7)	**0.050**
Saturated fatty acids (%)	8.2 (7.0–12.4)	10.4 (8.4–11.8)	0.327
Mono-unsaturated fatty acids (g)	21.5 (13.4–25.4)	37.5 (27.5–43.0)	**0.036**
Mono-unsaturated fatty acids (%)	17.3 (15.0–19.8)	16.6 (15.9–19.4)	0.575
Poli-unsaturated fatty acids (g)	4.7 (2.3–7.0)	7.3 (6.1–8.0)	0.161
Poli-unsaturated fatty acids (%)	3.5 (3.1–5.2)	3.5 (3.2–3.9)	0.401
Fiber (g)	14.9 (7.2–22.2)	22.6 (20.5–26.5)	**0.025**

* Proteins from the oral nutritional supplements were not included for this variable, since no information about animal and plant-based portions were available. %, percentage of kcal over the total daily energy intake. The Wilcoxon Signed Rank test was performed to compare patients' dietary intakes at T0 and T1. Statistical significance for $p < 0.05$ (in bold).

A significant increase in energy intake was observed. A significant increase in carbohydrates and intake of lipids (in grams) was also found, while the intake of proteins increased in grams but decreased in percentage. Sugar intake significantly increased in grams, but the percentage over the total energy intake did not. The intake of both saturated and mono-unsaturated fatty acids significantly increased (in grams). Finally, the amount of fiber significantly increased.

The median KIDMED score at T0 was 5.5 (3.0–8.5) and rose up to 10 (8.0–10.5) at T1 (p = 0.457), while the percentage of patients with a "low" MD adherence decreased from 37.5% to none (p = 0.083) (Figure 1). An increase in the percentage of patients eating vegetables, fish, grains, and dairy products for breakfast was observed between T0 and T1 (no significant results) (Figure 2). No correlation was found between the KIDMED score at T1 and the energy intake ($p = 0.663$) or the restoration of menses ($p = 0.882$) at T1.

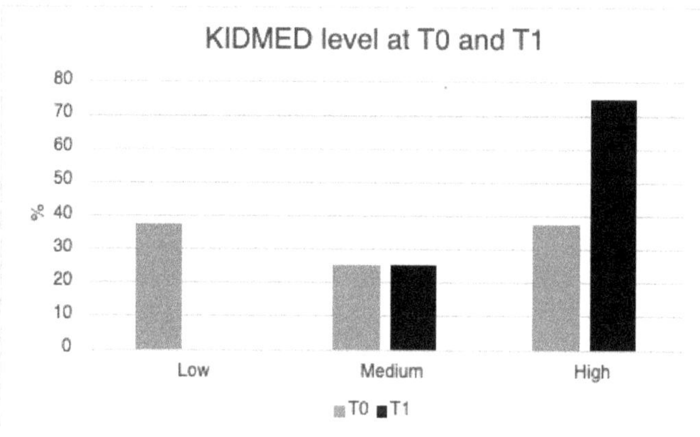

Figure 1. KIDMED level at T0 and T1. Low, medium, and high adherence to the Mediterranean Diet (MD).

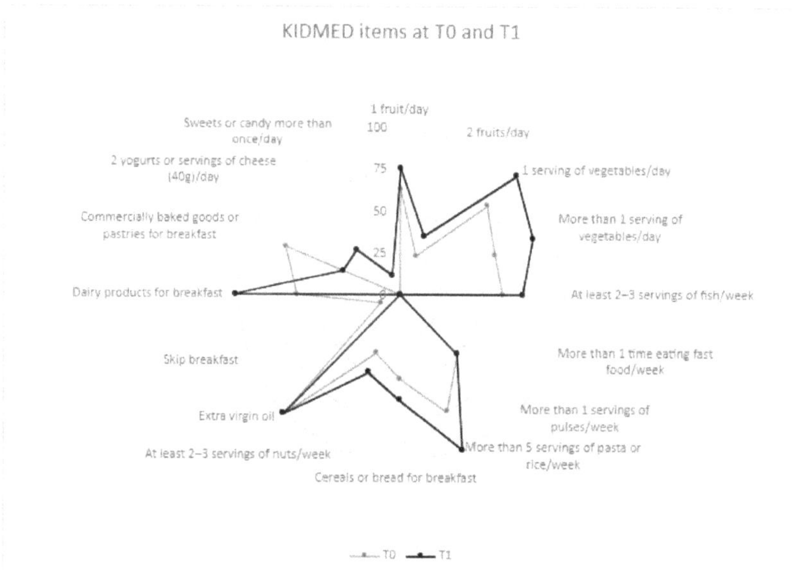

Figure 2. Compliance with items from KIDMED at T0 and T1. The radar chart plots the values of each item of the KIDMED questionnaire along a separate axis that starts in the centre of the chart (0% compliance) and ends at the outer ring (100% compliance). The values are the percentage of the population adherent to each recommendation.

3.3. Anthropometry and Body Composition

All anthropometrics improved between T0 and T1 after a mean of 6.7 months between the two visits (Table 2). Complete weight restoration (BMI > 10th percentile) was reached by five patients (62.5%).

Table 2. Anthropometric characteristics before (T0) and after (T1) the nutritional rehabilitation (n = 8).

	T0	T1	*p*
Height (cm)	157.3 (153.1–163.9)	158.4 (154.2–165.7)	**0.014**
Weight (kg)	38.1 (36.3–43.0)	46.7 (43.1–49.0)	**0.012**
BMI (kg/m^2)	15.8 (15.1–16.5)	17.8 (16.9–19.5)	**0.012**
BMI percentile	2.5 (1.2–3.9)	16.8 (5.2–37.8)	**0.012**
Waist circumference (cm)	57.9 (55.2–58.3)	61.5 (59.5–63.2)	**0.025**
Waist-to-height ratio	0.36 (0.35–0.37)	0.38 (0.37–0.40)	**0.036**
Abdomen circumference (cm)	68.9 (63.0–73.1)	71.9 (69.3–75.9)	**0.036**
Hip circumference (cm)	79.3 (76.3–82.0)	87.2 (83.6–89.7)	**0.017**
Mid Harm circumference (cm)	20.4 (19.9–21.0)	23.0 (22.2–24.6)	**0.017**
Mid-thigh circumference (cm)	39.6 (38.6–41.8)	43.0 (42.1–46.7)	**0.017**

Values are expressed as median and IQR (M [IQR]). The Wilcoxon Signed Rank test was performed to compare patients' anthropometric characteristics at T0 and T1. Statistical significance for $p < 0.05$ (in bold). BMI, body mass index.

No correlation was found between the KIDMED score at T1 and the Δ of weight (r = −0.540, p = 0.167) and Δ of BMI percentile (r = −0.417; p = 0.304). There was also no correlation between the KIDMED score at T1 and all measured circumferences. When using the KIDMED levels, a significantly higher increase in abdomen and hip circumferences was found in the group of patients with medium adherence compared with the high one (p = 0.046; p = 0.046).

Regarding body composition, at T1, a significant increase in the total body water, BCM, FFM, LBM, and LBMI at T1 was found. No significant improvement in FM amount was observed, with only three (37.5%) patients showing an FMI over the 10th percentile. A significant improvement in the REE was also detected (Table 3).

Table 3. Calorimetry, Bioimpedance Analysis, and Dual X-ray Analysis before and after the nutritional rehabilitation (n = 8).

		T0	T1	*p*
BIA	Rz Resistance	749.5 (711.5–767)	701.5 (682.5–755.5)	0.124
	Xc Reactance	70.0 (66.0–74.5)	69.5 (66.0–78.5)	0.779
	TBW (L)	25.4 (24.1–26.2)	27.0 (25.9–28.1)	**0.012**
	ECW (L)	11.4 (10.7–13.2)	12.0 (11.5–12.9)	0.161
	BCM (kg)	16.3 (15.0–17.2)	17.6 (16.7–21.1)	**0.042**
	BCMI (kg/m^2)	6.5 (6.1–6.9)	7.4 (6.7–8.0)	0.107
	PA (°)	5.3 (5.1–5.9)	5.8 (5.2–6.3)	0.622
DXA	FFM (kg)	31.59 (29.24–33.07)	34.41 (32.59–37.71)	**0.012**
	FM (kg)	8.57 (6.84–9.63)	10.09 (7.18–12.41)	0.161
	LBM (kg)	31.40 (28.50–34.51)	33.28 (32.00–35.73)	**0.036**
	FMpct (%)	21.2 (17.4–23.8)	21.5 (17.6–26.6)	0.575
	FMI (kg/m^2)	3.3 (2.9–3.7)	4.0 (2.9–4.9)	0.208
	LBMI (kg/m^2)	13.0 (11.8–13.0)	13.9 (12.8–14.2)	**0.050**
Calorimetry	VO_2 (mL/min)	137 (112.5–150.5)	161.5 (148.5–169)	**0.012**
	VCO_2 (mL/min)	122 (96.5–136)	146.5 (137–157)	**0.035**
	RER	0.88 (0.87–0.96)	0.90 (0.87–0.97)	0.575
	REE (kcal)	921 (781.5–1036.5)	1124.5 (1036–1154.5)	**0.012**

Values are expressed as median and IQR (M [IQR]). The Wilcoxon Signed Rank test was performed to compare patients' body composition variables at T0 and T1. Statistical significance for $p < 0.05$ (in bold). BIA, bioimpedance analysis; BCM, body cell mass; BCMI, body cell mass index; DXA, dual x-ray analysis; ECW, extracellular water; FFM, fat free mass; FM, fat mass; FMI, fat mass index; FMpct, percentage of fat mass; LBM, lean body mass; LBMI, lean body mass index; PA, phase angle; RER, Respiratory Exchange Ratio; Rz, Resistance; REE, resting energy expenditure; VCO_2, volumes of carbon dioxide; VO_2, volumes of oxygen; Xc, Reactance.

No correlation was found between the KIDMED score at T1 and BIA parameters, DXA parameters, and REE. In the DXA analysis, a significant difference between KIDMED medium and high level was found for FM, and, consequently, FMI increased (p = 0.045), resulting in a higher gain in the group with poorer MD adherence.

The strength measured through the handgrip increased from 18.7 (17.9–21.0) to 22.5 (20.2–23.9) (p = 0.069), and from 18.5 (17.4–20.7) to 21.4 (20.1–22.7) (p = 0.093) for the dominant and non-dominant arm, respectively. No correlation between the KIDMED score at T1 and the Δ of the handgrip measurements was found.

4. Discussion

The present observational pilot study aimed to describe adherence to a MD in outpatient adolescents diagnosed with AN. At baseline, the MD adherence was "medium", and it increased to "high" at T1, even if not significant, which demonstrates patients' compliance to the dietary intervention. The consumption of vegetables, fish, grains, nuts, and dairy products increased. The daily energy intake increased at T1 as well as the amount of all macronutrients and fiber. Conversely, the percentage of calories over the total energy intake from proteins decreased, leading to a better adherence to the national dietary reference values [22]. Finally, sugar intake significantly increased in grams, but the percentage over the total energy intake did not and remained under the recommendation of 15% [22]. Several studies have described how all these dietary characteristics have an antioxidant and anti-inflammatory effect, making the MD an optimal dietary pattern for the prevention and management of nutritional diseases [33,34].

During the six-month intervention, our patients gained weight and improved their BMI percentile as well as all of their anthropometrics, confirming what has been described in previous studies [8,35]. Even though the literature suggests caution in interpreting results of the BIA analysis in AN [36], a significant increase in the TBW was detected in our sample. This could be indicative of an improvement in patients' hydration status or could be associated with the increased amount of LBM, measured through the DXA analysis.

The circumferences of the upper and lower limbs were significantly increased as an indicator of muscle mass improvement, and this was confirmed by the increased amount of BCM, FFM, and LBM, measured through the BIA and DXA analyses, respectively. These results are in line with a previous study on adolescents [8]. Even though only a trend in the improvement of strength (handgrip) was observed, the improvement of LBM after the nutritional intervention is a clinically important factor [37], and it reflects the consequent increase in REE observed [37]. A recent study by Bou Khalil et al. [38] also showed that the FFM may be a better predictor of REE than weight and BMI. In patients with AN, the FFM is metabolically less active than in other malnourished individuals [38], and it is therefore possible to assume that for the same weight, the REE is lower than in malnourished but non-AN patients. Therefore, the increase in BCM, FFM, and LBM shown by our results may determine a further improvement in the metabolism rehabilitation of these patients.

Additionally, abdomen and hip circumferences, which are regions related to fat deposition, both increased, yet no significant increase in FM measured by the DXA analysis was detected. This contrasts with what was observed by El Ghoch et al. in 33 adolescent patients with AN, in which a significant increase in the total FM was detected. This difference could be related to the fact that their patients were followed for more than three months as inpatients and for only two months as outpatients [8]. The small sample size of the present study could also have affected the significance. When evaluating the waist-to-height ratio, a significant increase was observed. Since this ratio is one of the parameters used to measure central adiposity [39], this observation may confirm the hypothesis that short-term weight recovery in AN adolescent patients could lead to visceral fat redistribution [7,8]. Even if we did not find a significant increase in the total FM, almost 60% of our patients restored their periods.

In our sample, a complete weight recovery was not reached by all patients, with three of them still being underweight after six months. A longer follow-up, which was not possible due to COVID-19 restrictions, could have shown different results in weight and FM gain.

No association between the KIDMED score at T1 and the variation in anthropometrics and body composition parameters was detected. Although when considering the KIDMED level, the group of patients with a poorer adherence to the MD showed a larger increase in FM. Moreover, both abdomen and hip circumferences were higher in patients with poorer adherence. Conversely, there was no association between KIDMED and waist-to-height ratio in our sample. Further investigations with reference methods, such as the assessment of segmental FM in the android and truncal region, on a larger sample are needed to better understand if the MD could represent a dietary pattern reducing the metabolic risk in terms of visceral adiposity. In fact, even if FM restoration is extremely important in AN [40], understanding the amount and the distribution of the regained adipose tissue is essential, since it is related to the metabolic status of the patient [10]. Our main findings were the recovery of weight and major circumferences, confirmed by the improvement in lean mass evidenced by instrumental analysis (BIA and DXA) after the six–month intervention in which MD was chosen for the nutritional rehabilitation. In addition, contrary to what has already been described in the literature, increased dietary adherence resulted in a smaller increase in circumferences related to visceral fat accumulation. These data need to be confirmed with segmental analysis of body masses. Moreover, more than half of our patients have recovered their menstrual cycle. From this perspective, the MD could be a suitable dietary model to propose to patients and family members as it is ideal for good weight recovery, the maintenance of health status, and the prevention of relapses.

The present study has some limitations. Due to COVID-19 restrictions, not all of the enrolled patients were seen at T1 after 6 months, so the final sample size for the analysis was limited. Segmental parameters of body composition were also not available for all patients and, given the small sample size, they were not useful for statistical analysis. However, the novelty of our work is the investigation of MD adherence in AN patients before and after the nutritional rehabilitation.

5. Conclusions

This piece of work is an observational pilot study with a small sample size, hence the facts that the results cannot be generalized and it is only possible to speculate on them in order to imagine future research. To our knowledge, this is the first study describing adherence to the MD in a group of outpatient adolescents diagnosed with AN. A MD may be considered an excellent eating model for weight gain and nutritional restoration, even in patients with AN. It could lead to a proper weight restoration as well as an improvement in body composition and resting energy expenditure.

It is also worth highlighting that anthropometrics should not be considered the only aim of treatment of AN. Body composition and FM distribution in relation to the type of dietary pattern are key elements to monitor during the rehabilitation process.

Additional investigations are needed in this field to confirm these results and to better understand FM modification and distribution. The short- and long-term effects of a MD on patients' metabolism, microbiome, health, and psychological outcomes should be studied.

Author Contributions: Conceptualization, G.C.; methodology, G.C.; formal analysis, I.C. (Ileana Croci); investigation, G.C., G.L.D.S. and I.C. (Ilenia Chianello); data curation, G.C. and I.C. (Ileana Croci); writing—original draft preparation, G.C. and G.L.D.S.; writing—review and editing, G.C, G.L.D.S., K.P.M.; L.D.R., A.D.L., P.G., V.Z. and A.E.T.; supervision, L.D.R., A.D.L. and V.Z.; project administration, V.Z. All authors have read and agreed to the published version of the manuscript.

Funding: This work was supported also by the Italian Ministry of Health with Current Research funds.

Institutional Review Board Statement: The study was conducted in accordance with the Declaration of Helsinki, and approved by the Institutional Review Board (or Ethics Committee) of the Bambino Gesù Children Hospital (protocol code 1555_OPBG_2018, 20 November 2018).

Informed Consent Statement: Informed consent was obtained from all subjects involved in the study.

Data Availability Statement: The data presented in this study are available on reasonable request from the corresponding author. The data are not publicly available due to European data sharing policies.

Conflicts of Interest: The authors declare no conflict of interest.

References

1. Van Eeden, A.E.; van Hoeken, D.; Hoek, H.W. Incidence, Prevalence and Mortality of Anorexia Nervosa and Bulimia Nervosa. *Curr. Opin. Psychiatry* **2021**, *34*, 515. [CrossRef]
2. Kerruish, K.P.; O'Connor, J.; Humphries, I.R.J.; Kohn, M.R.; Clarke, S.D.; Briody, J.N.; Thomson, E.J.; Wright, K.A.; Gaskin, K.J.; Baur, L.A. Body Composition in Adolescents with Anorexia Nervosa. *Am. J. Clin. Nutr.* **2002**, *75*, 31–37. [CrossRef] [PubMed]
3. NICE. *NICE Guideline 69. Eating Disorders: Recognition and Treatment*; NICE: London, UK, 2017.
4. CREA; Centro di Ricerca Alimenti e Nutrizione. *Linee Guida per Una Sana Alimentazione—Revisione 2018*; CREA: Roma, Italy, 2019.
5. Hubel, C.; Yilmaz, Z.; Schaumberg, K.E.; Breithaupt, L.; Hunjan, A.; Horne, E.; Garcia-Gonzalez, J.; O'Reilly, P.F.; Bulik, C.M.; Breen, G. Body Composition in Anorexia Nervosa: Meta-Analysis and Meta-Regression of Cross-Sectional and Longitudinal Studies. *Int. J. Eat. Disord.* **2019**, *52*, 1205–1223. [CrossRef] [PubMed]
6. Franzoni, E.; Ciccarese, F.; Di Pietro, E.; Facchini, G.; Moscano, F.; Iero, L.; Monaldi, A.; Battista, G.; Bazzocchi, A. Follow-up of Bone Mineral Density and Body Composition in Adolescents with Restrictive Anorexia Nervosa: Role of Dual-Energy X-ray Absorptiometry. *Eur. J. Clin. Nutr.* **2014**, *68*, 247–252. [CrossRef] [PubMed]
7. El Ghoch, M.; Calugi, S.; Lamburghini, S.; Dalle Grave, R. Anorexia Nervosa and Body Fat Distribution: A Systematic Review. *Nutrients* **2014**, *6*, 3895–3912. [CrossRef]
8. El Ghoch, M.; Milanese, C.; Calugi, S.; Müller, M.J.; Pourhassan, M.; Ruocco, A.; Dalle Grave, R. Regional Fat Distribution in Adolescent and Adult Females with Anorexia Nervosa: A Longitudinal Study. *Clin. Nutr.* **2015**, *34*, 1224–1232. [CrossRef]
9. Ilyas, A.; Hübel, C.; Stahl, D.; Stadler, M.; Ismail, K.; Breen, G.; Treasure, J.; Kan, C. The Metabolic Underpinning of Eating Disorders: A Systematic Review and Meta-Analysis of Insulin Sensitivity. *Mol. Cell. Endocrinol.* **2019**, *497*, 110307. [CrossRef]
10. Prioletta, A.; Muscogiuri, G.; Sorice, G.P.; Lassandro, A.P.; Mezza, T.; Policola, C.; Salomone, E.; Cipolla, C.; Della Casa, S.; Pontecorvi, A.; et al. In Anorexia Nervosa, Even a Small Increase in Abdominal Fat Is Responsible for the Appearance of Insulin Resistance. *Clin. Endocrinol.* **2011**, *75*, 202–206. [CrossRef]
11. Karountzos, V.; Lambrinoudaki, I.; Tsitsika, A.; Deligeoroglou, E. The Role of Total Body Fat Mass and Trunk Fat Mass, Combined with Other Endocrine Factors, in Menstrual Recovery and Psychopathology of Adolescents with Anorexia Nervosa. *Gynecol. Endocrinol.* **2017**, *33*, 757–762. [CrossRef]
12. Eddy, K.T.; Dorer, D.J.; Franko, D.L.; Tahilani, K.; Thompson-Brenner, H.; Herzog, D.B. Diagnostic Crossover in Anorexia Nervosa and Bulimia Nervosa: Implications for DSM-V. *Am. J. Psychiatry* **2008**, *165*, 245–250. [CrossRef]
13. Willett, W.C.; Sacks, F.; Trichopoulou, A.; Drescher, G.; Ferro-Luzzi, A.; Helsing, E.; Trichopoulos, D. Mediterranean Diet Pyramid: A Cultural Model for Healthy Eating. *Am. J. Clin. Nutr.* **1995**, *61*, 1402S–1406S. [CrossRef]
14. Di Daniele, N.; Petramala, L.; Di Renzo, L.; Sarlo, F.; Della Rocca, D.G.; Rizzo, M.; Fondacaro, V.; Iacopino, L.; Pepine, C.J.; De Lorenzo, A. Body Composition Changes and Cardiometabolic Benefits of a Balanced Italian Mediterranean Diet in Obese Patients with Metabolic Syndrome. *Acta Diabetol.* **2013**, *50*, 409–416. [CrossRef]
15. Di Daniele, N.; Noce, A.; Vidiri, M.F.; Moriconi, E.; Marrone, G.; Annicchiarico-Petruzzelli, M.; D'Urso, G.; Tesauro, M.; Rovella, V.; De Lorenzo, A. Impact of Mediterranean Diet on Metabolic Syndrome, Cancer and Longevity. *Oncotarget* **2016**, *8*, 8947–8979. [CrossRef]
16. Di Renzo, L.; Gualtieri, P.; De Lorenzo, A. Diet, Nutrition and Chronic Degenerative Diseases. *Nutrients* **2021**, *13*, 1372. [CrossRef]
17. Funtikova, A.N.; Benítez-Arciniega, A.A.; Gomez, S.F.; Fitó, M.; Elosua, R.; Schröder, H. Mediterranean Diet Impact on Changes in Abdominal Fat and 10-Year Incidence of Abdominal Obesity in a Spanish Population. *Br. J. Nutr.* **2014**, *111*, 1481–1487. [CrossRef]
18. Bertoli, S.; Leone, A.; Vignati, L.; Bedogni, G.; Martínez-González, M.Á.; Bes-Rastrollo, M.; Spadafranca, A.; Vanzulli, A.; Battezzati, A. Adherence to the Mediterranean Diet Is Inversely Associated with Visceral Abdominal Tissue in Caucasian Subjects. *Clin. Nutr.* **2015**, *34*, 1266–1272. [CrossRef]
19. Romaguera, D.; Norat, T.; Mouw, T.; May, A.M.; Bamia, C.; Slimani, N.; Travier, N.; Besson, H.; Luan, J.; Wareham, N.; et al. Adherence to the Mediterranean Diet Is Associated with Lower Abdominal Adiposity in European Men and Women. *J. Nutr.* **2009**, *139*, 1728–1737. [CrossRef]
20. Leone, A.; Martínez-González, M.Á.; Lahortiga-Ramos, F.; Molero Santos, P.; Bertoli, S.; Battezzati, A.; Bes-Rastrollo, M. Adherence to the Mediterranean Dietary Pattern and Incidence of Anorexia and Bulimia Nervosa in Women: The SUN Cohort. *Nutrition* **2018**, *54*, 19–25. [CrossRef]
21. Ministero della Salute. *Linee di Indirizzo Nazionali per la Riabilitazione Nutrizionale Nei Disturbi dell'Alimentazione*; Ministero della Salut: Rome, Italy, 2017.
22. Società Italiana di Nutrizione Umana (SINU). LARN—Livelli di Assunzione di Riferimento per la Popolazione Italiana: ENERGIA. Fabbisogno Energetico Medio (AR) Nell'intervallo D'età 1–17 Anni. Available online: https://sinu.it/2019/07/09/fabbisogno-energetico-medio-ar-nellintervallo-deta-1-17-anni/ (accessed on 2 June 2021).
23. Buscemi, S.; Rosafio, G.; Vasto, S.; Massenti, F.M.; Grosso, G.; Galvano, F.; Rini, N.; Barile, A.M.; Maniaci, V.; Cosentino, L.; et al. Validation of a Food Frequency Questionnaire for Use in Italian Adults Living in Sicily. *Int. J. Food Sci. Nutr.* **2015**, *66*, 426–438. [CrossRef]
24. Atlante Fotografico delle Porzioni degli Alimenti per Adulti. Available online: https://www.scottibassani.it/atlante-fotografico-delle-porzioni-degli-alimenti/ (accessed on 15 June 2023).

25. Serra-Majem, L.; Ribas, L.; Ngo, J.; Ortega, R.M.; García, A.; Pérez-Rodrigo, C.; Aranceta, J. Food, Youth and the Mediterranean Diet in Spain. Development of KIDMED, Mediterranean Diet Quality Index in Children and Adolescents. *Public Health Nutr.* **2004**, *7*, 931–935. [CrossRef]
26. WHO. WHO Anthro Survey Analyser and Other Tools. Available online: https://www.who.int/tools/child-growth-standards/software (accessed on 15 June 2023).
27. Cole, T.J.; Flegal, K.M.; Nicholls, D.; Jackson, A.A. Body Mass Index Cut Offs to Define Thinness in Children and Adolescents: International Survey. *BMJ* **2007**, *335*, 194. [CrossRef] [PubMed]
28. Cole, T.J.; Lobstein, T. Extended International (IOTF) Body Mass Index Cut-Offs for Thinness, Overweight and Obesity. *Pediatr. Obes.* **2012**, *7*, 284–294. [CrossRef] [PubMed]
29. Weber, D.R.; Moore, R.H.; Leonard, M.B.; Zemel, B.S. Fat and Lean BMI Reference Curves in Children and Adolescents and Their Utility in Identifying Excess Adiposity Compared with BMI and Percentage Body Fat1234. *Am. J. Clin. Nutr.* **2013**, *98*, 49–56. [CrossRef] [PubMed]
30. De Lorenzo, A.; Di Renzo, L.; Morini, P.; de Miranda, R.C.; Romano, L.; Colica, C. New Equations to Estimate Resting Energy Expenditure in Obese Adults from Body Composition. *Acta Diabetol.* **2018**, *55*, 59–66. [CrossRef] [PubMed]
31. Weir, J.B.D.B. New Methods for Calculating Metabolic Rate with Special Reference to Protein Metabolism. *J. Physiol.* **1949**, *109*, 1–9. [CrossRef]
32. Pizzigalli, L.; Micheletti Cremasco, M.; LA Torre, A.; Rainoldi, A.; Benis, R. Hand Grip Strength and Anthropometric Characteristics in Italian Female National Basketball Teams. *J. Sports Med. Phys. Fit.* **2017**, *57*, 521–528. [CrossRef]
33. Di Renzo, L.; Gualtieri, P.; Romano, L.; Marrone, G.; Noce, A.; Pujia, A.; Perrone, M.A.; Aiello, V.; Colica, C.; De Lorenzo, A. Role of Personalized Nutrition in Chronic-Degenerative Diseases. *Nutrients* **2019**, *11*, 1707. [CrossRef]
34. Gouveri, E.T.; Tzavara, C.; Drakopanagiotakis, F.; Tsaoussoglou, M.; Marakomichelakis, G.E.; Tountas, Y.; Diamantopoulos, E.J. Mediterranean Diet and Metabolic Syndrome in an Urban Population: The Athens Study. *Nutr. Clin. Pract.* **2011**, *26*, 598–606. [CrossRef]
35. Misra, M.; Soyka, L.A.; Miller, K.K.; Grinspoon, S.; Levitsky, L.L.; Klibanski, A. Regional Body Composition in Adolescents with Anorexia Nervosa and Changes with Weight Recovery. *Am. J. Clin. Nutr.* **2003**, *77*, 1361–1367. [CrossRef]
36. Kyle, U.G.; Bosaeus, I.; De Lorenzo, A.D.; Deurenberg, P.; Elia, M.; Gómez, J.M.; Heitmann, B.L.; Kent-Smith, L.; Melchior, J.-C.; Pirlich, M.; et al. Bioelectrical Impedance Analysis—Part I: Review of Principles and Methods. *Clin. Nutr.* **2004**, *23*, 1226–1243. [CrossRef]
37. Rosa-Caldwell, M.E.; Eddy, K.T.; Rutkove, S.B.; Breithaupt, L. Anorexia Nervosa and Muscle Health: A Systematic Review of Our Current Understanding and Future Recommendations for Study. *Int. J. Eat. Disord.* **2023**, *56*, 483–500. [CrossRef]
38. Bou Khalil, R.; Sultan, A.; Seneque, M.; Richa, S.; Lefebvre, P.; Renard, E.; Courtet, P.; Maimoun, L.; Guillaume, S. Clinical Correlates of Measured and Predicted Resting Energy Expenditure in Patients with Anorexia Nervosa: A Retrospective Cohort Study. *Nutrients* **2022**, *14*, 2727. [CrossRef]
39. Moreira, C.; Santos, R.; Vale, S.; Santos, P.C.; Abreu, S.; Marques, A.I.; Soares-Miranda, L.; Mota, J. Ability of Different Measures of Adiposity to Identify High Metabolic Risk in Adolescents. *J. Obes.* **2011**, *2011*, 578106. [CrossRef]
40. Ayton, A. The Importance of Restoring Body Fat Mass in the Treatment of Anorexia Nervosa: An Expert Commentary. *J. Popul. Ther. Clin. Pharmacol.* **2019**, *26*, e9–e13. [CrossRef]

nutrients

MDPI

Article

Body Composition in Fussy-Eating Children, with and without Neurodevelopmental Disorders, and Their Parents, Following a Taste Education Intervention

Sigrun Thorsteinsdottir [1,*], Ragnar Bjarnason [2,3], Helga G. Eliasdottir [1] and Anna S. Olafsdottir [1]

[1] Faculty of Health Promotion, Sport and Leisure Studies, School of Education, University of Iceland, Stakkahlid, 105 Reykjavik, Iceland; helgag@gmail.com (H.G.E.); annaso@hi.is (A.S.O.)
[2] Faculty of Medicine, School of Health Sciences, University of Iceland, Laeknagardur 4th Floor, Vatnsmyrarvegur 16, 101 Reykjavik, Iceland; ragnarb@landspitali.is
[3] Department of Pediatrics, National University Hospital, Hringbraut, 101 Reykjavik, Iceland
[*] Correspondence: sthorsteinsdottir@hi.is; Tel.: +354-7705000

Abstract: Fussy eaters may have an increased risk of becoming overweight or obese as adolescents, with fussy eating and weight status also correlating with neurodevelopmental disorders (NDs) such as autism spectrum disorder (ASD) and attention deficit/hyperactivity disorder (ADHD). Further, maternal and children's weight status relationships are well-established. In this study, we analyzed the body composition of parent–child dyads using bioelectrical impedance analysis (BIA). Fifty-one children aged 8–12 years, with an ND (n = 18) and without (n = 33), and their parents, participated in a 7-week food-based Taste Education intervention with 6-month follow-up. The paired t-test was used to compare differences in body composition based on children's ND status. In logistic regression analysis, odds of children being in the overweight/obese or overfat/obese categories increased by a factor of 9.1 and 10.6, respectively, when having NDs, adjusting for parents' BMI (body mass index) or fat percentage (FAT%). Children with NDs and their parents had significantly higher mean BMI-SDS (BMI standard deviation score) and FAT% at pre-intervention than children without NDs and their parents. Mean BMI-SDS and FAT% lowered significantly between time points for children with NDs and their parents but not for children without NDs or their parents. The findings underline the need for additional exploration into the relationships between children's and parents' body composition based on children's ND status.

Keywords: BMI; standard deviation scores; fat percentage; body composition measurements; bioelectrical impedance analysis; neurodevelopmental disorders; fussy eating; autism spectrum disorder; ADHD; parent–child dyads

1. Introduction

In recent decades, the prevalence of overweight and obesity in children and adults has increased considerably worldwide [1–4]. Obesity is considered a chronic, relapsing, and progressive disease, affecting individuals in all environments and demographics, particularly those in the lower socioeconomic brackets [5–8].

The causes of obesity are multifaceted and complex and include environmental, physiological, genetic, and behavioral factors [8–10]. There is also evidence of parental feeding practices and obesity being tied to children's eating psychopathology and weight trajectories [11]. In one study, mothers who were overweight or had obesity were involved in less healthy feeding practices with their children than mothers in the healthy weight range [12]. Similar reports have been published on the positive correlations between parents' and children's weight status [13–15]. Other mechanisms affecting children's weight status may also be related to their eating behaviors, such as fussy eating and food neophobia, in which a limited diet may affect children's general health and growth [16–18]. Fussy eating is often seen in children with obesity [17,19,20], as fussy eaters may be at a higher risk for becoming overweight or have obesity as older children and adolescents, possibly due to a penchant for calorie-dense foods and sweet beverages, and rejection of fruits and vegetables [21]. However, some researchers have not been able to determine the association between children's increased weight status and fussy eating [22], with some studies even reporting the risk of underweight in fussy-eating children [23–28], especially in those who are not typically developing (TD).

1.1. Fussy Eating and Neurodevelopmental Disorders

Numerous interpretations exist regarding problematic eating behaviors, encompassing food neophobia (disinclination toward unfamiliar or unknown foods), fussy or selective eating (refusing a substantial portion of both new and familiar foods), exhibiting displeasure during mealtimes, and engaging in oppositional behaviors or tantrums [29–31]. Typically, fussy eating results in a limited diet, characterized by a notably low variety in consumed foods [16,32,33]. Given that fussy eating encompasses food neophobia, both terms are often collectively referred to as fussy eating.

Fussy eating and other selective eating behaviors in children are strongly correlated with neurodevelopmental disorders (NDs) such as autism spectrum disorder (ASD) and attention deficit/hyperactivity disorder (ADHD), as NDs may severely affect eating behaviors [34–38]. Significantly, NDs may be a mediating factor in children's weight status and fussy-eating behaviors [31,39,40], in which children with NDs, especially those with ASD rather than ADHD, may be hypersensitive to food textures, smells, and taste [38,41–44]. Sensory sensitivities may limit children's food variety, and although fussy eating often peaks between 2 and 6 years old, those with the most difficulties in accepting new foods and different sensory aspects of food will not grow easily out of their fussy eating [44]. Parents of fussy eaters, with and without NDs, frequently report their children refusing fruit and vegetables, whole grains seeds, and legumes, which may cause parental concern about the child's well-being [45–48] and weight increase as well as decrease [25,49,50]. In addition, parental worrying, and pressure to eat may cause stress in children, and exacerbate mealtime behavior problems, thus reducing mealtime enjoyment and food variety [31,46,51–56].

Despite ASD often receiving the stronger focus on challenging eating behaviors in children with NDs, a relatively recent study pointed to fussy eating being similar across NDs, where children with ADHD had similar problems to those with ASD [57]. Overconsuming calorie-rich food, sweets, and sugary drinks is common in ADHD [58–61]. This unhealthy eating behavior may translate into disordered eating, including binge-eating disorder, and higher BMI among men and women, including overweight and obesity [62–65]. The risk for disordered eating is especially high when ADHD symptoms are not treated with support measures or medication [59,63]. The prevalence of fussy eating is considerably higher in children with NDs than in TD children, impacting close to 80% of children with ASD [38,41,66] and up to 40% in children with ADHD [38,67].

1.2. Weight Status of Icelandic Children and Adults

During the past decades, childhood obesity has increased in Iceland, as it has globally [4,68–73]. The 2022 report from The Development Centre for Primary Healthcare in Iceland (DCPHI) stated there was 7.0% overall obesity in children aged 6, 9, 12, and 14 (n = 17,899), reporting data from all primary/elementary schools in Iceland. The rate is up from 6.5% (n = 17,533) in 2019–2020. Less than 1.3% of boys and girls in all age groups are reported as being underweight [72,73], with approximately 74% of children registered in the healthy weight range and 18% as overweight [72]. Icelandic children have some of the highest prevalence of obesity in Europe [74], corresponding with trends in Icelandic adults; according to a recent OECD survey (Organisation for Economic Co-operation and Development), Iceland now ranks highest in Europe for obesity in adults (27%) followed closely by Malta and Lithuania (both 26%), and the UK (21%) [75].

1.3. Body Composition Measurements

The BMI (body mass index, kg/m^2), adjusting for age and sex to categorize weight status in children, is one of the most widely used health indicators, despite its limitations [76,77]. For example, the BMI does not differentiate between fat-free mass (FFM) and fat mass [78], which makes measures of weight and height alone poor indicators of health, or as an index of adiposity, as substantial fat mass may lead to excessive fat accumulation in obesity [79,80]. Further, the BMI does not adjust for ethnic backgrounds, activity levels, or females' menarche status, which may affect body composition [79,81–86].

Body composition measurements in children are inherently challenging due to the precipitous growth-related changes in, for example, weight, height, fat mass, and FFM. Still, they are considered essential in clinical care [87]. Anthropomorphic measures are typically used as markers in the relationship between obesity and cardiovascular disease [81] and indicators of a heightened risk of several chronic diseases [69,88]. For example, rapid growth rates, especially during teenage years, may raise cancer risk later in life [89]. Further, chronic or cardiovascular disease indicators may include waist-to-height ratio, skinfold thickness, hip and waist circumference, and BMI [81].

Several body composition measurement techniques are available, such as dual-energy X-ray absorptiometry (DEXA), magnetic resonance imaging (MRI), and bioelectrical impedance analysis (BIA) [79,90]. Of the various techniques, BIA is considered the least invasive, quickest, safest, and one of the most reliable and cost-effective techniques, reproducible with <1% error on repeated measurements [90]. Furthermore, for its ease of use, it is also especially suitable for children. This technique is indicated for use for healthy children 5–17 years old and adults with active, moderately active, to inactive lifestyles [79,83,91–94]. The Tanita Body Composition Analyzer—Tanita MC-780 [83] is indicated for use in the measurement of weight and impedance and the estimation of BMI, total body fat percentage (FAT%) and segmental fat percentage, weight (fat mass, kg), bone mass (kg), and fat-free mass (FFM, kg). FAT% signifies the proportion of fat to the total body weight. Fat mass denotes the actual weight of fat within the body. FFM comprises tissue, bone, muscle, and water in the body [83,90]. The calculation of different components through BIA presumes that 73% of FFM is body water, a good electrical conductor, while fat mass is a poor conductor due to its lower hydration [94].

1.4. Relationships between Parents' and Children's Body Composition

Although the relationships between parents', especially maternal, and children's weight status are well-established [11,12,95–97], to the author's best knowledge, no study exists on the body composition of parents whose children have fussy eating, with or without NDs.

A deeper understanding of the body composition of children with and without NDs and the associations with their parents' body composition is essential, as deviations from a healthy status may be indicative of issues requiring further attention, such as poor nutrient profiles or stringent food choices. Problems affecting children's eating behaviors may, in the long term, increase weight-related difficulties for children and their parents, including decreased or increased weight in children [22] and reduced food variety [17,51], as well as increased parental stress and more negative mealtime experiences [98–101]. The factors underlying problematic eating behaviors may, individually or collectively, impact the weight trajectory of both parents and children [102]. In this study, we analyzed the body composition (BMI, BMI-SDS, and FAT% using BIA) of parents and children, with and without NDs, participating in a food-based intervention. The purpose of this study was to gain insight into differences and associations between parents' and fussy-eating children's body composition, based on ND status, i.e., based on children with or without neurodevelopmental disorders. To the best of our knowledge, body composition in a similar sample has not been investigated previously or in other food-based interventions.

2. Materials and Methods

The data used in this study were cross-sectional, comparing participants at pre-intervention and six months follow-up, based on a longitudinal, randomized controlled study of a Taste Education intervention. Parent–child dyads who completed both measurements were used in the study. For more detailed information on the original study's methods, see Thorsteinsdottir, Njardvik et al. [103].

2.1. Measures

Demographic information, including children's age, sex, and medication use, and parental education, occupation, and marital status, was obtained from the screening questionnaires developed by the researchers [103].

2.1.1. Anthropometric Measures

Height was measured to the nearest 0.1 cm using a portable stadiometer (Stadiometer, Ulm, Germany). Weight was measured to the closest tenth of a kilogram using an electronic weighing scale (Tanita MC-780 MA Multi Frequency Segmental Body Composition Analyzer) [83]. The children wore light clothing and were instructed to remove shoes and socks and empty all pockets before stepping on the scale. A correction for clothing weight was subtracted for participants: −1.0 kg for parents and −0.5 kg for children. Weight status (underweight, healthy weight, overweight, and obesity) was defined according to the International Task Force of Obesity [104]. BMI-SDS (body mass index standard deviation scores) were derived from BMI reference values for Swedish children adjusting for age and sex [105]. Participants were measured with an empty bladder, by the same team members, at the same time of day, and wearing similar clothes for both measurements. The team members had extensive experience measuring children and adults using the Tanita MC-780.

2.1.2. Measure of Fussy Eating

Children's fussy eating was evaluated by a parent-report measure, the Children's Eating Behavior Questionnaire (CEBQ) [106], containing 35 items each, rated on a five-point Likert scale ranging from 'never' to 'always'. CEBQ comprises eight scales: Food fussiness, Slowness in eating, Food responsiveness, Emotional over-eating, Emotional under-eating, Enjoyment of food, Desire to drink and Satiety responsiveness. The psychometric properties of the instrument have been previously reported [106,107]. Further, the psychometric properties of the Icelandic version [108] have suggested good correspondence to Wardle and colleagues' original research [106]. An average of the items for each subscale was calculated. A high score on food fussiness indicates high levels of fussy eating. A high score for enjoyment of food suggests high levels of enjoyment. Both subscales were the focus of the current study. Internal reliability coefficients (Cronbach's alpha) for all subscales ranged from good (0.71) for satiety responsiveness to very good for emotional over-eating (0.86). In this present study, Cronbach's alpha was very good for food fussiness (0.85) and enjoyment of food (0.85).

Parents answered questions regarding the CEBQ at the start of the intervention, with follow-up at six months (Figure 1). Questionnaires were administered and stored online using Qualtrics software (Qualtrics, Provo, UT, USA).

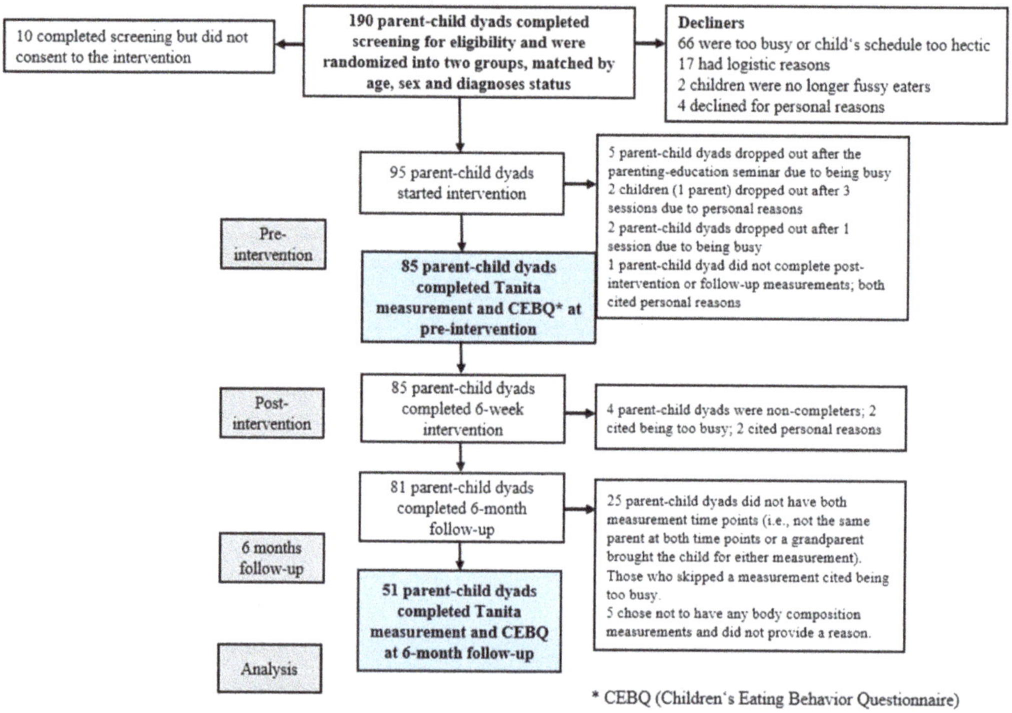

Figure 1. Flow diagram of intervention by stages of the study showing Tanita body composition and CEBQ (Children's Eating Behavior Questionnaire) measure points in blue.

2.1.3. Tanita Body Composition Analyzer

For analysis, the patient's sex, date of birth, and height were entered into the Tanita software. The 'standard' body type was selected for all participants as none were professional athletes, or training in heavy weightlifting or bodybuilding. All participants were asked to stand on the device platform and to keep their hands by their sides while gripping the machine's handles. Each measurement took less than one minute.

2.2. Participants

The participants in this study were children aged between 8–12 years old and their parents. To ensure that children's ADHD and ASD diagnoses were valid, all were required to have been diagnosed by one of the three main Icelandic diagnostic centers, which all utilize standardized diagnostic protocols and instruments. Of the 81 parent–child dyads that completed the Taste Education intervention [103], 51 completed two body composition analysis measurements, at baseline and six months follow-up (Table 1). Twenty-five parent–child dyads did not have both measurement time points (i.e., not the same parent at both time points or a grandparent brought the child for either measurement). Those who skipped a measurement cited being too busy. Five chose not to have any body composition measurements and did not provide a reason (Figure 1). There were no significant differences in any of the background measures for parents or children between the 51 participants who received both measurements and the 30 that had either one measurement or chose not to have any.

Table 1. Characteristics of children and parents participating in the study, at pre-intervention (n = 51).

Child	
Children's age in years, Mean (SD)	10.0 (1.44)
Female, *n* (%)	21 (41.2)
Anthropomorphic measures, Mean (SD)	
Height (cm)	143.0 (11.5)
Weight (kg)	37.3 (12.3)
BMI (kg/m^2)	17.9 (3.5)
BMI-SDS	0.27 (1.21)
Diagnoses, *n* (%)	
Without ND	33 (64.7)
ND (ADHD, Autism, or both)	18 (35.3)
ADHD, primarily	4 (7.8)
ASD, primarily	4 (7.8)
Anxiety	10 (19.6)
Other	4 (7.8)
Parent	
Parents' age in years, Mean (SD)	42.2 (4.94)
Mother, *n* (%)	42 (82.3)
Education, *n* (%)	
No higher education	3 (5.9)
Vocational education	11 (21.6)
University level	37 (72.5)
Single parent household, *n* (%)	5 (9.8)
Occupational status, *n* (%)	
Full-time occupation	34 (66.7)
Part-time occupation	6 (11.8)
Student	4 (7.8)
Other	7 (13.7)
Anthropomorphic measures, Mean (SD)	
Height (cm)	169.4 (7.9)
Weight (kg)	76.6 (16.9)
BMI (kg/m^2)	26.9 (5.1)

Abbreviations: SD, standard deviation; BMI, body mass index; BMI-SDS, BMI standard deviation score; ND, neurodevelopmental disorder; ADHD, attention deficit/hyperactive disorder; ASD, autism spectrum disorder.

The majority of parents were mothers, and all participants were Icelandic and spoke Icelandic. The participants in the study were invited via email lists in collaboration with the Icelandic ASD and ADHD societies and through advertisements published on a website set up expressly for the study. All children attended mainstream schooling. Inclusion criteria encompassed Icelandic-speaking participants and fussy-eating children 8–12 years of age [103]. Descriptive characteristics of the participants at pre-intervention are provided in Table 1.

2.3. Procedures

Parents volunteered to partake in the study and were invited to answer a screening questionnaire online about themselves and their children for consent and eligibility. Participants were not financially rewarded for participating in the study, although the children received a graduation certification and were gifted a tote bag for completing the Taste Education program. The sessions took place at a home economics teaching kitchen, within the School of Education at the University of Iceland, from 2018 to 2019. The Taste Education program was tailored as an after-school program being delivered midweek, at the same time of day for all participants. The intervention was divided into two components, i.e., (a) two parenting-education sessions, two hours each, prior to the first session with the children, and (b) six kitchen sessions, 90 min each, comprising food preparation skills and games as a base for sensory and taste education in the teaching kitchen with parent–child dyads (for further details of the kitchen sessions see Thorsteinsdottir et al. [103]). The sensory-based education centred on food-themed games, introducing texture-based exercises, sounds of food in the mouth, and cooking and baking simple recipes (re-introducing the now familiar ingredients). Each session built upon the previous one with food items used previously, re-introduced in the following session. Exercises were based on repeated exposures (repetition of seeing foods, handling them, and tasting). For details on the foods introduced in the Taste Education intervention, and changes in acceptance, see Thorsteinsdottir et al. [103].

2.4. Statistical Analyzes

Data were analyzed using R Studio 4.2.2 [109]. Descriptive statistics were calculated and are presented as *n* (%) and mean (SD). Cases with missing data were excluded listwise, and only parent–child dyads with two body composition measurements were included in the analyses.

Parents' BMI status was divided into four groups, adjusting for age and sex: underweight, healthy weight, overweight, and obesity [110]. Likewise, children were classified into four categories based on their BMI status adjusting for age and sex: underweight (less than the 5th percentile), healthy weight (5th percentile to <85th percentile), overweight (85th percentile to <95th percentile), and obesity (95th percentile or greater) [104].

Body fat percentages were based on body fat ranges, with cut-offs to define underfat, normal, overfat, and obesity, adjusting for age and sex set at the 2nd, 85th, and 95th centiles for children [111]. Parents' body fat percentage was also divided into four groups, adjusting for age and sex [83,112].

The paired t-test was used to compare differences in Tanita body composition measurements based on children's ND status and between parents based on their children's ND status. To retain statistical power, categories for BMI and FAT% were collapsed into binary variables; BMI: underweight/healthy weight vs. overweight/obese (underweight/healthy < 18.5–24.99, adjusted for age and sex) [110] and FAT%: underfat/healthy vs. overfat/obese (underfat/healthy < 16.0–34.99%, adjusted for age and sex) [112].

A comparison between children's and parents' body composition is presented using boxplots, crosstabs, paired- and independent samples *t*-test, and the chi-square or Fisher's exact test where applicable. Multivariable associations between children's ND status and children's BMI or FAT% status were assessed using binary logistic regression, adjusting for parents' BMI or FAT% status. Estimated associations were described with odds ratios and 95% confidence intervals (CIs). *p*-values of <0.05 were considered statistically significant. Although multiple hypotheses tests were conducted, unadjusted alphas were reported [113,114].

3. Results

3.1. Sample Characteristics

The demographic characteristics of the 51 participants are presented in Table 1. More than a third of the children (35.3%) had an ND. The mean age of participating children was 10.0 (SD = 1.4; range 7–13 years), and 41.2% were female. Two of the 18 children with an ND were female (11.1%). The mean BMI-SDS for the children was 0.27 (SD = 1.21). The majority of parents were mothers (82.3%), 66.7% had a full-time occupation, and 72.5% had obtained a university education. The mean age of parents was 42.2 (SD = 4.9; range 31–52 years old), and the mean parental BMI was 26.9 (SD = 5.1). Two of the 18 parents whose children had an ND were fathers (11.1%).

3.2. Body Compositions Based on Sex

Although not the focus of the present study, differences in body compositions based on sex were calculated before analyzing measures based on ND (Table 2). For children, the proportion of boys with an ND (88.9%) was significantly higher than for girls ($\chi^2(1, N = 51) = 8.55, p = 0.003$), so analyses for children's measures were run separately before examining measures based on ND (Table 2). There were no significant differences between girls and boys based on age ($t(34) = 1.286, p = 0.207$), weight ($t(49) = 0.975, p = 0.334$), height ($t(39) = 1.910$, $p = 0.063$), BMI ($t(48) = -0.055$, $p = 0.956$), fat mass ($t(45) = 0.162$, $p = 0.872$), FAT% ($t(49) = 0.253$, $p = 0.802$), or FFM ($t(48) = 1.485$, $p = 0.144$). The only significant difference between girls and boys was for bone mass: boys had higher bone mass ($M = 1.61$ kg, $SD = 0.36$) than girls ($M = 1.39$ kg, $SD = 0.31$), ($t(47) = 2.273$, $p = 0.028$).

Table 2. Differences in body composition measurements of parents and children, based on children's ND status (with or without an ND), at pre-intervention.

Children's body composition measurements, based on ND status				
ND Status	Without ND ($n = 33$)	ND ($n = 18$)	t-test or χ^2 (1)	p
Measures, Mean (SD) or n (%)				
Age in years	10.0 (1.55)	10.2 (1.25)	−0.492	0.624
Weight (kg)	34.8 (9.26)	41.9 (15.81)	−1.711	0.139
Height (cm)	141.2 (12.13)	146.2 (9.63)	−1.610	0.053
BMI (kg/m^2)	17.2 (2.39)	19.2 (4.77)	−1.684	0.049
BMI-SDS	−0.1 (1.05)	0.9 (1.27)	−2.773	0.005
Overweight/obese	2 (6.1)	8 (44.4)	8.587	0.003
Fat mass (kg)	7.8 (3.34)	10.8 (8.06)	−1.508	0.067
FAT%	21.2 (4.39)	26.6 (6.71)	−3.074	0.001
Overfat/obese	3 (9.1)	10 (55.5)	10.906	0.001
FFM (kg)	27.0 (6.44)	30.9 (8.37)	−1.742	0.066
Bone mass (kg) *	1.4 (0.32)	1.7 (0.39)	−2.156	0.026
Parents' body composition measurements, based on children's ND status				
ND Status	Without ND ($n = 33$)	ND ($n = 18$)	t-test or χ^2 (1)	p
Measures, Mean (SD) or n (%)				
Age in years	43.6 (4.97)	39.6 (3.75)	3.278	0.004
Weight (kg)	72.6 (13.60)	84.0 (20.21)	−2.137	0.021
Height (cm)	169.1 (7.83)	170.1 (8.21)	−0.435	0.661
BMI (kg/m^2)	25.5 (3.31)	29.9 (6.38)	−2.893	0.001
Overweight/obese	15 (45.5)	14 (77.8)	3.774	0.045
Fat mass (kg)	21.0 (7.28)	29.4 (11.01)	−2.916	0.002
FAT%	28.7 (7.01)	34.3 (7.07)	−2.700	0.009
Overfat/obese	12 (36.4)	12 (66.7)	3.163	0.046
FFM (kg)	51.6 (10.62)	55.1 (11.55)	−1.065	0.280
Bone mass (kg)	2.6 (0.50)	2.8 (0.54)	−1.100	0.266

Abbreviations: SD, standard deviation; BMI, body mass index; BMI-SDS, BMI standard deviation score; FAT%, fat percentage; FFM, fat-free mass. All p-values from t-test, χ^2 test or Fisher's exact test. Unadjusted alphas are reported. * Boys had significantly higher bone mass than girls.

Since the proportion of parents' sex did not differ by their children's ND status, ($\chi^2(1, N = 51) = 0.27$, $p = 0.603$), parents' measures were run based on ND status (Table 2).

3.3. Multivariable Associations between Children's BMI or Fat Percentage (FAT%) and ND Status

A logistic regression analysis was conducted containing children's BMI status at pre-intervention as the dependent variable (overweight/obese versus underweight/healthy weight) and ND status (ND versus not having ND) as the independent variable, adjusting for parents' BMI status (Table 3a). When analyzing the unadjusted results, the odds of children being in the overweight/obese category increased by a factor of 12.4 in the crude analysis when having an ND (95% CI: 2.53–68.26, $p = 0.003$) compared to those who did not have an ND. When adjusting for parents' BMI status, the odds of children being in the overweight/obese category lowered to 9.08 (95% CI: 1.56–52.72, $p = 0.014$) when having an ND.

Table 3. (**a**) Multivariable associations between children's BMI status at pre-intervention; overweight/obese category versus underweight/healthy weight, and ND status (with or without ND), using binary logistic regression analysis (unadjusted and adjusted analysis), $n = 51$. (**b**) Multivariable associations between children's fat percentage (FAT%) status at pre-intervention; overfat/obese category, versus underfat/healthy, and ND status (with or without ND), using binary logistic regression analysis (unadjusted and adjusted analysis), $n = 51$.

Multivariable Associations Using Binary Logistic Regression							
			(**a**)				
	n	β	Unadjusted OR (95% CI)	p	β	Adjusted OR (95% CI)	p
Parents' BMI category	51						
Underweight/healthy	22						
vs							
Overweight/Obese	29				2.24	9.45 (1.10–81.49)	0.040
ND status	51						
Without ND	33						
vs							
ND	18	2.52	12.4 (2.53–68.26)	0.003	2.21	9.08 (1.56–52.72)	0.014
			(**b**)				
	n	β	Unadjusted OR (95% CI)	p	β	Adjusted OR (95% CI)	p
Parents' FAT% category	51						
Underfat/healthy	27						
vs							
Overfat/Obese	24				0.91	2.12 (0.46–81.50)	0.334
ND status	51						
Without ND	33						
vs							
ND	18	2.53	12.5 (3.04–66.70)	0.001	2.36	10.56 (2.27–49.20)	0.003

Abbreviations: BMI, body mass index; ND, neurodevelopmental disorders; CI, confidence intervals; OR, odds ratio.

A logistic regression analysis was also conducted containing children's FAT% status at pre-intervention as the dependent variable (overfat/obese versus underfat/healthy) and ND status (ND versus not having ND) as the independent variable, adjusting for parents' FAT% status (Table 3b). When analyzing the unadjusted results, the odds of children being in the overfat/obese category increased by a factor of 12.5 in the crude analysis when having an ND (95% CI: 3.04–66.70, $p = 0.001$) compared to those who did not have an ND. When adjusting for parents' FAT% status, the odds of children being in the overweight/obese category remained significant, with an OR of 10.56 (95% CI: 2.27–49.20, $p = 0.003$) when having an ND.

3.4. Changes in Children's BMI-SDS and Parents' BMI and Fat Percentage (FAT%), Based on ND Status Comparing Changes between Time Points

When analyzing the distribution and changes in children's BMI-SDS and parents' BMI and FAT%, it was evident that children with an ND had significantly higher mean BMI-SDS ($M = 0.9$, $SD = 1.27$) at pre-intervention compared with children without an ND ($M = -0.1$, $SD = 1.05$) ($t(17) = 6.041$, $p < 0.001$) (Figure 2). The mean BMI-SDS lowered significantly between time points for children with an ND ($t(17) = 4.408$, $p < 0.001$), with no significant changes for children without an ND ($t(32) = -1.893$, $p = 0.243$). Similarly, parents of children with an ND had higher mean BMI ($M = 29.9$, $SD = 6.38$) at pre-intervention than parents whose children did not have an ND ($M = 25.5$, $SD = 3.31$). The BMI of parents whose children had an ND lowered significantly between time points ($t(17) = 3.355$, $p = 0.003$) but did not change significantly for parents whose children did not have an ND ($t(32) = -1.189$, $p = 0.243$).

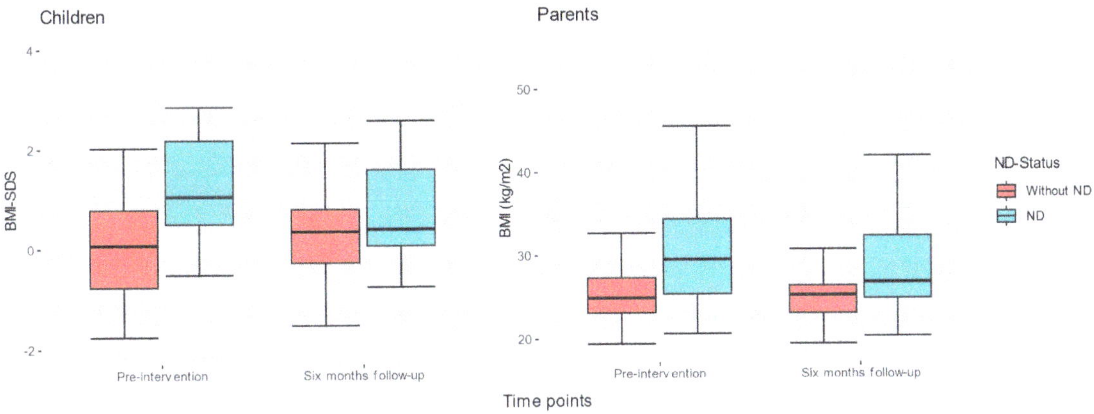

Figure 2. Distribution and changes in children's BMI-SDS and parents' BMI, based on ND status between baseline and six months follow-up.

Figure 3 shows the distribution of children's and parents' FAT%. Children with an ND had significantly higher mean FAT% ($M = 26.6$, $SD = 6.71$) at pre-intervention compared with children without an ND ($M = 21.2$, $SD = 4.39$) ($t(25) = -3.074$, $p = 0.005$). The mean FAT% lowered significantly between time points for children with an ND ($t(17)$, 2.646, $p = 0.017$) and increased significantly for children without an ND ($t(32) = -2.223$, $p = 0.033$). Similarly, parents of children with an ND had significantly higher mean FAT% ($M = 34.3$, $SD = 7.07$) compared with parents whose children did not have an ND ($M = 28.7$, $SD = 7.01$) ($t(35) = -2.699$, $p = 0.011$). The FAT% of parents whose children had an ND did not change significantly between time points ($t(17)$, 0.702, $p = 0.492$) and did not lower significantly for parents whose children did not have an ND ($t(32) = 0.041$, $p = 0.968$).

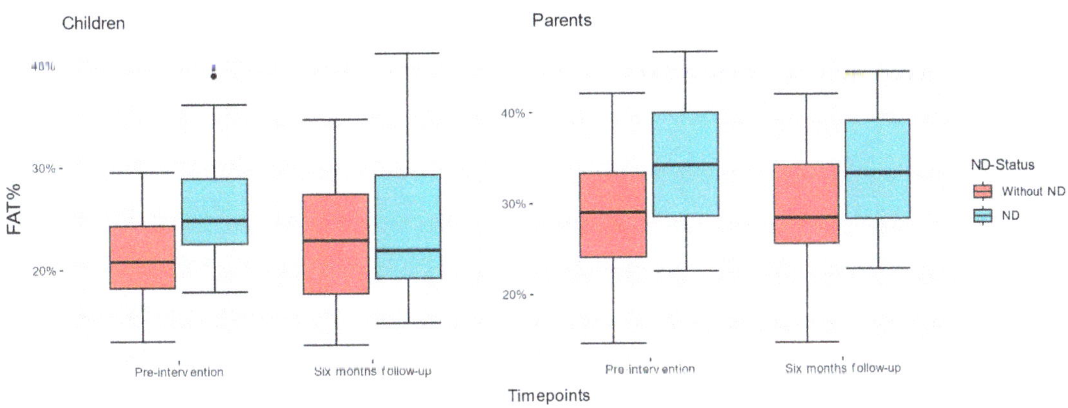

Figure 3. Distribution and changes in children's and parents' fat percentage (FAT%) between both time points, based on children's ND status.

4. Discussion

This study aimed to analyze the body composition of parents and children, with and without an ND, participating in a food-based Taste Education intervention. To the best of our knowledge, body composition in a similar parent–child dyad sample has not been investigated previously or in other food-based interventions. Our study found that at pre-intervention children with an ND had significantly higher BMI, BMI-SDS, and FAT% measures than children without an ND. In addition, parents whose children had an ND were significantly younger and had higher BMI, fat mass, and FAT% than those whose children were without an ND.

Although some studies have pointed to the protective aspect of fussy eating against over-eating due to a greater dislike of certain foods [23,32,115], we did not find evidence of this in our study [103], as only two children were identified as being underweight and underfat. Further, as one child had an ND and one did not, we were not able to find evidence of children with an ND being more likely to be underweight, as identified in some studies [23–28]. On the contrary, the odds of children being in the overweight/obese category versus underweight/healthy weight were raised over nine times when adjusting for parents' BMI status. Similarly, the odds of children being in the overfat/obese category versus underfat/healthy were raised almost 11 times for children with an ND after adjusting for parents' FAT% status. Unfortunately, studies are scarce on body composition in fussy-eating children. We could only identify one study where fussy-eating children had a lower fat-free mass at six years old than non-fussy eaters [26], which might point to a trajectory toward increased weight. Fussy eating may be a learned behavior, as parents' adaptation to the food environment in which the children with fussy eating, with and without an ND, perhaps influences parents' food choices. This has been noted in studies on maternal overweight and obesity and children's control of food intake, where increased maternal weight was associated with children's increased control over intake and food choices [11]. Further, parents may use food as a soothing mechanism for children with difficult temperaments [11] and as a reward or punishment system for children's behavior, especially those who exhibit behavioral problems around mealtimes [14,31,116]. Studies have also shown that parents are more likely to use food as a reward if they perceive their child as a fussy eater, which may lead to selective eating behaviors and limited food choices [14,102,116,117].

Studies have indicated that parents with their own eating or weight concerns are more likely to control their child's feeding environment and food intake [98,99], which may impact several mechanisms of weight and fussy eating. In our study, the relationships between children's ND status and increased weight might have caused worries for parents about their children's weight trajectory, or about their children heading towards obesity, and therefore sought out assistance in terms of our food intervention.

It may also be helpful to compare our present results to a study on 104 Icelandic children with obesity (mean age; 12.0, *SD* = 3.5, mean BMI-SDS; 3.5, *SD* = 0.9), where almost half of the parents considered their child a fussy eater. In addition, nearly half of the children had a diagnosed disorder, including ASD with or without ADHD [20]. Approximately 8% of the children in our sample had obesity, which is slightly higher compared with recent estimates of 7% from The Development Centre for Primary Healthcare in Iceland (DCPHI) for overall obesity in children aged 6, 9, 12, and 14 years old [72]. However, of those children who had an ND, four had obesity (22.2%), and none of the 33 children that did not have an ND had obesity. Just under a third of the parents in our study had obesity, similar to obesity levels in Icelandic adults [75]. Therefore, the results raise concerns about the health status of Icelandic children with NDs.

Children with an ND had significantly higher BMI-SDS and FAT% at pre-intervention than children without an ND. For the older children without an ND, there was a shift from healthy weight towards being overweight and increased FAT%, and as they may have been on the cusp of puberty, this might affect their weight status [105]. Although we did not record the amount of food that the children consumed in our intervention, we saw evidence of children eating a more varied diet and an indication of increased enjoyment of eating as measured by the Children's Eating Behavior Questionnaire (CEBQ) [103], which might have influenced the older children who, based on age, have more autonomy regarding food choices. Similarly, parents whose children had an ND had significantly higher BMI and FAT% at pre-intervention than those with children without an ND. However, BMI-SDS and FAT% lowered significantly between pre-intervention and six months follow-up for children who had an ND while increasing significantly between time points for children without an ND. Parents of children with an ND participating in our study may have been worried about their children's diets, as some already had obesity, motivating them more firmly to use the tools on fussy eating we provided in our intervention. There were no differences based on children's ND status on the variety of fruit, vegetables, and other foods in our intervention [103], so it is unclear if the amount consumed was less. It is also unclear whether or which aspects of our Taste Education program affected the children's weight status. However, studies have shown that improved eating behaviors may positively impact children's weight status [14,28], possibly through parents' reduced worry or stress [15,24,53,98,99]. In other papers recently published by the authors of the present study, the children from this sample decreased problematic mealtime behaviors [118], increased food variety, and decreased fussy eating [103] following our Taste Education intervention. Further, improved dietary variety, especially in terms of wholegrains, fruits, vegetables, and legumes emphasized in our Taste Education program, generally benefits children's weight status, health, and overall well-being [18,24,25,40,97].

The strength and limitations of our recent Taste Education study have been detailed elsewhere [48,103,118]. The present study has many strengths. Primarily, the study is the first to investigate the body composition of a sample of fussy-eating children with and without an ND, and their parents, following a Taste Education intervention. Further strengths include objective body composition measurements using a Tanita Body Composition Analyzer—Tanita MC-780 [83] performed at two time points at six-month intervals and by the same team members with extensive experience. Some studies have found that in children, BIA may slightly overestimate change in FAT% with increased error in measurement with further changes in FAT% [119]. Thus, although the BIA technology is a considerably better measurement tool than relying on BMI alone, further examination of whether BIA can adequately measure changes in body composition over time is essential in larger samples of children from less homogenous groups.

The current study also had some limitations. The sample size was small as only 51 parent–child dyads were available for both measurements, with wide confidence intervals (CIs) for the multivariable regression analysis. Although there were no significant differences in background characteristics between those who received both measurements and those who did not, we could not rule out factors such as reluctance to participate, for example, due to weight concerns or increased weight between time points. There was no evidence of parents of children with an ND not wanting to attend both measurements, even though those children were more likely to be overweight or have obesity than TD children. Further, although care was taken to measure the participants at the same time of day at both time points, with an empty bladder, it was not possible to control the food or fluid intake right before the measurements. No comparison group was available for this study regarding children without fussy eating, and these data are unavailable in Iceland. Therefore, as the findings were temporal, no causal inference was possible as we were not able to isolate the effects of fussy eating on body composition. Although the sample of children represented a school classroom in Iceland well (i.e., a combination of children with and without an ND and being inclusive of other diagnoses), there was a very high proportion of well-educated parents in full-time work living in two-parent homes. The parents' status indicates a high socioeconomic standing, so the results may not replicate lower socioeconomic circumstances; even more so, the high rate of obesity among participating children and parents is rather alarming. Finally, the increase in family-wise error across the reported statistical analyses was not controlled. Generally, we decided to report unadjusted alphas [113,114] as we consider this data analysis introductory, and not meant for intervention purposes, and we would like to emphasize replication with larger samples.

5. Conclusions

The findings from this study underline the need for additional exploration into the relationships between children's and parents' body composition, and reasons for differences between BMI-SDS and FAT% of children with and without an ND, and similarly for the differences in BMI and FAT% between parents whose children had an ND and those who did not. Notably, there are no previously published studies on the associations between body compositions of fussy-eating children with and without an ND and their parents. The findings of the current study may be helpful as a step towards improving awareness of the weight status of children with an ND and fussy eating and possible associations between parents' weight status.

Author Contributions: Conceptualization, S.T. and A.S.O.; Data curation, S.T.; Formal analysis, S.T.; Funding acquisition, S.T. and A.S.O.; Investigation, S.T.; Methodology, S.T. and A.S.O.; Project administration, A.S.O.; Resources, R.B. and A.S.O.; Supervision, A.S.O.; Visualization, S.T. and A.S.O.; Writing—original draft, S.T.; Writing—review and editing, S.T., R.B., H.G.E. and A.S.O. All authors have read and agreed to the published version of the manuscript.

Funding: This research was funded by the University of Iceland's Research fund (research grant and doctoral fund) and the Public Health Fund of the Directorate of Health.

Institutional Review Board Statement: The study was conducted according to the guidelines of the Declaration of Helsinki and approved by the Icelandic National Bioethics Committee and the Data Protection Authority ((VSNb2017110020/03.01), 9 January 2018).

Informed Consent Statement: Informed consent was obtained from all subjects involved in the study. Parents signed consent for children under 12 years old.

Data Availability Statement: The datasets generated during and/or analyzed during the current study are available from the corresponding author upon reasonable request.

Acknowledgments: We thank the University of Iceland's Research fund (doctoral fund and research grant) and the Public Health Fund of the Directorate of Health for their support. We also thank Marta Ólafsdóttir for assisting with the Tanita body composition measurements. Further, we are grateful to the Pediatric Department of the Landspítali University Hospital for the loan of their Tanita MC-780. Finally, we would like to express our deep gratitude to all the participants in our study and our assistant taste educators.

Conflicts of Interest: The authors declare no conflict of interest. The funders had no role in the design of the study; in the collection, analyses, or interpretation of data; in the writing of the manuscript; or in the decision to publish the results.

References

1. Wabitsch, M.; Moss, A.; Kromeyer-Hauschild, K. Unexpected plateauing of childhood obesity rates in developed countries. *BMC Med.* **2014**, *12*, 17. [CrossRef] [PubMed]
2. Weghuber, D.; Barrett, T.; Barrientos-Pérez, M.; Gies, I.; Hesse, D.; Jeppesen, O.K.; Kelly, A.S.; Mastrandrea, L.D.; Sørrig, R.; Arslanian, S. Once-Weekly Semaglutide in Adolescents with Obesity. *N. Engl. J. Med.* **2022**, *387*, 2245–2257. [CrossRef]
3. Hampl, S.E.; Hassink, S.G.; Skinner, A.C.; Armstrong, S.C.; Barlow, S.E.; Bolling, C.F.; Avila Edwards, K.C.; Eneli, I.; Hamre, R.; Joseph, M.M.; et al. Clinical Practice Guideline for the Evaluation and Treatment of Children and Adolescents With Obesity. *Pediatrics* **2023**, *151*, e2022060640. [CrossRef] [PubMed]
4. Abarca-Gómez, L.; Abdeen, Z.A.; Hamid, Z.A.; Abu-Rmeileh, N.M.; Acosta-Cazares, B.; Acuin, C.; Adams, R.J.; Aekplakorn, W.; Afsana, K.; Aguilar-Salinas, C.A.; et al. Worldwide trends in body-mass index, underweight, overweight, and obesity from 1975 to 2016: A pooled analysis of 2416 population-based measurement studies in 128·9 million children, adolescents, and adults. *Lancet* **2017**, *390*, 2627–2642. [CrossRef] [PubMed]
5. Bharti, B.; Malhi, P. Psychiatric Comorbidities in Adolescents with Obesity: A Wake-Up Call for Life Course and Multisectoral Interventions. *Indian J. Pediatr.* **2021**, *88*, 215–216. [CrossRef]
6. Inchley, J.; Currie, D.; Jewell, J.; Breda, J.; Barnekow, V. *Adolescent Obesity and Related Behaviours: Trends and Inequalities in the WHO European Region, 2002–2014: Observations from the Health Behaviour in School-Aged Children (HBSC) WHO Collaborative Cross-national Study*; World Health Organization, Regional Office for Europe: Copenhagen, Denmark, 2017; viii + 87p.

7. Chung, A.; Backholer, K.; Wong, E.; Palermo, C.; Keating, C.; Peeters, A. Trends in child and adolescent obesity prevalence in economically advanced countries according to socioeconomic position: A systematic review. *Obes. Rev.* **2016**, *17*, 276–295. [CrossRef]
8. Wyse, C.; Case, L.; Walsh, Ó.; Shortall, C.; Jordan, N.; McCrea, L.; O'Malley, G. Evaluating 12 Years of Implementing a Multidisciplinary Specialist Child and Adolescent Obesity Treatment Service: Patient-Level Outcomes. *Front. Nutr.* **2022**, *9*, 895091. [CrossRef]
9. Tully, L.; Arthurs, N.; Wyse, C.; Browne, S.; Case, L.; McCrea, L.; O'Connell, J.M.; O'Gorman, C.S.; Smith, S.M.; Walsh, A.; et al. Guidelines for treating child and adolescent obesity: A systematic review. *Front. Nutr.* **2022**, *9*, 902865. [CrossRef]
10. Chung, Y.L.; Rhie, Y.-J. Severe Obesity in Children and Adolescents: Metabolic Effects, Assessment, and Treatment. *JOMES* **2021**, *30*, 326–335. [CrossRef]
11. Patel, C.; Karasouli, E.; Shuttlewood, E.; Meyer, C. Food Parenting Practices among Parents with Overweight and Obesity: A Systematic Review. *Nutrients* **2018**, *10*, 1966. [CrossRef]
12. Haycraft, E.; Karasouli, E.; Meyer, C. Maternal feeding practices and children's eating behaviours: A comparison of mothers with healthy weight versus overweight/obesity. *Appetite* **2017**, *116*, 395–400. [CrossRef]
13. Niec, L.N.; Todd, M.; Brodd, I.; Domoff, S.E. PCIT-Health: Preventing Childhood Obesity by Strengthening the Parent–Child Relationship. *Cogn. Behav. Pract.* **2020**, *29*, 335–347. [CrossRef]
14. Jansen, P.W.; Derks, I.P.M.; Mou, Y.; van Rijen, E.H.M.; Gaillard, R.; Micali, N.; Voortman, T.; Hillegers, M.H.J. Associations of parents' use of food as reward with children's eating behaviour and BMI in a population-based cohort. *Pediatr. Obes.* **2020**, *15*, e12662. [CrossRef]
15. Liang, J.; Matheson, B.E.; Rhee, K.E.; Peterson, C.B.; Rydell, S.; Boutelle, K.N. Parental control and overconsumption of snack foods in overweight and obese children. *Appetite* **2016**, *100*, 181–188. [CrossRef] [PubMed]
16. DeCosta, P.; Moller, P.; Frost, M.B.; Olsen, A. Changing children's eating behaviour—A review of experimental research. *Appetite* **2017**, *113*, 327–357. [CrossRef]
17. Taylor, C.M.; Emmett, P.M. Picky eating in children: Causes and consequences. *Proc. Nutr. Soc.* **2019**, *78*, 161–169. [CrossRef] [PubMed]
18. Taylor, C.M.; Wernimont, S.M.; Northstone, K.; Emmett, P.M. Picky/fussy eating in children: Review of definitions, assessment, prevalence and dietary intakes. *Appetite* **2015**, *95*, 349–359. [CrossRef] [PubMed]
19. Gibson, E.L.; Cooke, L. Understanding Food Fussiness and Its Implications for Food Choice, Health, Weight and Interventions in Young Children: The Impact of Professor Jane Wardle. *Curr. Obes. Rep.* **2017**, *6*, 46–56. [CrossRef] [PubMed]
20. Thorsteinsdottir, S.; Olafsdottir, A.S.; Brynjolfsdottir, B.; Bjarnason, R.; Njardvik, U. Odds of fussy eating are greater among children with obesity and anxiety. *Obes. Sci. Pract.* **2022**, *8*, 91–100. [CrossRef]
21. Finistrella, V.; Manco, M.; Ferrara, A.; Rustico, C.; Presaghi, F.; Morino, G. Cross-sectional exploration of maternal reports of food neophobia and pickiness in preschooler-mother dyads. *J. Am. Coll. Nutr.* **2012**, *31*, 152–159. [CrossRef]
22. Brown, C.L.; Vander Schaaf, E.B.; Cohen, G.M.; Irby, M.B.; Skelton, J.A. Association of Picky Eating and Food Neophobia with Weight: A Systematic Review. *Child. Obes.* **2016**, *12*, 247–262. [CrossRef]
23. Carruth, B.R.; Skinner, J.D. Revisiting the picky eater phenomenon: Neophobic behaviors of young children. *J. Am. Coll. Nutr.* **2000**, *19*, 771–780. [CrossRef]
24. Galloway, A.T.; Fiorito, L.; Lee, Y.; Birch, L.L. Parental pressure, dietary patterns, and weight status among girls who are "picky eaters". *J. Am. Diet. Assoc.* **2005**, *105*, 541–548. [CrossRef]
25. Kozioł-Kozakowska, A.; Piórecka, B.; Schlegel-Zawadzka, M. Prevalence of food neophobia in pre-school children from southern Poland and its association with eating habits, dietary intake and anthropometric parameters: A cross-sectional study. *Public Health Nutr.* **2018**, *21*, 1106–1114. [CrossRef]
26. de Barse, L.M.; Tiemeier, H.; Leermakers, E.T.M.; Voortman, T.; Jaddoe, V.W.V.; Edelson, L.R.; Franco, O.H.; Jansen, P.W. Longitudinal association between preschool fussy eating and body composition at 6 years of age: The Generation R Study. *Int. J. Behav. Nutr. Phys. Act.* **2015**, *12*, 153. [CrossRef]
27. Ekstein, S.; Laniado, D.; Glick, B. Does Picky Eating Affect Weight-for-Length Measurements in Young Children? *Clin. Pediatr.* **2009**, *49*, 217–220. [CrossRef]
28. Xue, Y.; Lee, E.; Ning, K.; Zheng, Y.; Ma, D.; Gao, H.; Yang, B.; Bai, Y.; Wang, P.; Zhang, Y. Prevalence of picky eating behaviour in Chinese school-age children and associations with anthropometric parameters and intelligence quotient. A cross-sectional study. *Appetite* **2015**, *91*, 248–255. [CrossRef]
29. Lim, P.S.; Balistreri, K.A.; Silverman, A.H.; Davies, W.H. Disrupted mealtime interactions are associated with stress and internalizing symptoms in caregivers of school-age children. *Child. Health Care* **2021**, *50*, 432–451. [CrossRef]
30. Dovey, T.M.; Kumari, V.; Blissett, J. Eating behaviour, behavioural problems and sensory profiles of children with avoidant/restrictive food intake disorder (ARFID), autistic spectrum disorders or picky eating: Same or different? *Eur. Psychiatry* **2019**, *61*, 56–62. [CrossRef] [PubMed]
31. Ledford, J.R.; Whiteside, E.; Severini, K.E. A systematic review of interventions for feeding-related behaviors for individuals with autism spectrum disorders. *Res. Autism Spectr. Disord.* **2018**, *52*, 69–80. [CrossRef]
32. Dovey, T.M.; Staples, P.A.; Gibson, E.L.; Halford, J.C. Food neophobia and 'picky/fussy' eating in children: A review. *Appetite* **2008**, *50*, 181–193. [CrossRef] [PubMed]

33. Olsen, A. Reflections on current practice for taste learning in children. *Int. J. Gastron. Food Sci.* **2019**, *15*, 26–29. [CrossRef]
34. Barnhill, K.; Gutierrez, A.; Ghossainy, M.; Marediya, Z.; Devlin, M.; Sachdev, P.; Marti, C.N.; Hewitson, L. Dietary status and nutrient intake of children with autism spectrum disorder: A case-control study. *Res. Autism Spectr. Disord.* **2018**, *50*, 51–59. [CrossRef]
35. Cermak, S.A.; Curtin, C.; Bandini, L.G. Food selectivity and sensory sensitivity in children with autism spectrum disorders. *J. Am. Diet. Assoc.* **2010**, *110*, 238–246. [CrossRef]
36. Evans, E.W.; Must, A.; Anderson, S.E.; Curtin, C.; Scampini, R.; Maslin, M.; Bandini, L. Dietary patterns and body mass index in children with autism and typically developing children. *Res. Autism Spectr. Disord.* **2012**, *6*, 399–405. [CrossRef]
37. Hubbard, K.L.; Anderson, S.E.; Curtin, C.; Must, A.; Bandini, L.G. A comparison of food refusal related to characteristics of food in children with autism spectrum disorder and typically developing children. *J. Acad. Nutr. Diet* **2014**, *114*, 1981–1987. [CrossRef]
38. Mayes, S.D.; Zickgraf, H. Atypical eating behaviors in children and adolescents with autism, ADHD, other disorders, and typical development. *Res. Autism Spectr. Disord.* **2019**, *64*, 76–83. [CrossRef]
39. Wentz, E.; Bjork, A.; Dahlgren, J. Neurodevelopmental disorders are highly over-represented in children with obesity: A cross-sectional study. *Obesity* **2017**, *25*, 178–184. [CrossRef] [PubMed]
40. Shmaya, Y.; Eilat-Adar, S.; Leitner, Y.; Reif, S.; Gabis, L. Nutritional deficiencies and overweight prevalence among children with autism spectrum disorder. *Res. Dev. Disabil.* **2015**, *38*, 1–6. [CrossRef]
41. Mayes, S.D.; Calhoun, S.L.; Mayes, R.D.; Molitoris, S. Autism and ADHD: Overlapping and discriminating symptoms. *Res. Autism Spectr. Disord.* **2012**, *6*, 277–285. [CrossRef]
42. Nadon, G.; Feldman, D.; Gisel, E. Feeding Issues Associated with the Autism Spectrum Disorders. In *Recent Advances in Autism Spectrum Disorders*; Fitzgerald, M., Ed.; IntechOpen: London, UK, 2013; Volume 1.
43. Nadon, G.; Feldman, D.; Dunn, W.; Gisel, E. Mealtime problems in children with Autism Spectrum Disorder and their typically developing siblings: A comparison study. *Autism Int. J. Res. Pract.* **2011**, *15*, 98–113. [CrossRef]
44. Manning-Courtney, P.; Murray, D.; Currans, K.; Johnson, H.; Bing, N.; Kroeger-Geoppinger, K.; Sorensen, R.; Bass, J.; Reinhold, J.; Johnson, A.; et al. Autism Spectrum Disorders. *Curr. Probl. Pediatr. Adolesc. Health Care* **2013**, *43*, 2–11. [CrossRef]
45. de Barse, L.M.; Jansen, P.W.; Edelson-Fries, L.R.; Jaddoe, V.W.V.; Franco, O.H.; Tiemeier, H.; Steenweg-de Graaff, J. Infant feeding and child fussy eating: The Generation R Study. *Appetite* **2017**, *114*, 374–381. [CrossRef]
46. Margari, L.; Marzulli, L.; Gabellone, A.; de Giambattista, C. Eating and Mealtime Behaviors in Patients with Autism Spectrum Disorder: Current Perspectives. *Neuropsychiatr. Dis. Treat.* **2020**, *16*, 2083–2102. [CrossRef]
47. Sharp, W.G.; Jaquess, D.L.; Lukens, C.T. Multi-method assessment of feeding problems among children with autism spectrum disorders. *Res. Autism Spectr. Disord.* **2013**, *7*, 56–65. [CrossRef]
48. Thorsteinsdottir, S.; Olsen, A.; Olafsdottir, A.S. Fussy Eating among Children and Their Parents: Associations in Parent-Child Dyads, in a Sample of Children with and without Neurodevelopmental Disorders. *Nutrients* **2021**, *13*, 2196. [CrossRef] [PubMed]
49. Antoniou, E.E.; Roefs, A.; Kremers, S.P.; Jansen, A.; Gubbels, J.S.; Sleddens, E.F.; Thijs, C. Picky eating and child weight status development: A longitudinal study. *J. Hum. Nutr. Diet* **2016**, *29*, 298–307. [CrossRef] [PubMed]
50. Hayes, J.F.; Altman, M.; Kolko, R.P.; Balantekin, K.N.; Holland, J.C.; Stein, R.I.; Saelens, B.E.; Welch, R.R.; Perri, M.G.; Schechtman, K.B.; et al. Decreasing Food Fussiness in Children with Obesity Leads to Greater Weight Loss in Family-Based Treatment. *Obesity* **2016**, *24*, 2158–2163. [CrossRef]
51. Fraser, K.; Markides, B.R.; Barrett, N.; Laws, R. Fussy eating in toddlers: A content analysis of parents' online support seeking. *Matern. Child. Nutr.* **2021**, *17*, e13171. [CrossRef] [PubMed]
52. Searle, B.-R.E.; Harris, H.A.; Thorpe, K.; Jansen, E. What children bring to the table: The association of temperament and child fussy eating with maternal and paternal mealtime structure. *Appetite* **2020**, *151*, 104680. [CrossRef]
53. Wolstenholme, H.; Heary, C.; Kelly, C. Fussy eating behaviours: Response patterns in families of school-aged children. *Appetite* **2019**, *136*, 93–102. [CrossRef] [PubMed]
54. Fries, L.R.; Martin, N.; van der Horst, K. Parent-child mealtime interactions associated with toddlers' refusals of novel and familiar foods. *Physiol. Behav.* **2017**, *176*, 93–100. [CrossRef]
55. Finnane, J.M.; Jansen, E.; Mallan, K.M.; Daniels, L.A. Mealtime Structure and Responsive Feeding Practices Are Associated With Less Food Fussiness and More Food Enjoyment in Children. *J. Nutr. Educ. Behav.* **2017**, *49*, 11–18.e11. [CrossRef]
56. Curtin, C.; Hubbard, K.; Anderson, S.E.; Mick, E.; Must, A.; Bandini, L.G. Food selectivity, mealtime behavior problems, spousal stress, and family food choices in children with and without autism spectrum disorder. *J. Autism Dev. Disord.* **2015**, *45*, 3308–3315. [CrossRef] [PubMed]
57. Smith, B.; Rogers, S.L.; Blissett, J.; Ludlow, A.K. The relationship between sensory sensitivity, food fussiness and food preferences in children with neurodevelopmental disorders. *Appetite* **2020**, *150*, 104643. [CrossRef]
58. Cortese, S.; Tessari, L. Attention-Deficit/Hyperactivity Disorder (ADHD) and Obesity: Update 2016. *Curr. Psychiatry Rep.* **2017**, *19*, 4. [CrossRef]
59. Cortese, S.; Angriman, M.; Maffeis, C.; Isnard, P.; Konofal, E.; Lecendreux, M.; Purper-Ouakil, D.; Vincenzi, B.; Bernardina, B.D.; Mouren, M.-C. Attention-Deficit/Hyperactivity Disorder (ADHD) and Obesity: A Systematic Review of the Literature. *Crit. Rev. Food Sci. Nutr.* **2008**, *48*, 524–537. [CrossRef] [PubMed]
60. Nederkoorn, C.; Dassen, F.C.; Franken, L.; Resch, C.; Houben, K. Impulsivity and overeating in children in the absence and presence of hunger. *Appetite* **2015**, *93*, 57–61. [CrossRef] [PubMed]

61. Leventakou, V.; Micali, N.; Georgiou, V.; Sarri, K.; Koutra, K.; Koinaki, S.; Vassilaki, M.; Kogevinas, M.; Chatzi, L. Is there an association between eating behaviour and attention-deficit/hyperactivity disorder symptoms in preschool children? *J. Child. Psychol. Psychiatry* **2016**, *57*, 676–684. [CrossRef] [PubMed]
62. Ptacek, R.; Kuzelova, H.; Stefano, G.B.; Raboch, J.; Sadkova, T.; Goetz, M.; Kream, R.M. Disruptive patterns of eating behaviors and associated lifestyles in males with ADHD. *Med. Sci. Monit.* **2014**, *20*, 608–613. [CrossRef]
63. Altfas, J.R. Prevalence of attention deficit/hyperactivity disorder among adults in obesity treatment. *BMC Psychiatry* **2002**, *2*, 9. [CrossRef] [PubMed]
64. El Archi, S.; Cortese, S.; Ballon, N.; Réveillère, C.; De Luca, A.; Barrault, S.; Brunault, P. Negative Affectivity and Emotion Dysregulation as Mediators between ADHD and Disordered Eating: A Systematic Review. *Nutrients* **2020**, *12*, 3292. [CrossRef]
65. Hanson, J.A.; Phillips, L.N.; Hughes, S.M.; Corson, K. Attention-deficit hyperactivity disorder symptomatology, binge eating disorder symptomatology, and body mass index among college students. *J. Am. Coll. Health* **2020**, *68*, 543–549. [CrossRef]
66. Mari-Bauset, S.; Zazpe, I.; Mari-Sanchis, A.; Llopis-Gonzalez, A.; Morales-Suarez-Varela, M. Food selectivity in autism spectrum disorders: A systematic review. *J. Child. Neurol.* **2014**, *29*, 1554–1561. [CrossRef]
67. Råstam, M.; Täljemark, J.; Tajnia, A.; Lundström, S.; Gustafsson, P.; Lichtenstein, P.; Gillberg, C.; Anckarsäter, H.; Kerekes, N. Eating Problems and Overlap with ADHD and Autism Spectrum Disorders in a Nationwide Twin Study of 9- and 12-Year-Old Children. *Sci. World J.* **2013**, *2013*, 7. [CrossRef]
68. Chu, D.-T.; Minh Nguyet, N.T.; Nga, V.T.; Thai Lien, N.V.; Vo, D.D.; Lien, N.; Nhu Ngoc, V.T.; Son, L.H.; Le, D.-H.; Nga, V.B.; et al. An update on obesity: Mental consequences and psychological interventions. *Diabetes Metab. Syndr.Clin. Res. Rev.* **2019**, *13*, 155–160. [CrossRef]
69. Di Cesare, M.; Sorić, M.; Bovet, P.; Miranda, J.J.; Bhutta, Z.; Stevens, G.A.; Laxmaiah, A.; Kengne, A.-P.; Bentham, J. The epidemiological burden of obesity in childhood: A worldwide epidemic requiring urgent action. *BMC Med.* **2019**, *17*, 212. [CrossRef]
70. McGirr, J.; O'Malley, G.; Walsh, O. Identification and management of children and adolescents with obesity referred to a general paediatric outpatient department. *Ir. Med. J.* **2022**, *114*, 416.
71. Eiðsdóttir, S.Þ.; Kristjánsson, Á.L.; Sigfúsdóttir, I.D.; Garber, C.E.; Allegrante, J.P. Trends in Body Mass Index among Icelandic Adolescents and Young Adults from 1992 to 2007. *Int. J. Environ. Res. Public Health* **2010**, *7*, 2191–2207. [CrossRef] [PubMed]
72. DCPHI. *School Health Annual Report: Overweight and Obesity 2021–2022 in Children 6–14 Years Old [Heilsuvernd Skólabarna Ársskýrsla 2021–2022]*; Development Centre for Primary Healthcare in Iceland: Reykjavík, Iceland, 2023; Unpublished report.
73. DCPHI. *School Health Annual Report: Overweight and Obesity 2019–2020 in Children 6–14 Years Old [Heilsuvernd Skólabarna Ársskýrsla 2019–2020]*; Development Centre for Primary Healthcare in Iceland: Reykjavík, Iceland, 2021; Unpublished report.
74. World Health Organization. *WHO European Regional Obesity Report 2022*; World Health Organization: Copenhagen, Denmark, 2022.
75. OECD. *The Heavy Burden of Obesity*; OECD: Paris, France, 2019. [CrossRef]
76. Freedman, D.S.; Khan, L.K.; Serdula, M.K.; Dietz, W.H.; Srinivasan, S.R.; Berenson, G.S. The relation of childhood BMI to adult adiposity: The Bogalusa Heart Study. *Pediatrics* **2005**, *115*, 22–27. [CrossRef] [PubMed]
77. McCarthy, H.D. Measuring growth and obesity across childhood and adolescence. *Proc. Nutr. Soc.* **2014**, *73*, 210–217. [CrossRef] [PubMed]
78. Ellis, K.J.; Shypailo, R.J.; Abrams, S.A.; Wong, W.W. The reference child and adolescent models of body composition. A contemporary comparison. *Ann. N. Y. Acad. Sci.* **2000**, *904*, 374–382. [CrossRef] [PubMed]
79. Gutiérrez-Marín, D.; Escribano, J.; Closa-Monasterolo, R.; Ferré, N.; Venables, M.; Singh, P.; Wells, J.C.; Muñoz-Hernando, J.; Zaragoza-Jordana, M.; Gispert-Llauradó, M.; et al. Validation of bioelectrical impedance analysis for body composition assessment in children with obesity aged 8–14y. *Clin. Nutr.* **2021**, *40*, 4132–4139. [CrossRef] [PubMed]
80. Wells, J. A Hattori chart analysis of body mass index in infants and children. *Int. J. Obes.* **2000**, *24*, 325–329. [CrossRef] [PubMed]
81. Talma, H.; Chinapaw, M.J.; Bakker, B.; HiraSing, R.A.; Terwee, C.B.; Altenburg, T.M. Bioelectrical impedance analysis to estimate body composition in children and adolescents: A systematic review and evidence appraisal of validity, responsiveness, reliability and measurement error. *Obes. Rev. Off. J. Int. Assoc. Study Obes.* **2013**, *14*, 895–905. [CrossRef] [PubMed]
82. Phillips, S.M.; Bandini, L.G.; Compton, D.V.; Naumova, E.N.; Must, A. A longitudinal comparison of body composition by total body water and bioelectrical impedance in adolescent girls. *J. Nutr.* **2003**, *133*, 1419–1425. [CrossRef] [PubMed]
83. Tanita Corporation. *Tanita Body Composition Analyzer: Instruction Manual*; Tanita Corporation: Amsterdam, The Netherlands, 2014; pp. 1–39.
84. Olafsdottir, A.S.; Torfadottir, J.E.; Arngrimsson, S.A. Health Behavior and Metabolic Risk Factors Associated with Normal Weight Obesity in Adolescents. *PLoS ONE* **2016**, *11*, e0161451. [CrossRef]
85. Hinriksdóttir, G.; Tryggvadóttir, Á.; Ólafsdóttir, A.S.; Arngrímsson, S.Á. Fatness but Not Fitness Relative to the Fat-Free Mass Is Related to C-Reactive Protein in 18 Year-Old Adolescents. *PLoS ONE* **2015**, *10*, e0130597. [CrossRef] [PubMed]
86. Arngrimsson, S.B.; Richardsson, E.E.; Jonsson, K.; Olafsdottir, A.S. Body composition, aerobic fitness, physical activity and metabolic profile among 18 year old Icelandic high-school students. *Icel. J. Med.* **2012**, *98*, 277–282. [CrossRef]
87. Kyle, U.G.; Earthman, C.P.; Pichard, C.; Coss-Bu, J.A. Body composition during growth in children: Limitations and perspectives of bioelectrical impedance analysis. *Eur. J. Clin. Nutr.* **2015**, *69*, 1298–1305. [CrossRef]

88. Dhawan, D.; Sharma, S. Abdominal obesity, adipokines and non-communicable diseases. *J. Steroid Biochem. Mol. Biol.* **2020**, *203*, 105737. [CrossRef]
89. Haraldsdottir, A.; Steingrimsdottir, L.; Maskarinec, G.; Adami, H.-O.; Aspelund, T.; Valdimarsdottir, U.A.; Bjarnason, R.; Thorsdottir, I.; Halldorsson, T.I.; Gunnarsdottir, I.; et al. Growth Rate in Childhood and Adolescence and the Risk of Breast and Prostate Cancer: A Population-Based Study. *Am. J. Epidemiol.* **2021**, *191*, 320–330. [CrossRef]
90. Kreissl, A.; Jorda, A.; Truschner, K.; Skacel, G.; Greber-Platzer, S. Clinically relevant body composition methods for obese pediatric patients. *BMC Pediatr.* **2019**, *19*, 84. [CrossRef]
91. Wang, L.; Hui, S.S.-c. Validity of Four Commercial Bioelectrical Impedance Scales in Measuring Body Fat among Chinese Children and Adolescents. *BioMed Res. Int.* **2015**, *2015*, 614858. [CrossRef]
92. Haroun, D.; Croker, H.; Viner, R.M.; Williams, J.E.; Darch, T.S.; Fewtrell, M.S.; Eaton, S.; Wells, J.C. Validation of BIA in obese children and adolescents and re-evaluation in a longitudinal study. *Obesity* **2009**, *17*, 2245–2250. [CrossRef]
93. Orkin, S.; Yodoshi, T.; Romantic, E.; Hitchcock, K.; Arce-Clachar, A.C.; Bramlage, K.; Sun, Q.; Fei, L.; Xanthakos, S.A.; Trout, A.T.; et al. Body composition measured by bioelectrical impedance analysis is a viable alternative to magnetic resonance imaging in children with nonalcoholic fatty liver disease. *J. Parenter. Enter. Nutr.* **2022**, *46*, 378–384. [CrossRef]
94. Chula de Castro, J.A.; Lima, T.R.d.; Silva, D.A.S. Body composition estimation in children and adolescents by bioelectrical impedance analysis: A systematic review. *J. Bodyw. Mov. Ther.* **2018**, *22*, 134–146. [CrossRef]
95. Danielzik, S.; Langnase, K.; Mast, M.; Spethmann, C.; Muller, M.J. Impact of parental BMI on the manifestation of overweight 5–7 year old children. *Eur. J. Nutr.* **2002**, *41*, 132–138. [CrossRef] [PubMed]
96. Gunnarsdottir, T.; Njardvik, U.; Olafsdottir, A.S.; Craighead, L.; Bjarnason, R. Childhood obesity and co-morbid problems: Effects of Epstein's family-based behavioural treatment in an Icelandic sample. *J. Eval. Clin. Pr.* **2012**, *18*, 465–472. [CrossRef] [PubMed]
97. Rhee, K. Childhood overweight and the relationship between parent behaviors, parenting style and family functioning. *Ann. Am. Acad. Political. Soc. Sci.* **2008**, *615*, 12–37. [CrossRef]
98. Blissett, J.; Haycraft, E. Parental eating disorder symptoms and observations of mealtime interactions with children. *J. Psychosom. Res.* **2011**, *70*, 368–371. [CrossRef]
99. Blissett, J.; Meyer, C.; Haycraft, E. Maternal and paternal controlling feeding practices with male and female children. *Appetite* **2006**, *47*, 212–219. [CrossRef]
100. Baughcum, A.E.; Powers, S.W.; Johnson, S.B.; Chamberlin, L.A.; Deeks, C.M.; Jain, A.; Whitaker, R.C. Maternal feeding practices and beliefs and their relationships to overweight in early childhood. *J. Dev. Behav. Pediatr.* **2001**, *22*, 391–408. [CrossRef]
101. Francis, L.A.; Hofer, S.M.; Birch, L.L. Predictors of maternal child-feeding style: Maternal and child characteristics. *Appetite* **2001**, *37*, 231–243. [CrossRef]
102. Jansen, P.W.; Tharner, A.; van der Ende, J.; Wake, M.; Raat, H.; Hofman, A.; Verhulst, F.C.; van Ijzendoorn, M.H.; Jaddoe, V.W.; Tiemeier, H. Feeding practices and child weight: Is the association bidirectional in preschool children? *Am. J. Clin. Nutr.* **2014**, *100*, 1329–1336. [CrossRef]
103. Thorsteinsdottir, S.; Njardvik, U.; Bjarnason, R.; Haraldsson, H.; Olafsdottir, A.S. Taste education—A food-based intervention in a school setting, focusing on children with and without neurodevelopmental disorders and their families. A randomized controlled trial. *Appetite* **2021**, *167*, 105623. [CrossRef] [PubMed]
104. Lobstein, T.; Baur, L.; Uauy, R. Obesity in children and young people: A crisis in public health. *Obes. Rev.* **2004**, *5* (Suppl. S1), 4–104. [CrossRef]
105. Wikland, K.A.; Luo, Z.C.; Niklasson, A.; Karlberg, J. Swedish population-based longitudinal reference values from birth to 18 years of age for height, weight and head circumference. *Acta Paediatr.* **2002**, *91*, 739–754. [CrossRef] [PubMed]
106. Wardle, J.; Guthrie, C.A.; Sanderson, S.; Rapoport, L. Development of the Children's Eating Behaviour Questionnaire. *J. Child. Psychol. Psychiatry* **2001**, *42*, 963–970. [CrossRef]
107. Ashcroft, J.; Semmler, C.; Carnell, S.; van Jaarsveld, C.H.; Wardle, J. Continuity and stability of eating behaviour traits in children. *Eur. J. Clin. Nutr.* **2008**, *62*, 985–990. [CrossRef] [PubMed]
108. Klar, E.K. *The Psychometric Properties of the Icelandic Version of the Child Eating Behaviour Questionnaire (CEBQ)*; University of Iceland: Reykjavik, Iceland, 2012.
109. R:CoreTeam. *R: A Language and Environment for Statistical Computing*; R Foundation for Statistical Computing: Vienna, Austria, 2023.
110. CDC—National Center for Health Statistics. *Defining Adult Overweight & Obesity*; CDC: Atlanta, GA, USA, 2023.
111. McCarthy, H.D.; Cole, T.J.; Fry, T.; Jebb, S.A.; Prentice, A.M. Body fat reference curves for children. *Int. J. Obes.* **2006**, *30*, 598–602. [CrossRef] [PubMed]
112. Gallagher, D.; Heymsfield, S.B.; Heo, M.; Jebb, S.A.; Murgatroyd, P.R.; Sakamoto, Y. Healthy percentage body fat ranges: An approach for developing guidelines based on body mass index. *Am. J. Clin. Nutr.* **2000**, *72*, 694–701. [CrossRef] [PubMed]
113. Nakagawa, S. A farewell to Bonferroni: The problems of low statistical power and publication bias. *Behav. Ecol.* **2004**, *15*, 1044–1045. [CrossRef]
114. Cabin, R.J.; Mitchell, R.J. To Bonferroni or not to Bonferroni: When and how are the questions. *Bull. Ecol. Soc. Am.* **2000**, *81*, 246–248.
115. Jacobi, C.; Agras, W.S.; Bryson, S.; Hammer, L.D. Behavioral validation, precursors, and concomitants of picky eating in childhood. *J. Am. Acad. Child. Adolesc. Psychiatry* **2003**, *42*, 76–84. [CrossRef]

116. Piazza, C.C.; Fisher, W.W.; Brown, K.A.; Shore, B.A.; Patel, M.R.; Katz, R.M.; Sevin, B.M.; Gulotta, C.S.; Blakely-Smith, A. Functional analysis of inappropriate mealtime behaviors. *J. Appl. Behav. Anal.* **2003**, *36*, 187–204. [CrossRef]
117. Jansen, P.W.; de Barse, L.M.; Jaddoe, V.W.V.; Verhulst, F.C.; Franco, O.H.; Tiemeier, H. Bi-directional associations between child fussy eating and parents' pressure to eat: Who influences whom? *Physiol. Behav.* **2017**, *176*, 101–106. [CrossRef]
118. Thorsteinsdottir, S.; Njardvik, U.; Bjarnason, R.; Olafsdottir, A.S. Changes in Eating Behaviors Following Taste Education Intervention: Focusing on Children with and without Neurodevelopmental Disorders and Their Families: A Randomized Controlled Trial. *Nutrients* **2022**, *14*, 4000. [CrossRef]
119. Elberg, J.; McDuffie, J.R.; Sebring, N.G.; Salaita, C.; Keil, M.; Robotham, D.; Reynolds, J.C.; Yanovski, J.A. Comparison of methods to assess change in children's body composition. *Am. J. Clin. Nutr.* **2004**, *80*, 64–69. [CrossRef] [PubMed]

nutrients

MDPI

Article

Mediterranean Diet Adherence and Its Relationship to Metabolic Markers and Body Composition in Portuguese University Students

Sofia Lopes, Tatiana Fontes, Regina Menezes, Luís Monteiro Rodrigues and Cíntia Ferreira-Pêgo *

CBIOS—Universidade Lusófona's Research Center for Biosciences and Health Technologies, Av. Campo Grande 376, 1749-024 Lisbon, Portugal; f6775@ulusofona.pt (S.L.); f6776@ulusofona.pt (T.F.); regina.menezes@ulusofona.pt (R.M.); monteiro.rodrigues@ulusofona.pt (L.M.R.)

* Correspondence: cintia.pego@ulusofona.pt

Abstract: Background: Transitioning to university involves several changes, which might affect dietary habits. The present study aimed to assess the potential relationships involving adherence to the MedDiet, body composition, and metabolic markers within a Portuguese university sample. Methods: A cross-sectional study involved 70 participants, 52 women, and 18 men (23.00 ± 7.00 years old and a BMI of 21.99 ± 2.79 kg/m^2). The average MedDiet adherence of participants was 9.23 points, as evaluated by the 14 point validated questionnaire, with classifications of low and high (under or over 9 points, respectively). Body composition was assessed using X-ray dual densitometry (DXA), and metabolic markers were collected from capillary blood. Results: Statistically significant differences in HDL cholesterol and the total/HDL cholesterol ratio were found between groups. Lower levels ($p < 0.05$) of visceral (VAT) and subcutaneous adipose tissue (SAT), BMI, and waist circumference were found in the higher MedDiet adherence group. Those measures were negatively correlated ($p < 0.05$) with the adherence scores to the MedDiet. Conclusion: Higher adherence to MedDiet seemed to have a favorable and important impact on lipid profiles, primarily HDL-c. A positive relationship between MedDiet adherence and body composition distribution was also described, mostly due to the influence of higher adherence to MedDiet at lower levels of VAT and SAT in Portuguese university students.

Keywords: Mediterranean diet; university students; body composition; adipose tissue; metabolic markers

1. Introduction

The Mediterranean diet (MedDiet), commonly associated with southern Europe and Mediterranean areas [1], is characterized by high consumption of fresh fruits, vegetables, extra-virgin olive oil, nuts, whole grains, and legumes, moderate consumption of fish and dairy products (mainly fermented), and low intake of red meat or processed foods [2–4]. These characteristics were recorded on the representative list of the Intangible Cultural Heritage of Humanity (UNESCO) in 2021 [5]. MedDiet has been referred to as effective in controlling obesity, a pandemic currently challenging health systems worldwide [3,4,6]. In this line, it has been associated with a risk reduction for multiple chronic diseases, including cardiovascular, metabolic, neurodegenerative, and some types of cancer, among others [2,6–10]. This might result from the high anti-inflammatory activity of MedDiet components related to the consumption of short-chain fatty acids, polyunsaturated fatty acids, (poly)phenols [11,12], and antioxidants [1,9]. In spite of several mechanisms that have been suggested to explain these impacts, many doubts still persist. Without doubt, MedDiet has been clearly linked to an improved quality of life [3], influencing both physical and mental well-being [3], and consequently decreasing morbidity and mortality of all causes [2,13]. These beneficial effects might also be related to and influenced by the positive relationship between increased MedDiet adherence and lower body composition, as higher adherence to MedDiet has been associated with a decrease in fat mass (FM) [10] and an increase in fat-free mass (FFM) [14]. Studies have shown a positive impact of the MedDiet on metabolic health, likely due to its high consumption of plant-based foods, which are high in antioxidants, fiber, and other nutrients [1,9]. The MedDiet is associated with lower inflammation [15], lower blood pressure, lower levels of total cholesterol and low-density lipoprotein (LDL) [16], and higher levels of high-density lipoprotein (HDL) [17]. Overall, the research data points to the possibility that following the MedDiet can improve metabolic indicators and be beneficial in the prevention and treatment of many chronic diseases [15,18].

The lifestyle shifts for young adults when entering university are known to determine multiple changes [2,10,13], including an increase in FM and Body Mass Index (BMI) [14,19]. Currently, the eating habits of college students resemble a Western eating pattern since there is a higher consumption of "fast", processed, and industrialized food and products with high energy content [10,13], which might directly relate to mass gain and metabolic risk [2,13,19].

In this context, we decided to investigate a group of university students at a Portuguese university where the MedDiet is a reference to better understand potential relationships among MedDiet adherence, body composition, and relevant metabolic markers.

2. Materials and Methods

2.1. Study Design and Population

A cross-sectional observational study was designed. Recruitment took place on the University Campus of the Lisbon Metropolitan Area between January 2022 and February 2023, resulting in a final sample of 70 individuals of both sexes, aged between 18 and 39 (23.00 $\pm$ 7.00) years old, who were pursuing a bachelor's, a master's, or a doctoral degree. Non-inclusion criteria were being underage, regular consumption of any medicines, being (or suspecting to be) pregnant and/or breastfeeding, being/feeling sick, and not being a university student. All participants were Caucasian, and data were collected by trained nutritionists in a face-to-face interview. All participants provided signed, informed written consent. Procedures followed all principles of good clinical practice adopted for human research studies, as described in the Helsinki Declaration and its further amendments [20]. The study was previously approved by the Institutional Ethics Committee (CE.ECTS/P05-21).

2.2. Participants' Characterization and Instruments

General characterization data, such as sex, age, area of residence (urban or rural), and place of residence according to the division of the Nomenclature of Territorial Units for Statistics (NUTS) II [21], were collected for all participants. Lifestyle data such as smoking or other habits, medication, supplementation, hours, and quality of sleep according to the Pittsburgh sleep quality index study [22], as well as other personal and familiar information of interest, were also registered. Physical activity was evaluated using the short version of the validated International Physical Activity Questionnaire (IPAQ) [23,24]. Mass was measured by an electronic scale [0.1 kg (0.1–200 kg) accuracy], wearing light clothing and no shoes. Height was a self-reported variable used to calculate Body Mass Index (BMI) according to Quetelet's formula [body mass (kg)/height (m)^2] [25]. The waist circumference was measured using a tape at the midpoint between the last rib and the iliac crest after full exhalation of air. Dual-energy X-ray absorptiometry (DXA) (Lunar Prodigy Advance–General Electric Healthcare®, Chicago, IL, USA) was used to measure bone mass, fat mass, lean mass, tissue mass, fat-free mass, total mass, and visceral and subcutaneous adipose tissue. Before each whole-body scan, the DXA was calibrated according to the manufacturer's instructions using a standard calibration block. All measurements were collected under the same atmospheric conditions by the same researcher. To assess MedDiet adherence, participants were given a validated 14 item questionnaire [26,27]. This consisted of 12 questions on food consumption frequency and 2 questions on food intake habits considered characteristic of the Mediterranean diet. Each question was scored 0 (if the condition was not met) or 1 (if the condition was met). The final score ranged from 0 to 14 points. Using this score, MedDiet adherence was classified into two categories: low (<9 points) and high (≥9 points). A portable automatic testing device, the LINX DUO (Menarini Diagnostics®), was used to assess metabolic markers such as glycated hemoglobin (HbA1c), the lipid profile (triglycerides, total cholesterol, HDL), and blood glucose. Taking these variables into consideration, LDL cholesterol, very-low-density lipoprotein (VLDL), total cholesterol/HDL ratio, and non-HDL cholesterol were also quantified. For the blood extraction process, a puncture device (OneTouch Ultra Soft with Microlet 23 gauge lancet) was used. An automatic monitor (Tensoval–HARTMANN®) was used to measure the three components of blood pressure: systolic, diastolic, and heart rate. Before the measurement, the volunteer rested for 5 min and sat upright with the back supported, both feet flat on the floor, and the upper arm supported at heart level. All measurements were taken in the non-dominant arm, with the middle of the cuff positioned with its midsection over the brachial artery. Measurements were performed with at least 12 h of fasting (including no water, caffeine sources, diuretics, and/or alcoholic beverage consumption) and no exercise in the previous 24 h to ensure proper hydration conditions. All participants were also asked to empty their bladders prior to measurements.

2.3. Statistical Analysis

Statistical analysis was performed using IBM SPSS Statistics version 22 (SPSS Inc., Chicago, IL, USA). Parametric tests were used when the sample presented a normal distribution, and non-parametric tests when the sample presented a non-normal distribution. The Kolmogorov–Smirnov normality test was used when $n > 50$ and the Shapiro–Wilk normality test when $n \leq 50$. Nominal variables were shown as percentages (frequencies) and continuous variables as mean (standard deviation, SD) or median (interquartile range, IQR), depending on the type of variable. For the comparison between two categorical variables, the chi-squared, Fisher's exact, and Monte Carlo tests were used as appropriate. The Student's *t*-test and Mann–Whitney U test were used between categorical and scale variables. The Pearson or Spearman's rank correlation coefficients were used to examine the relationship between the MedDiet score, metabolic indicators, and body composition values. All statistical tests were two-tailed, and the significance level was set at $p < 0.05$.

3. Results

The participants in our study had MedDiet adherence scores ranging from 5 to 13, with a mean score of 9.23. Twenty-three participants out of seventy (32.86%) presented low adherence, and forty-seven (67.14%) had high adherence. The general characteristics of the study population are shown in Table 1. The mean age was 23.00 ± 7.00 years old, and the average BMI was 21.99 ± 2.79 kg/m^2. The mean height was 1.67 ± 0.08 m, and the median body mass was 59.40 ± 14.00 kg. Participants with low adherence showed significantly higher values of BMI and waist circumference.

Table 1. Sociodemographic characteristics of Portuguese university students according to categories of Mediterranean diet adherence.

	Total Population (n = 70)	Low Adherence (n = 23)	High Adherence (n = 47)	p-Value
Sex, % (n)				
Male	25.70 (18)	39.10 (9)	19.10 (9)	0.072 ^{c}
Female	74.30 (52)	60.90 (14)	80.9 (38)	
Age, years	23.00 (7.00)	24.00 (7.00)	23.00 (7.00)	0.598 ^{b}
Height, m	1.67 (0.08)	1.68 (0.72)	1.66 (0.85)	0.500 ^{a}
Mass, kg	59.40 (14.00)	63.80 (20.80)	57.10 (13.60)	0.138 ^{b}
BMI, kg/m^2	21.99 (2.79)	23.10 (3.34)	21.44 (2.32)	0.018 ^{a}

Table 1. *Cont.*

	Total Population (n = 70)	Low Adherence (n = 23)	High Adherence (n = 47)	p-Value
Waist Circumference, cm	70.95 (14.00)	76.00 (16.50)	68.00 (7.30)	0.004 [b]
Liquid Ingestion, L/day	2.00 (1.00)	2.00 (1.00)	2.00 (1.00)	0.749 [b]
Monthly Family Income, % (n)				
Under EUR 1000	8.60 (6)	8.70 (2)	8.50 (4)	
EUR 1000–3000	65.70 (46)	65.20 (15)	66.00 (31)	1.000 [d]
EUR > 3000	25.70 (18)	26.10 (6)	25.50 (12)	
Smoking Status, % (n)				
Smoker	11.40 (8)	17.40 (4)	8.50 (4)	
Ex-Smoker	11.40 (8)	13.00 (3)	10.60 (5)	0.564 [d]
Non-Smoker	77.10 (54)	69.60 (16)	80.90 (38)	
Academic course, % (n)				
Health	62.90 (44)	60.90 (14)	63.80 (30)	0.810 [c]
Other	37.1 (26)	39.10 (9)	36.20 (17)	
Home Living, % (n)				
Parents' home	48.60 (34)	56.50 (13)	44.70 (21)	
With other students	17.10 (12)	13.00 (3)	19.10 (9)	0.590 [c]
Partner	18.60 (13)	21.70 (5)	17.00 (8)	
Alone	15.70 (11)	8.70 (2)	19.10 (9)	

Data are expressed as a percentage (n), mean (SD), or median (IQR) for categorical and continuous variables, as appropriate. p-values for group comparisons were tested by [a] Student's t-test/ [b] Mann–Whitney U test or [c] chi-squared/ [d] Monte Carlo test, as appropriate. Abbreviations: BMI, Body Mass Index.

Metabolic markers for each MedDiet adherence category are presented in Table 2. Low-adherence individuals had significantly lower values of HDL cholesterol and higher values of the total cholesterol/HDL ratio compared to participants in the high-adherence categories. Noteworthy, high-adherence individuals presented lower glycemia values compared to the other group; however, these results were not statistically significant (p = 0.057).

Table 2. Metabolic markers according to categories of Mediterranean diet adherence.

	Total Population (n = 70)	Low Adherence (n = 23)	High Adherence (n = 47)	p-Value
Hemoglobin A1c, %	5.23 (0.40)	5.19 (0.39)	5.26 (0.40)	0.530 [a]
Triglycerides, mg/dL	93.50 (68.00)	89.00 (73.00)	98.00 (70.00)	0.822 [b]
Total Cholesterol, mg/dL	169.24 (32.09)	167.30 (36.57)	170.19 (30.04)	0.726 [a]
HDL, mg/dL	60.77 (15.61)	53.87 (9.90)	64.15 (22.00)	0.009 [a]
Glucose, mg/dL	89.50 (15.00)	94.00 (14.00)	88.00 (12.00)	0.057 [b]
LDL, mg/dL	82.00 (27.45)	90.50 (40.00)	81.00 (28.00)	0.210 [a]
VLDL, mg/dL	19.00 (13.00)	17.50 (14.00)	20.00 (14.00)	0.523 [a]
TC/HDL ratio, mg/dL	2.75 (0.84)	3.06 (1.07)	2.65 (0.74)	0.017 [a]
Non-HDL, mg/dL	105.00 (30.00)	111.50 (44.00)	105.00 (26.00)	0.460 [a]
Systolic Blood Pressure, mm Hg	110.00 (12.06)	113.13 (10.57)	108.47 (12.55)	0.130 [a]
Diastolic Blood Pressure, mm Hg	70.50 (14.00)	70.00 (13.00)	71.00 (15.00)	0.131 [b]
Heart Rate, bpm	68.00 (14.00)	66.00 (13.00)	69.00 (17.00)	0.381 [b]

Data are expressed as a mean (SD) or median (IQR). p-values for group comparisons were tested by [a] Student's t-test or [b] Mann–Whitney U test, as appropriate; Abbreviations: HDL, High-Density Lipoprotein; LDL, Low-Density Lipoprotein; VLDL, Very-Low-Density Lipoprotein; TC/HDL, Total Cholesterol/High-Density Lipoprotein; NHDL, Non-High-Density Lipoprotein; bpm, beats per minute.

Table 3 shows body composition distribution according to MedDiet adherence categories. Participants with lower adherence had significantly higher Subcutaneous Adipose Tissue (SAT) content (1076.61 $\pm$ 603.05 cm^3 vs. 751.58 $\pm$ 379.03 cm^3) and Visceral Adipose Tissue (VAT) content (267.00 $\pm$ 334.00 cm^3 vs. 106.00 $\pm$ 155.00 cm^3), compared to individuals with higher adherence to the MedDiet.

Table 3. Body composition distribution according to categories of Mediterranean diet adherence.

	Total Population (n = 70)	Low Adherence (n = 23)	High Adherence (n = 47)	p-Value
Total BMD, %	1.94 (0.24)	1.86 (0.23)	1.98 (0.24)	0.060 [a]
Total BMC, %	3.88 (0.33)	3.81 (0.29)	3.91 (0.35)	0.229 [a]
Fat Mass, %	27.88 (6.90)	28.76 (7.88)	27.45 (6.41)	0.460 [a]
Lean Mass, %	68.23 (6.73)	67.41 (7.72)	68.63 (6.24)	0.481 [a]
Fat-Free Mass, %	72.11 (6.89)	71.22 (7.88)	72.54 (6.39)	0.455 [a]
VAT, cm^3	141.50 (238.00)	267.00 (334.00)	106.00 (155.00)	0.005 [a]
SAT, cm^3	858.37 (485.16)	1076.61 (603.05)	751.58 (379.03)	0.008 [b]

Data are expressed as a mean (SD) or median (IQR). p-values for group comparisons were tested by [a] Student's t-test or [b] Mann–Whitney U test, as appropriate. Abbreviations: BMD, Bone Mineral Density; BMC, Bone Mineral Content; VAT, Visceral Adipose Tissue; SAT, Subcutaneous Adipose Tissue.

Average MedDiet adherence scores according to demographic characteristics can be observed in Table 4. Out of a range of 0–14 points, the mean adherence scores for men and women were 8.78 and 9.38, respectively. There were no significant differences, but participants in the 2nd year of their bachelor's course presented a mean of 10.20 points, higher than the rest of the study years (p = 0.051).

Table 4. Mediterranean diet adherence scores by demographic characteristics.

	Mean (SD)	p-Value [a]
Gender		
Male	8.78 (1.63)	0.221
Female	9.38 (1.85)	
Academic course		
Health	9.25 (1.87)	0.898
Other	9.19 (1.72)	
Student Worker		
Yes	9.21 (1.98)	0.904
No	9.26 (1.59)	
Grade Level		
Bachelor's	9.33 (1.86)	0.543
Master's	8.82 (1.43)	
PhD	9.57 (2.30)	
Year Coursing—Bachelor's		
1st	8.33 (1.75)	0.051
2nd	10.20 (2.17)	
3rd	9.83 (1.63)	
4th	8.36 (1.86)	
Type of housing		
Family	9.12 (1.84)	0.620
Friends/Partner/Alone	9.33 (1.79)	
Residence		
Urban	9.07 (1.71)	0.104
Rural	10.00 (2.13)	
Monthly Family Income		
Up to EUR 1000	8.67 (1.51)	0.697
EUR 1000–3000	9.33 (1.71)	
EUR > 3000	9.17 (2.15)	
Smoking Status. % (n)		
Smoker	8.25 (1.74)	0.224
Ex-Smoker	9.00 (2.00)	
Non-Smoker	9.41 (1.74)	
PAL		
Low	9.18 (2.27)	0.413
Medium	9.47 (1.78)	
High	8.76 (1.25)	

Data are expressed as mean (SD); [a] statistical significance $p \leq 0.05$. Abbreviations: PAL, Physical Activity Level.

Mediterranean diet adherence scores, BMI, anthropometric measurements, and fat tissue correlations are shown in Figure 1 as scatter plots. Higher adherence scores significantly correlate with lower values of BMI, waist circumference, VAT, and SAT.

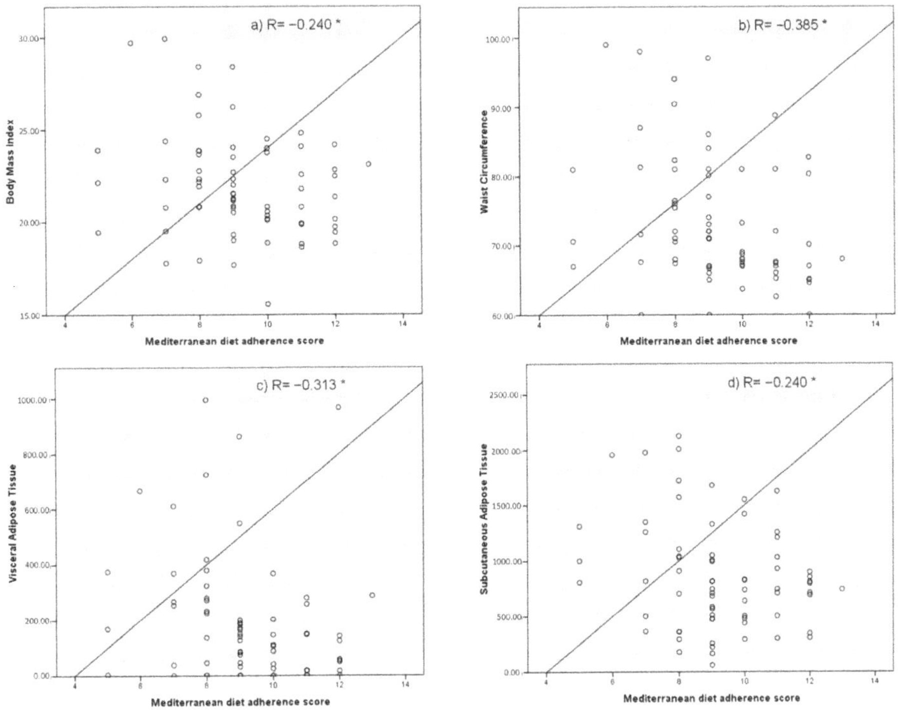

Figure 1. Scatter charts evaluated the correlation (R) between Mediterranean Adherence Score and (**a**) Body Mass Index; (**b**) Waist Circumference; (**c**) Visceral Fat Tissue and (**d**) Subcutaneous Fat Tissue. * Statistical significance $p \leq 0.05$.

Table 5 shows the agreement with the dietary recommendations based on the 14 item MedDiet adherence questionnaire according to sex, course, house living, and income. Low adherence was observed for each of the items. Additionally, volunteers enrolled in a course not related to health sciences presented a higher percentage of agreement with a portion of legumes than those studying a health sciences-related course ($p = 0.002$). Participants living with parents had higher adherence scores than those living with friends. Individuals with monthly incomes between EUR 1000 and 3000 tended to comply more with the MedDiet adherence criteria than other income levels.

Table 5. Agreement with the recommendations based on each item of MEDAS-14 by category.

	Recommendation	Compliance by Sex			Compliance by Course			Compliance by Living Arrangement			Compliance by Income Level			
		Men	Women	p-Value [a]	Health	Other	p-Value [a]	Friends	Family	p-Value [a]	EUR < 1000	EUR 1000–3000	EUR > 3000	p-Value [a]
1. Do you use olive oil as a main culinary fat?	Yes	94.40	94.20	0.973	95.50	92.30	0.584	100.00	88.90	0.045	100.00	93.50	94.40	0.811
2. How much olive oil do you consume in a given day (including the oil used for frying. salads. out-of-house meals. etc.)?	≥4 tbsp	22.20	34.60	0.329	36.40	23.10	0.247	38.20	25.00	0.233	83.30	28.30	22.20	0.015
3. How many vegetable servings do you consume per day? (1 serving: 200 g consider side dishes as half a serving))	≥2 (≥1 portion raw or as a salad)	72.20	73.10	0.944	72.70	73.10	0.975	67.60	77.80	0.341	100.00	76.10	55.60	0.074
4. How many fruit units (including natural fruit juices) do you consume per day?	≥3	61.10	48.10	0.340	50.00	53.80	0.756	55.90	47.20	0.469	16.70	58.70	44.40	0.121
5. How many servings of red meat. hamburger. or meat products (ham. sausage. etc.) do you consume per day? (1 serving: 100–150 g)	<1	66.70	86.50	0.062	81.80	80.80	0.913	76.50	86.10	0.300	100.00	80.40	77.80	0.459
6. How many servings of butter. margarine. or cream you consume per day? (1 serving: 12 g)	<1	72.20	80.80	0.446	77.30	80.80	0.730	73.50	83.30	0.318	66.70	71.70	100.00	0.035
7. How many sweet or carbonated beverages do you drink per day?	<1	88.90	92.30	0.655	90.90	92.30	0.840	88.20	94.40	0.354	66.70	93.50	94.40	0.076
8. How much wine do you drink per week?	≥7 glasses	5.60	7.70	0.762	6.80	7.70	0.891	8.80	5.60	0.596	0.00	4.30	16.70	0.177
9. How many servings of legumes do you consume per week? (1 serving: 150 g)	≥3	66.70	59.60	0.596	47.70	84.60	0.002	44.10	77.80	0.004	66.70	58.70	66.70	0.809

Table 5. *Cont.*

	Recommendation	Compliance by Sex			Compliance by Course			Compliance by Living Arrangement			Compliance by Income Level			
		Men	Women	*p*-Value [a]	Health	Other	*p*-Value [a]	Friends	Family	*p*-Value [a]	EUR < 1000	EUR 1000–3000	EUR > 3000	*p*-Value [a]
10. How many servings of fish or shellfish do you consume per week? (1 serving of 100–150 g of fish or 4–5 units or 200 g of shellfish)	≥3	27.80	73.10	0.001	72.70	42.30	0.012	70.60	52.80	0.126	33.30	67.40	55.60	0.229
11. How many times per week do you consume commercial sweets or pastries (not homemade). such as cakes. cookies. biscuits. or custard?	<3	88.90	67.30	0.076	72.70	73.10	0.975	61.80	83.30	0.043	33.30	78.30	72.20	0.066
12. How many servings of nuts (including peanuts) do you consume per week? (1 serving 30 g)	≥3	55.60	55.80	0.987	56.80	53.80	0.809	47.10	63.90	0.157	33.30	63.00	44.40	0.207
13. Do you preferentially consume chicken. turkey. or rabbit meat instead of veal. pork. hamburger. or sausage?	Yes	61.10	73.10	0.340	77.30	57.70	0.084	79.40	61.10	0.095	50.00	71.70	72.20	0.535
14. How many times per week do you consume vegetables. pasta. rice. or other dishes seasoned with sofrito (sauce made with tomato and onion. leek. or garlic and simmered with olive oil)?	≥2	83.30	86.50	0.738	81.80	92.30	0.226	88.20	88.30	0.558	100.00	82.60	88.90	0.470

Data are expressed as a mean (SD); [a] statistical significance $p \leq 0.05$. Abbreviations: PAL, Physical Activity Level; tbsp, tablespoon.

4. Discussion

The present study was designed to provide a more thorough assessment of the relationship between adherence to MedDiet, body composition, and metabolic markers in a cohort of healthy Portuguese university students. Recent surveys have produced slightly different results regarding the prevalence of MedDiet adherence [28]. It appears that adherence is largely influenced by cultural heritage, but it is unclear why adherence is lost over time [28]. The use of different questionnaires and cut-off points to measure adherence might contribute to this result's variability [3]. The globalization of markets has led to a "Westernization" of the overall European diet, with younger generations leaving traditional dietary patterns [28] as they have more access to non-Mediterranean food groups such as animal fats, vegetable oils (other than olive oil), sugar, and red meat [3,28]. Overall, studies [3,29] show low rates of adherence to the MedDiet, particularly among young people who tend to move away from healthy lifestyle habits. This seems to be influenced by emotional, physiological, and environmental changes [30] experienced during this life period, leading to changes in their dietary patterns [31], including an increase in fast food consumption [29].

Regarding metabolic markers, the HDL cholesterol and total cholesterol/HDL ratio were statistically more favorable in those students with higher MedDiet adherence. Low HDL and high LDL cholesterol levels are known to be the main determinants of cardiovascular risk [32,33]. The MedDiet has been suggested to improve cardiovascular health due to the high omega-3 and omega-6 content of extra-virgin olive oil and nuts [17,32]. Healthier levels of other lipid profile variables, such as triglycerides, LDL, and non-HDL cholesterol, were observed in the higher adherence category, although differences were not statistically significant. These differences have been previously observed and may be explained by the higher consumption of water-soluble fiber associated with this dietary pattern [14,32].

Concerning body composition distribution, our study has shown that higher MedDiet compliance led to significantly lower levels of VAT and SAT. Similar results have been published [14,34], but the evidence regarding the relationship between MedDiet and VAT is still not clear [3]. Although both VAT and SAT contribute to overall body fat mass, they have distinct characteristics [35,36]. VAT surrounds the abdominal organs, including the liver, pancreas, and gut, and is more metabolically active than SAT, rather than being associated with insulin resistance, inflammation, and other metabolic disorders [37]. On the other hand, SAT is located directly beneath the skin and serves as a primary energy reserve for the body [36]. Unlike VAT, however, SAT does not seem to be associated with metabolic dysfunction and disorders [37]. Participants who are living with their parents seem to have higher adherence to the MedDiet. This may be due to the fact that older people generally demonstrate greater adherence levels as compared to younger individuals [28]. Given that family and environment are crucial in shaping dietary habits and food preferences [38], parents, grandparents, and older siblings have a significant impact on establishing "healthy" eating habits in their children [39]. In the case of the MedDiet, family-based food traditions and practices could be a vital element in encouraging adherence to this dietary pattern [40]. Participants with low socioeconomic levels seem to follow fewer items related to healthier MedDiet adherence than those with a higher socioeconomic level. It may be that individuals with lower socioeconomic status tend to have less accessibility to fresh fruits and vegetables, which are usually more expensive than processed foods [31]. This can make it difficult to follow a diet rich in these foods, such as MedDiet. The results of our study indicate that the consumption of olive oil was statistically higher among participants with low incomes, and similar results were found for all the groups analyzed (EUR < 1000, EUR 1000–3000, and EUR > 3000). The countries situated in the Mediterranean region, including Portugal, provide olive oil at comparatively lower prices, which may further explain its increased usage among these participants [3]. Our correlation analysis seems to be in line with recent observations suggesting that higher adherence to the MedDiet was statistically related to lower values of VAT and SAT [14,32,41], and with lower BMI and waist circumference [42,43], as seen before. These observations may be explained by the composition of the typical Mediterranean diet, which includes many foods, such as fruits and vegetables, with low energy densities and high water and fiber contents [42]. These foods increase the feeling of satiety, as they require more chewing and take longer to digest than foods with high energy density, which can lead to reduced energy intake, resulting in weight loss [43]. The adoption of an unhealthy lifestyle, similar to a more Western dietary pattern, is common during this time of transition, as previously mentioned [2]. A Western-style diet has been linked to the development of several non-communicable chronic diseases [2,44], such as obesity, cardiovascular disorders, Type II diabetes mellitus, and even mental health, as a result of fatigue and a lack of energy caused by a lack of essential nutrients [45]. Even though the young participants analyzed in our study appeared to be in "good health", our results showed that those in the low MedDiet adherence group had statistically unhealthier values for metabolic markers associated with cardiovascular health and for body composition associated with metabolic dysfunction and disorders. Although young people (generally) appear to have strong health and resistance to disease conditions, the effects of poor adherence to this dietary pattern can be cumulative [45], resulting in poor long-term quality of life and the possible development of the aforementioned health problems [45]. Thus, it is important to promote healthy eating habits in younger adult populations, including increased adherence to MedDiet. This can be achieved through nutrition education, beginning by promoting healthy eating environments within colleges and universities themselves [28].

To the best of our knowledge, this is the first study developed in a university student population demonstrating that higher adherence to the MedDiet was related to more favorable body composition distribution and metabolic marker levels. Our conclusions are well supported by the assessment technologies used. DXA is one of the most specific methods of body composition assessment [46]. Metabolic markers were assessed using a minimally invasive method.

Some limitations should be assumed in the present study. The reduced sample size and the cross-sectional design do not allow the establishment of a causal effect. Self-reported height may be a limitation, as it affects BMI calculations. In our study, the values were confirmed by comparison with the values registered on the participants citizen card. Several studies have already demonstrated the reliability and accuracy of using the values from a citizen's card to obtain some anthropometric measurements [45]. Another limitation can be attributed to the fact that the validated questionnaire on MedDiet adherence is not adapted to the gastronomic differences of each country [3]. As an example, high consumption of vegetable soup has been identified in Portugal; however, this is not specifically evaluated in the questionnaire. Further, the question regarding wine consumption (seven glasses/week) may be inappropriate for the age group investigated since young adults usually do not drink wine to the same extent as older adults. Additionally, the binary scoring system for different food items does not allow for the assessment of the degree of proximity to the optimal consumption of a particular item [47].

5. Conclusions

The present study demonstrated for the first time that higher MedDiet adherence seems to lead to favorable metabolic marker levels in young Portuguese university students, showing healthier values of HDL-c and the TC/HDL-c ratio and also being related to healthier body composition due to the reduced levels of SAT and VAT. Poor adherence to MedDiet may have future negative impacts on health and quality of life and may affect physical and mental well-being. Given that this study presented a cross-sectional design, the implementation of programs that encourage adherence to MedDiet in young adults is important to maybe help prevent some non-communicable chronic diseases and improve quality of life in the long term.

Author Contributions: Conceptualization, L.M.R., R.M. and C.F.-P.; methodology, S.L. and T.F.; software, S.L. and T.F.; validation, L.M.R., R.M. and C.F.-P.; formal analysis, S.L.; investigation, S.L, T.F., R.M. and C.F.-P.; resources, L.M.R., R.M. and C.F.-P.; data curation, S.L. and T.F.; writing—original draft preparation, S.L.; writing—review and editing, R.M., L.M.R. and C.F.-P.; visualization, R.M., L.M.R. and C.F.-P.; supervision, R.M., L.M.R. and C.F.-P.; project administration, R.M., L.M.R. and C.F.-P.; funding acquisition, R.M., L.M.R. and C.F.-P. All authors have read and agreed to the published version of the manuscript.

Funding: This research was funded by national funds through FCT—Foundation for Science and Technology, I.P. (Portugal), under the [UIDB/04567/2020] and [UIDP/04567/2020] projects, and by COFAC/ILIND—Cooperativa De Formação e Animação Cultural CRL/Instituto Lusófono de Investigação e Desenvolvimento (grant COFAC/ILIND/CBIOS/2/2021). C.F.-P. is funded by the FCT—Foundation for Science and Technology, I.P. (Portugal) Scientific Employment Stimulus contract [reference number CEEC/CBIOS/NUT/2018]. R.M. is funded by the FCT—Foundation for Science and Technology, I.P. (Portugal) Scientific Employment Stimulus contract [reference number CEEC/04567/CBIOS/2020].

Institutional Review Board Statement: The study was conducted in accordance with the Declaration of Helsinki and approved by the Institutional Ethics Committee of the School of Sciences and Health Technologies (protocol code CE.ECTS/P05-21).

Informed Consent Statement: Informed consent was obtained from all participants involved in the study.

Data Availability Statement: Data is unavailable due to privacy or ethical restrictions.

Acknowledgments: The authors acknowledge all the participants.

Conflicts of Interest: The authors declare no conflict of interest.

References

1. Mistretta, A.; Marventano, S.; Antoci, M.; Cagnetti, A.; Giogianni, G.; Nolfo, F.; Rametta, S.; Pecora, G.; Marranzano, M. Mediterranean diet adherence and body composition among Southern Italian adolescents. *Obes. Res. Clin. Pract.* **2017**, *11*, 215–226. [CrossRef] [PubMed]
2. Zulet Fraile, P.; Lizancos Castro, A.; Andía Melero, V.; González Antigüedad, C.; Monereo Megías, S.; Calvo Revilla, S. Relación de La Composición Corporal Medida Por DEXA Con El Estilo de Vida y La Satisfacción Con La Imagen Corporal En Estudiantes Universitarios. *Nutr. Hosp.* **2019**, *36*, 919–925. [CrossRef] [PubMed]
3. Cobo-Cuenca, A.I.; Garrido-Miguel, M.; Soriano-Cano, A.; Ferri-Morales, A.; Martínez-Vizcaíno, V.; Martín-Espinosa, N.M. Adherence to the Mediterranean Diet and Its Association with Body Composition and Physical Fitness in Spanish University Students. *Nutrients* **2019**, *11*, 2830. [CrossRef] [PubMed]
4. Galan-Lopez, P.; Sánchez-Oliver, A.J.; Ries, F.; González-Jurado, J.A. Mediterranean Diet, Physical Fitness and Body Composition in Sevillian Adolescents: A Healthy Lifestyle. *Nutrients* **2019**, *11*, 2009. [CrossRef] [PubMed]
5. UNESCO—Falconry, a Living Human Heritage. Available online: https://ich.unesco.org/en/RL/falconry-a-living-human-heritage-01708 (accessed on 9 March 2023).
6. Galan-Lopez, P.; Ries, F.; Gisladottir, T.; Domínguez, R.; Sánchez-Oliver, A.J. Healthy Lifestyle: Relationship between Mediterranean Diet, Body Composition and Physical Fitness in 13 to 16-Year Old Icelandic Students. *Int. J. Environ. Res. Public Health* **2018**, *15*, 2632. [CrossRef]
7. Silveira, E.A.; Barbosa, L.S.; Rodrigues, A.P.S.; Noll, M.; De Oliveira, C. Body fat percentage assessment by skinfold equation, bioimpedance and densitometry in older adults. *Arch. Public Health* **2020**, *78*, 65. [CrossRef]
8. Murphy, R.A.; Reinders, I.; Register, T.C.; Ayonayon, H.N.; Newman, A.B.; Satterfield, S.; Goodpaster, B.H.; Simonsick, E.M.; Kritchevsky, S.B.; Harris, T.B. Associations of BMI and adipose tissue area and density with incident mobility limitation and poor performance in older adults. *Am. J. Clin. Nutr.* **2014**, *99*, 1059–1065. [CrossRef]
9. Ortega, F.B.; Sui, X.; Lavie, C.J.; Blair, S.N. Body Mass Index, the Most Widely Used But Also Widely Criticized Index: Would a Gold-Standard Measure of Total Body Fat Be a Better Predictor of Cardiovascular Disease Mortality? *Mayo Clin. Proc.* **2016**, *91*, 443–455. [CrossRef]
10. Ferreira-Pêgo, C.; Rodrigues, J.; Costa, A.; Sousa, B. Adherence to the Mediterranean Diet in Portuguese University Students. *Biomed. Biopharm. Res. J.* **2019**, *16*, 41–49. [CrossRef]
11. Leri, M.; Scuto, M.; Ontario, M.L.; Calabrese, V.; Calabrese, E.J.; Bucciantini, M.; Stefani, M. Healthy Effects of Plant Polyphenols: Molecular Mechanisms. *Int. J. Mol. Sci.* **2020**, *21*, 1250. [CrossRef]
12. Castro-Barquero, S.; Lamuela-Raventós, R.M.; Doménech, M.; Estruch, R. Relationship between Mediterranean Dietary Polyphenol Intake and Obesity. *Nutrients* **2018**, *10*, 1523. [CrossRef]

13. da Silva, T.R.; Martins, C.C.; Ferreira, L.L.; Spritzer, P.M. Mediterranean diet is associated with bone mineral density and muscle mass in postmenopausal women. *Climacteric* **2019**, *22*, 162–168. [CrossRef] [PubMed]
14. Kalkuz, S.; Demircan, A. Effects of the Mediterranean diet adherence on body composition, blood parameters and quality of life in adults. *Postgrad. Med. J.* **2021**, *97*, 798–802. [CrossRef] [PubMed]
15. Sood, S.; Feehan, J.; Itsiopoulos, C.; Wilson, K.; Plebanski, M.; Scott, D.; Hebert, J.R.; Shivappa, N.; Mousa, A.; George, E.S.; et al. Higher Adherence to a Mediterranean Diet Is Associated with Improved Insulin Sensitivity and Selected Markers of Inflammation in Individuals Who Are Overweight and Obese without Diabetes. *Nutrients* **2022**, *14*, 4437. [CrossRef] [PubMed]
16. Hernáez, Á.; Castañer, O.; Goday, A.; Ros, E.; Pintó, X.; Estruch, R.; Salas-Salvadó, J.; Corella, D.; Arós, F.; Serra-Majem, L.; et al. The Mediterranean diet decreases LDL atherogenicity in high cardiovascular risk individuals: A randomized controlled trial. *Mol. Nutr. Food Res.* **2017**, *61*, 1601015. [CrossRef]
17. Rees, K.; Takeda, A.; Martin, N.; Ellis, L.; Wijesekara, D.; Vepa, A.; Das, A.; Hartley, L.; Stranges, S. Mediterranean-style diet for the primary and secondary prevention of cardiovascular disease. *Cochrane Database Syst. Rev.* **2019**, *2019*, CD009825. [CrossRef]
18. Bakaloudi, D.R.; Chrysoula, L.; Leonida, I.; Kotzakioulafi, E.; Theodoridis, X.; Chourdakis, M. Impact of the level of adherence to the Mediterranean diet on blood pressure: A systematic review and meta-analysis of observational studies. *Clin. Nutr.* **2021**, *40*, 5771–5780. [CrossRef]
19. Manzano-Carrasco, S.; Felipe, J.L.; Sanchez-Sanchez, J.; Hernandez-Martin, A.; Gallardo, L.; Garcia-Unanue, J. Physical Fitness, Body Composition, and Adherence to the Mediterranean Diet in Young Football Players: Influence of the 20 mSRT Score and Maturational Stage. *Int. J. Environ. Res. Public Health* **2020**, *17*, 3257. [CrossRef]
20. World Medical Association. World Medical Association Declaration of Helsinki Ethical Principles for Medical Research Involving Human Subjects. *Bull. World Health Organ.* **2001**, *70*, 373–374.
21. Instituto da Gestão do Fundo Social Europeu Nomenclatura Das Unidades Territoriais Para Fins Estatísticos (NUTS). Available online: http://www.igfse.pt/st_glossario.asp?startAt=2&categoryID=309 (accessed on 15 January 2023).
22. Buysse, D.J.; Reynolds, C.F.; Monk, T.H.; Berman, S.R.; Kupfer, D.J. The Pittsburgh sleep quality index: A new instrument for psychiatric practice and research. *Psychiatry Res.* **1989**, *28*, 193–213. [CrossRef]
23. Craig, C.L.; Marshall, A.L.; Sjöström, M.; Bauman, A.E.; Booth, M.L.; Ainsworth, B.E.; Pratt, M.; Ekelund, U.L.; Yngve, A.; Sallis, J.F.; et al. International Physical Activity Questionnaire: 12-Country Reliability and Validity. *Med. Sci. Sport. Exerc.* **2003**, *35*, 1381–1395. [CrossRef] [PubMed]
24. Ekelund, U.; Sepp, H.; Brage, S.; Becker, W.; Jakes, R.; Hennings, M.; Wareham, N.J. Criterion-related validity of the last 7-day, short form of the International Physical Activity Questionnaire in Swedish adults. *Public Health Nutr.* **2006**, *9*, 258–265. [CrossRef] [PubMed]
25. Garrow, J.S.; Webster, J. Quetelet's index (W/H2) as a measure of fatness. *Int. J. Obes.* **1985**, *9*, 147–153. [PubMed]
26. Martínez-González, M.Á.; Corella, D.; Salas-Salvadó, J.; Ros, E.; Covas, M.I.; Fiol, M.; Wärnberg, J.; Arós, F.; Ruíz-Gutiérrez, V.; Lamuela-Raventós, R.M.; et al. Cohort Profile: Design and methods of the PREDIMED study. *Int. J. Epidemiol.* **2012**, *41*, 377–385. [CrossRef] [PubMed]
27. Mediterranean Diet Adherence in the Mediterranean Healthy Eating, Aging and Lifestyle (MEAL) Study Cohort—PubMed. Available online: https://pubmed.ncbi.nlm.nih.gov/28562120/ (accessed on 9 March 2023).
28. Karam, J.; Bibiloni, M.d.M.; Serhan, M.; Tur, J.A. Adherence to Mediterranean Diet among Lebanese University Students. *Nutrients* **2021**, *13*, 1264. [CrossRef]
29. García-Meseguer, M.J.; Burriel, F.C.; García, C.V.; Serrano-Urrea, R. Adherence to Mediterranean diet in a Spanish university population. *Appetite* **2014**, *78*, 156–164. [CrossRef]
30. Baydemir, C.; Ozgur, E.G.; Balci, S. Evaluation of adherence to Mediterranean diet in medical students at Kocaeli University, Turkey. *J. Int. Med. Res.* **2018**, *46*, 1585–1594. [CrossRef]
31. Tuttolomondo, A.; Simonetta, I.; Daidone, M.; Mogavero, A.; Ortello, A.; Pinto, A. Metabolic and Vascular Effect of the Mediterranean Diet. *Int. J. Mol. Sci.* **2019**, *20*, 4716. [CrossRef]
32. Carr, S.S.; Hooper, A.J.; Sullivan, D.R.; Burnett, J.R. Non-HDL-cholesterol and apolipoprotein B compared with LDL-cholesterol in atherosclerotic cardiovascular disease risk assessment. *Pathology* **2019**, *51*, 148–154. [CrossRef]
33. Bendall, C.L.; Mayr, H.; Opie, R.; Bes-Rastrollo, M.; Itsiopoulos, C.; Thomas, C.J. Central obesity and the Mediterranean diet: A systematic review of intervention trials. *Crit. Rev. Food Sci. Nutr.* **2018**, *58*, 3070–3084. [CrossRef]
34. Boivin, A.; Brochu, G.; Marceau, S.; Marceau, P.; Hould, F.-S.; Tchernof, A. Regional differences in adipose tissue metabolism in obese men. *Metabolism* **2007**, *56*, 533–540. [CrossRef]
35. Sam, S. Differential effect of subcutaneous abdominal and visceral adipose tissue on cardiometabolic risk. *Horm. Mol. Biol. Clin. Investig.* **2018**, *33*, 20180014. [CrossRef]
36. Lotta, L.A.; Abbasi, A.; Sharp, S.J.; Sahlqvist, A.-S.; Waterworth, D.; Brosnan, J.M.; Scott, R.A.; Langenberg, C.; Wareham, N.J. Definitions of Metabolic Health and Risk of Future Type 2 Diabetes in BMI Categories: A Systematic Review and Network Meta-analysis. *Diabetes Care* **2015**, *38*, 2177–2187. [CrossRef]
37. Scaglioni, S.; De Cosmi, V.; Ciappolino, V.; Parazzini, F.; Brambilla, P.; Agostoni, C. Factors Influencing Children's Eating Behaviours. *Nutrients* **2018**, *10*, 706. [CrossRef]
38. The Influence of Peers' and Siblings' on Children's and Adolescents' Healthy Eating Behavior. A Systematic Literature Review—PubMed. Available online: https://pubmed.ncbi.nlm.nih.gov/31927070/ (accessed on 16 March 2023).

39. Iaccarino Idelson, P.; Scalfi, L.; Valerio, G. Adherence to the Mediterranean Diet in children and adolescents: A systematic review. *Nutr. Metab. Cardiovasc. Dis.* **2017**, *27*, 283–299. [CrossRef]
40. Mendonça, N.; Gregório, M.J.; Salvador, C.; Henriques, A.R.; Canhão, H.; Rodrigues, A.M. Low Adherence to the Mediterranean Diet Is Associated with Poor Socioeconomic Status and Younger Age: A Cross-Sectional Analysis of the EpiDoC Cohort. *Nutrients* **2022**, *14*, 1239. [CrossRef]
41. Kastorini, C.-M.; Milionis, H.J.; Esposito, K.; Giugliano, D.; Goudevenos, J.A.; Panagiotakos, D.B. The Effect of Mediterranean Diet on Metabolic Syndrome and Its Components: A Meta-Analysis of 50 Studies and 534,906 Individuals. *J. Am. Coll. Cardiol.* **2011**, *57*, 1299–1313. [CrossRef]
42. Agnoli, C.; Sieri, S.; Ricceri, F.; Giraudo, M.T.; Masala, G.; Assedi, M.; Panico, S.; Mattiello, A.; Tumino, R.; Giurdanella, M.C.; et al. Adherence to a Mediterranean diet and long-term changes in weight and waist circumference in the EPIC-Italy cohort. *Nutr. Diabetes* **2018**, *8*, 22. [CrossRef]
43. Tosti, V.; Bertozzi, B.; Fontana, L. Health Benefits of the Mediterranean Diet: Metabolic and Molecular Mechanisms. *J. Gerontol. Ser. A* **2018**, *73*, 318–326. [CrossRef]
44. Ventriglio, A.; Sancassiani, F.; Contu, M.P.; Latorre, M.; Di Slavatore, M.; Fornaro, M.; Bhugra, D. Mediterranean Diet and Its Benefits on Health and Mental Health: A Literature Review. *Clin. Pract. Epidemiol. Ment. Health* **2020**, *16*, 156–164. [CrossRef]
45. Bazzocchi, A.; Ponti, F.; Albisinni, U.; Battista, G.; Guglielmi, G. DXA: Technical aspects and application. *Eur. J. Radiol.* **2016**, *85*, 1481–1492. [CrossRef] [PubMed]
46. Rumbo-Rodríguez, L.; Sánchez-SanSegundo, M.; Ferrer-Cascales, R.; García-D'urso, N.; Hurtado-Sánchez, J.A.; Zaragoza-Martí, A. Comparison of Body Scanner and Manual Anthropometric Measurements of Body Shape: A Systematic Review. *Int. J. Environ. Res. Public Health* **2021**, *18*, 6213. [CrossRef] [PubMed]
47. Chiriacò, M.; Tubili, C.; Bo, S.; Parillo, M.; Vetrani, C.; Mazzotti, A.; Pistis, D.; Marelli, G.; Grandone, I.; Natali, A. Critical evaluation of the questionnaires assessing adherence to the Mediterranean diet that are based on servings. *Nutr. Metab. Cardiovasc. Dis. NMCD* **2023**, *33*, 724–736. [CrossRef] [PubMed]

nutrients

MDPI

Article

Healthy Eating in the Spanish University Community: A Case Study

Ángeles Arjona Garrido *, Montserrat Monserrat Hernández and Juan Carlos Checa Olmos

Laboratory of Social and Cultural Anthropology, University of Almeria, 04120 Almeria, Spain; mmh548@ual.es (M.M.H.); jcheca@ual.es (J.C.C.O.)

* Correspondence: arjona@ual.es

Abstract: The Mediterranean Diet (MedD), which UNESCO recognizes as an Intangible Cultural Heritage, constitutes a healthy eating pattern that helps prevent illness. The aim of this work is to know how well the university community of Almeria (Spain) adheres to MedD as a healthy lifestyle standard. For this purpose, the authors administered a survey to students, teachers, and administrative and service personnel at the University of Almeria. The sample for the survey comprised 610 people. Of whom, 64.7% were women; 23% were Teaching, and Research Staff (PDI); 17.3% were Administration and Services Staff (PAS); and 59.7% were students. The average age was 32 years. Results show an average level of MedD adherence overall in the university community, although 40.9% have a low adherence level. The most representative MedD adherent can be profiled as a young Spanish female, who values sustainability, reads the labels of the products she consumes, exercises regularly, cooks healthy food, and recycles waste. We suggest [to the University authorities] to advertise the benefits of the Mediterranean Diet among the university community and offer menus based on the MedD in the university canteen.

Keywords: food; eating behaviour; Mediterranean diet; University of Almeria

1. Introduction

Eating behavior is influenced by numerous factors that do not always correspond to healthy patterns. Moreover, nutritional value does not tend to be the main motivation for choosing a food product. Cultural, psychological, economic, climatic, social, and geographic factors, among others, mold the dietary profile [1–4]. A healthy diet protects against nutritional deficiencies and non-communicable diseases: diabetes, heart disease, stroke, and cancer [1], but it requires particular nutritional practices. The Food and Agriculture Organization of the United Nations (FAO) and the World Health Organization (WHO) established dietary standards based on three general assumptions: caloric intake must be balanced with caloric expenditure. Keep salt consumption below 5 g per day (equivalent to less than 2 g of sodium per day). In addition, keep fat consumption to less than 30% of daily caloric intake. Unsaturated fats are preferable to saturated fats. Saturated fats should be <10% of total Kcal and trans fats < 1%. To these, we will add multiple dietary guidelines specific to the trends and habits of the locality (The Spanish Food Safety Agency (AESAN) [5] is the government body in charge of maintaining Spaniards' food safety) and period of the year.

Widely recommended as healthy, the Mediterranean Diet (MedD) is a culturally transmitted eating pattern consisting of variables such as climate, attitudes, and consumption of certain products [5–7]. The Mediterranean Diet was recognized by UNESCO as Intangible Cultural Heritage and a healthy eating pattern by public policy and health professionals [8–10]. The MedD emphasizes the consumption of plant-based foods such as vegetables, fruits, whole grains, nuts, and pulses (legumes). The diet also includes protein from small amounts of fish, poultry, and lean cuts of beef. Olive oil is the primary source of fat. In terms of cooking methods, MedD recommends stewing, grilling, or consuming raw vegetables and fruits in salads. Processed sauces, sugar, and salt should be avoided or limited [11].

Abundant scientific evidence supports the health benefits of this diet. International research shows that it improves life expectancy and protects against diseases such as Alzheimer's, cardiorespiratory diseases, cancer, and more [12–18]. However, studies examining global trends in adherence to MedD show that European countries in the Mediterranean region have experienced a significant decline in adherence over the past 70 years, which has been attributed to the increased consumption of popular (junk) food from Northern Europe and the United States. For instance, Greece, which was at the top of the MedD adherence ranking in the 1960s, has dropped to the tenth position in recent years, while Spain has dropped to the eighteenth position. In contrast, countries such as Denmark have shown improvement, moving from the 40th to the 32nd position, and Morocco has risen to the second position in recent years. North America, on the other hand, has the lowest adherence to the Mediterranean Diet worldwide [19]. This trend is especially pronounced among young people [20].

New data show a worldwide rise in unhealthy eating habits [1,2]. The Spanish National Institute of Statistics [15], for example, found that in 2022 young Spaniards between the ages of 15 and 17 consumed a diet high in fast food that requires little preparation, such as sandwiches, pizzas, pasta, hamburgers, meats, etc. Research shows an increase in poor nutrition among young people in recent years. However, during the COVID-19 pandemic, data on the eating habits of young people are unclear. While some studies show healthier habits than previous years [21], others show the opposite [22]. International research on this topic has also reported mixed results [23,24]. This variability in results may be due to several factors, including the phase of the pandemic during which the measurements were taken, the geographical area of residence, and other sociodemographic factors.

These habits translate into an unhealthy age group of overweight (249,500) and obese (40,600) young people, which represent 16% and 2.6%, respectively, of the 1,530,209 people in the 15–17 age group in Spain [25].

The new life cycle that starts with tertiary education means, for many, leaving the family home, moving to a new city, time pressure, food vendors that offer unhealthy menus, and economic factors that can influence the choice of unhealthy food [26,27], even when the individual internalized healthy eating habits in childhood. The goal of this work is to know the adherence of the university community of Almeria (Spain) to the Mediterranean Diet. According to our hypothesis, sociodemographic factors and consuming habits explain why a high percentage of the university community does not adhere to the Mediterranean diet, particularly students living alone.

2. Materials and Methods

Research for this article was carried out at the University of Almeria (UAL) during the academic year 2021/2022 (September–November). Our selection of the UAL community was based on two factors. (1) The community was already interested in the topic. To promote healthy eating habits on campus, the university's Vice-Rectorate for Sports, Sustainability, and a Healthy University funded the diagnostic survey, "Nutritional Habits, Health, and Environmental Engagement in the University Community", that we designed, conducted, and analyzed for this paper. (2) This university community belongs to the province of Almeria, where abundant, high-quality food choices are widely available. Often called the orchard of Europe, Almeria is the largest fruit and vegetable producer in Europe, and it provides fresh seafood along 217 kilometers of coastline. Therefore, healthy foods are plenty and at hand in the vicinity of the university campus.

2.1. Participants

The scope of the study covers a university community of 15,268 people. We assumed an error $\pm$ 3.9, resulting in 610 completed surveys. Of this sample, 64.7% were women, 34.1% were men, and 1.3% preferred not to say. Further, 23% were Teaching and Research

Staff (PDI), and 17.3% were Administration and Services Staff (PAS) (These professionals work in different services: Rectorate, Vice Rectorates, Faculties or Schools, libraries, etc. In addition, they have different professional scales. We grouped them under the heading Management and Administration Services) and 59.7% were students. The average age was 32 years. In total, 92.5% are Spaniards (see Table 1).

Table 1. Sample characteristics.

		%
Sex	Women	64.7
	Men	34.1
Origin	Spanish	92.5
	International	7.5
Role or profession	Students	59.7
	Professors	23
	Administration and services personnel	17.3
Work or study center	School of Engineering	6.4
	Faculty of Education	14.8
	Faculty of Health Sciences	14.8
	Faculty of Economics and Business Sciences	9.8
	Faculty of Experimental Sciences	14.1
	Faculty of Law	6.2
	Faculty of Humanities	4.9
	Faculty of Psychology	11.5
	International School of Doctoral Programmes	9.2
	Management and Administration Services	8.4

Source: Authors' elaboration.

2.2. Instrument

The questionnaire, entitled "Nutritional Habits, Health and Environmental Engagement in the University Community", had four sections: respondents' informed consent, consumption behavior, food and sustainability knowledge, and lifestyle and sociodemographic data.

To ascertain the level of adherence to the MedD, we used the Mediterranean Diet Score 2 Tool (T-MDS) [11]. The T-MDS index is calculated by assigning a value of 0 or 1 to nine components of daily intake. A value of 1 is assigned if the respondents' daily consumption of protective MedD foods is equal to or greater than the average intake of these foods and 0 if consumption is lower. The score evaluates the daily intake of nine components:

- The ratio of monounsaturated fatty acids to saturated fatty acids (MUFA/SFA according to the Spanish Food Composition Database (BEDCA) [28].
- High consumption of vegetables, legumes, fruit and nuts, cereals, and fish.
- Moderate consumption of alcohol, milk, and dairy products.
- Low consumption of meat and derivatives.

To obtain more detailed information on respondents' eating habits, we also questioned them about the types of foods they consumed in four intake categories: dairy products (skimmed, semi, or whole milk), cereals (whole or white), fish (white or blue), and meat (red or white).

Following the methods outlined by Giménez [29], we calculated our respondents' average intake of each dietary element. For each of the components, individuals receive a positive point if their intake is higher than the sample's average for components understood as "protective" (vegetables, legumes, fruits, nuts, cereals, and fish) and zero if their intake is lower than the average for "non-protective" components (meat and dairy). For the ratio of monounsaturated fats to saturated fats, we scored 1 for above the median and 0 otherwise.

We assessed the frequency of consumption for each specific type of food or beverage using a table with single-response boxes, coded in appropriate amounts (grams and/or servings), and with eight possible answers (from 0 to 7 days a week). For weekly reference foods and for daily reference foods such as water, dairy, cereals, vegetables, and fruits, we provided 4 possible answers (from 0 to more than 3 servings/day) [30] (To standardize the servings, participants were shown a fact sheet based on the recommended energy and nutrient intake in the European Union, specifying the amount that corresponded to each serving and for each food (for example, 1 serving of white meat = 150 gr; or 1 serving of olive oil = 1 tablespoon) [31]). The reference period about which respondents were questioned was within the last month.

In general, the sum of points from all components ranges from 0 to 9, where "0" means no adherence to the MedD and "9" means the maximum level of adherence to the MedD. We rated 7–9 points as "good" adherence [17,29,30].

2.3. Procedure

We obtained our sample in stages. First, we sent an email to the entire university community. Recipients who decided to participate in the study could access the survey through a link attached to the email. Second, we sent another email asking participants to complete a stratified sample according to their role in UAL (Students, Administration and Services Staff, Teaching and Research Staff) [see Figure 1].

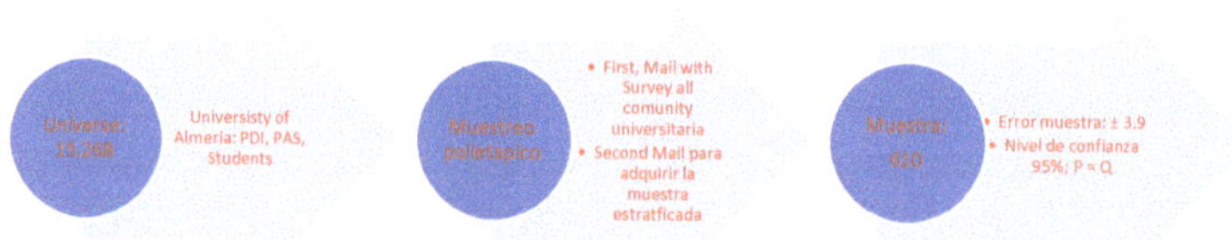

Figure 1. Survey Datasheet. Source: Author's elaboration.

For data analysis, we used the statistical package SPSS 25.0.0 from IBM Statistics. For the linear regression, we had SPSS convert ordinal and nominal variables into dummy variables, choosing the Faculty of Education Sciences as the SPSS "reference category" for the "study and work center" variable because it had the largest number of UAL students.

3. Results and Discussion

In general, 78.2% of those surveyed considered their lifestyle to be healthy or very healthy, 21.3% unhealthy, and 0.6% not at all healthy. Those who believed that their lifestyle was healthy related it mostly to healthy eating ("eating healthy", "a varied diet", "low consumption of fats and sugars", "following the Mediterranean Diet") (Spontaneous answers to an open-ended question), along with physical exercise and adequate rest. A total of 71.8% of the university community indicated that they always or almost always maintained a healthy diet, 21.9% sometimes, and 6.2% almost never or never.

However, in line with the aims of this study, we investigated actual food intake to check the correspondence between respondents' perception of their healthy eating habits and the parameters for healthy eating as defined by the Mediterranean Diet. Data in Table 2 show that respondents met the recommendations for eating vegetables but were deficient in critical areas: the recommended consumption of cereals, nuts, and seeds, low intake of water and fruit, and excessive consumption of processed foods, salt, and sweets, counter to the recommendations of the AESAN [5]. This could be due to choosing a convenient substitute between meals or snacks. We see a similar outcome in other studies of Spaniards' eating habits [32,33].

Table 2. Relationship between MedD recommendations and survey results.

Food Group	Servings Recommended (BEDCA *)	% Surveyed Who Follow Recommendations (Total)
Water	1.5 to 2 L of water per day.	8.8%
Vegetables	Minimum 2 servings per day.	90.7%
Cereals	1–2 servings per day, preferably the whole-grain variety.	42.2%
Olive oil	2–3 servings per day.	56.4%
Fruit	2–3 servings per day.	24.7%
Dairy products	2–3 servings per day.	63.8%
Nuts and seeds	1–2 servings per day.	67.6%
Fish	2–3 servings per week. **	64.5% oily fish; 83.4% white fish
White meat	2 servings per week.	58.2%
Red meat	No more than 2 servings per week.	93.55%
Salt	To reduce consumption or avoid it by substituting it with spices.	46%
Processed food	Less than once per week.	40.2%
Sweets	Less than 2 servings per week.	23.9%
Wine	With moderation and respecting customs.	46%

* BEDCA (Base Española de Datos y Composición de Alimentos). ** The recommended guidelines do not distinguish between blue or white fish (this study separated them due to curiosity about the consumption of polyunsaturated fatty acids in the population surveyed). Source: Authors' elaboration.

When we used these data to test the MedD index, we verified that (1) no one had no adherence at all (value 0) nor total adherence (value 9) (see Table 3); (2) we found the highest percentage (25.1%) for value 1 on the scale. In other words, 1 out of every 4 people in the Almeria University community eats almost no MedD-recommended foods.

Table 3. Adherence to the Mediterranean Diet.

Score	N	%
1.00	153	25.1
2.00	34	5.6
3.00	62	10.2
4.00	92	15.1
5.00	105	17.2
6.00	90	14.8
7.00	48	7.9
8.00	26	4.3
Total	610	100.0

Source: Authors' elaboration.

More specifically, after grouping the results into three summary blocks, we found that 40.9% had low adherence, 47% had intermediate adherence, and 12.1% had high adherence (see Figure 2).

Collating the level of MedD adherence with respondents' sociodemographic characteristics, we found that women had a higher adherence rate, 17%, compared to 7.1% for men. Spaniards had higher adherence rates than non-Spaniards, more than half of whom scored at a low level of adherence (see Table 4).

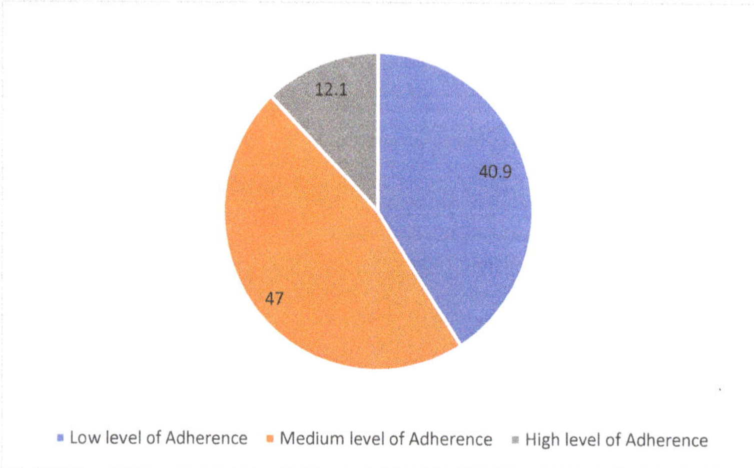

Figure 2. Adherence to the Mediterranean Diet (%). Source: Authors' elaboration.

Table 4. Level of adherence by origin and individual variables (%).

		Low Level of Adherence	Medium Level of Adherence	High Level of Adherence
Sex	Woman	31.2%	51.8%	17.0%
	Man	40.4%	52.5%	7.1%
Origin	Spanish	38.6%	48.4%	13.0%
	International	53.3%	42.2%	4.4%
Age	18–20	41.0%	44.0%	15.0%
	21–25	32.2%	57.5%	10.3%
	26–30	39.3%	44.6%	16.1%
	31–35	28.1%	53.1%	18.8%
	36–40	32.3%	51.6%	16.1%
	41–45	25.8%	51.6%	22.6%
	46–50	26.2%	59.5%	14.3%
	51–55	36.4%	50.9%	12.7%
	56–60	30.8%	64.1%	5.1%
	>60	50.0%	38.9%	11.1%
Role or activity	Students	42.3%	46.3%	11.5%
	Professors	27.9%	55.9%	16.2%
	Administration and services personnel	32.4%	54.1%	13.5%
Centre of study or work	School of Engineering	64.1%	28.2%	7.7%
	Faculty of Education	47.8%	41.1%	11.1%
	Faculty of Health Sciences	25.6%	56.7%	17.8%
	Faculty of Economics and Business Sciences	66.7%	28.3%	5.0%
	Faculty of Experimental Sciences	33.7%	51.2%	15.1%
	Faculty of Law	47.4%	36.8%	15.8%
	Faculty of Humanities	33.3%	46.7%	20.0%
	Faculty of Psychology	45.7%	44.3%	10.0%
	International School of Doctoral Programmes	30.4%	58.9%	10.7%
	Management and Administration Services	23.5%	68.6%	7.8%

Source: Authors' elaboration.

Taking age into account, we found that no age group showed a high level of MedD adherence. Among people between 41 and 45 years of age, 22.6% was the highest value. The 56 to 60 age group had the lowest, only 5.1%. Therefore, our data mostly showed low adherence, especially among those over 60 years of age and those between 18 and 20 years of age, with medium adherence primarily among those between 51 and 60 years of age (see Table 4).

By role at the university, UAL students showed the lowest adherence to the Mediterranean diet: 42.3% scored low, compared to 27.9% of teaching and research staff and 32.4% of administrative and service staff.

We found similar results in other studies in Spain [34–40] and internationally [41,42], which confirm that students consume more fats, proteins, sweets, and snacks than the MedD recommends, and that, as we also observed, they consume lesser quantities of legumes, nuts, fruits, vegetables, and olive oil. This may be due to low economic capital [30], little disposable time for cooking [37], or the novelty of living more independently from their families [35].

Moreover, the lack of MedD adherence among students is not exclusive to Almeria University. We see it in other Spanish universities. At the University of Alicante, for example, no group of students presented a satisfactory intake of the fundamental MedD foods [34]. At the Miguel Hernández University of Elche (Alicante), one in four students had low or very low adherence to MedD [43]. At the University of Granada [27], more than 77% of respondents needed to improve their diets, and only 22.8% had adequate eating habits.

In our opinion, these results are primarily because of the "student lifestyle" and activity-filled university life outweigh education and information about health issues [44]. Second, education alone is not enough without a capacity for analysis and critical thinking. In this regard, the pilot study of Sánchez et al. [38] showed that providing specific information exclusive to MedD led to higher adherence scores.

However, a few studies present more encouraging data on student adherence. A survey at the Soria campus of the University of Valladolid showed that 11.7% of students had low adherence to MedD (compared to our 42.3%); 46.8%, average; and 41.1%, optimal [43]. In addition, student adherence was generally higher at the University of Extremadura, with an average MedD score of 5.72 [45], compared to 3.9 at the University of Almeria.

On the other hand, teaching, research, and administrative staff have higher rates of adherence to the MedD than students because of their higher incomes and more structured schedules, which allow them to buy fresh foods in greater variety and schedule time for cooking. By center (studies and work), the Faculty of Humanities has the largest percentage of high MedD adherence (20%), followed by the Faculty of Health Sciences (17.8%). On the low end, the Faculty of Economics and Business Sciences scored only 5% for high-level adherence. Overall, 66.7% showed low adherence to the Mediterranean Diet (see Table 4 and Figure 3).

To identify possible predictors of MedD variability, we performed four linear regression models (see Table 5):

In Model 1, we introduced individual and demographic variables. Clearly, the most predictive variable is sex (female), followed by Spanish citizenship and, on the negative side, living alone. In other words, Spanish women who live with family members have greater MedD adherence. The variables of student status and young age are negative predictors of MedD adherence. Therefore, the diet of professionals (teaching and research staff, and administrative and service staff) shows the most MedD eating. Youth and being a student correspond to less MedD eating. In short, the combination of sociodemographic variables that predict high scores on MedD adherence suggests the profile of a woman of Spanish nationality, living with her family, not a student, and not young.

In Model 2, we introduced consumption-habit variables. The first thing we note is that only the personal variable of being a woman has more explanatory weight than consumption habits. Secondly, reading labels and regular exercise are positively related to

MedD. Therefore, informing oneself about the products one consumes, avoiding snacks between meals, and regular exercise are the consumption habits that define MedD in our sample.

In Model 3, we added variables of knowledge and information about healthy eating. This allowed us to observe a significant positive relationship between high MedD values and participants' knowledge of what constitutes a Healthy Dish. Other critical information, however, was not significant in predicting MedD variability, namely, awareness of which foods contain monounsaturated and polyunsaturated fatty acids, knowledge of how to read food labels and knowledge of the glycaemic index and what it tells us about foods.

In this model, personal variables and consumption habits have greater explanatory power for MedD adherence than information about food.

Finally, in Model 4, we introduced variables of sustainability. We see that throwing food away is a negative predictor of MedD adherence, and recycling waste is a positive predictor. Specifically, people who do not throw food away or recycle waste follow MedD guidelines more closely.

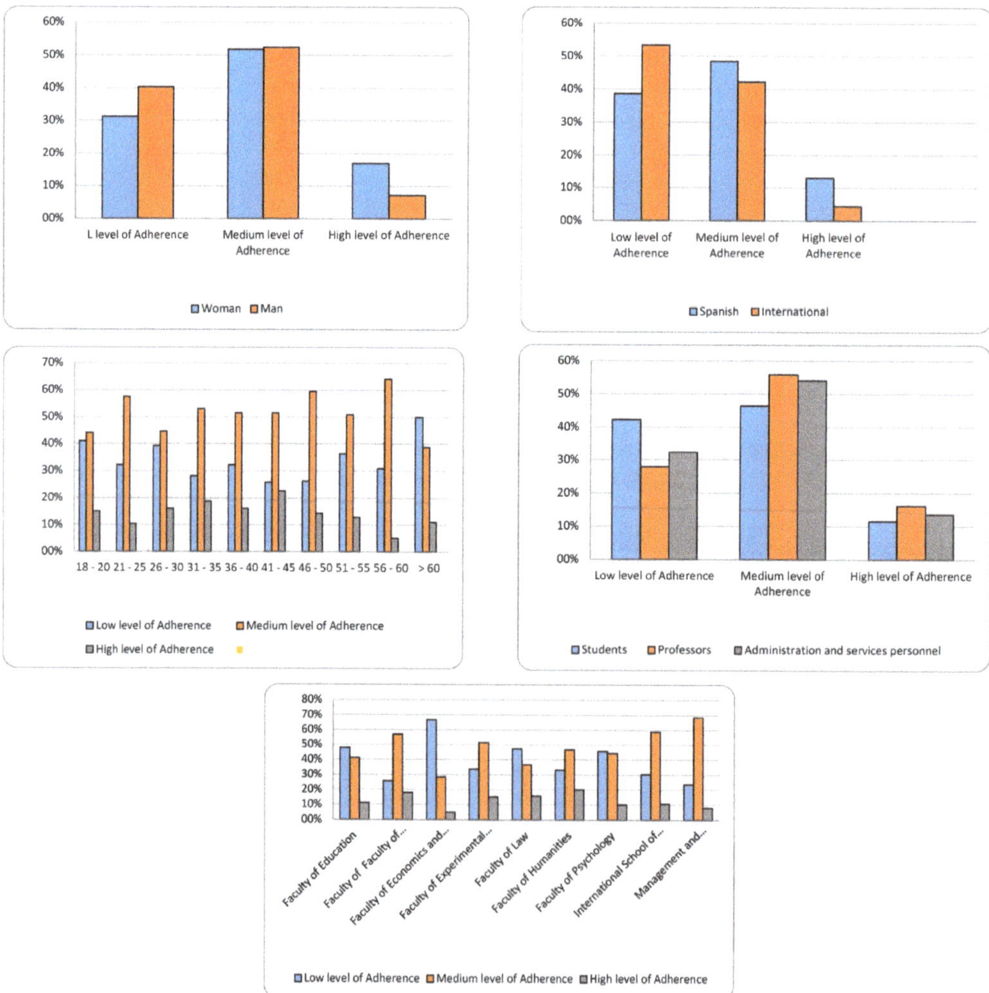

Figure 3. Level of adherence by origin and individual variables (%). Source: Author's elaboration.

Table 5. Models explaining the degree of MedD.

	Personal Variables	Model 1	Model 2	Model 3	Model 4
	Sex (female)	0.295 *	0.257 *	0.254 *	0.264
	Household type (alone)	−0.144 **	−0.123 **	−0.096 **	−0.103
	Origin (Spanish)	0.179 *	0.148 *	0.154 *	0.141
	Role (student)	−0.097 **	−0.083 **	0.044 ***	0.038
	Age	−0.054 **	−0.050 **	−0.155 **	−0.141 **
	School of Engineering	0.065 ***	0.065 ***	0.064 ***	0.067
	Faculty of Health Sciences	0.011 ***	0.039 ***	0.030 ***	0.064 ***
	Faculty of Economics and Business Sciences	0.106 ***	0.131 ***	0.135 ***	0.162 ***
	Faculty of Experimental Sciences	−0.004 ***	−0.011 ***	0.003 ***	0.27 ***
	Faculty of Law	−0.069 ***	−0.037 ***	−0.044 ***	−0.029 ***
	Faculty of Humanities	0.019 ***	0.040 ***	0.035 ***	0.054 ***
	Faculty of Psychology	−0.090 ***	−0.042 ***	−0.036 ***	−0.035 ***
	International School of Doctoral Programmes	−0.006 ***	−0.044 ***	−0.056 ***	−0.045 ***
	Management and Administration Services	−0.058 ***	−0.043 ***	−0.040 ***	−0.034 ***
Consumption habits	Read the labels		0.159 *	0.155 *	0.129 *
	I like cooking		0.097 **	0.089 **	0.095 **
	Snacking between meals		−0.123 **	−0.128 **	−0.122 **
	Plan a meal		0.030 ***	0.026 ***	0.016 ***
	Regular exercise		0.149 *	0.140 *	0.132 *
Knowledge/ awareness	Healthy Dish			0.123 **	0.015 **
	Omega-rich salmon			0.084 ***	0.080 ***
	High GI egg			0.019 ***	0.015 ***
	Healthy Labelling			0.041 ***	0.024 ***
Sustainability	Throwing food away				−0.108 **
	Interest in learning about the environment				0.007 ***
	Recycle waste				0.121 **
	Type of bags I use				−0.92 ***
	Coefficient/ratio R^2	0.241	0.309	0.318	0.344

Source: own elaboration. * $p < 0.01$; ** $p < 0.05$; *** $p > 0.05$.

In summary, Model 4, which encompasses all the variables (individual, consumption habits, Knowledge/awareness, and Sustainability), shows that being a woman and exercising regularly implies greater adherence to MedD, as the international research shows [46–48].

In all societies, women are mainly responsible for shopping and food preparation. Women are taught culinary skills and abilities as part of their socialization more often than men, and they are responsible for the culture of beauty [49,50]. As our data confirm, women are more careful with their diet than men. In addition, Spanish women and those living with Spanish relatives—compared to foreign students living away from their family homes—show a higher MedD adherence because of their culinary socialization. The manner of eating with family who shares the same food standards, and the practices of sitting around a table together and carrying on a conversation without digital devices, help to maintain healthy eating patterns [51,52].

Consumption and recreation habits also factor into the MedD score. Consumers who read labels to find out about the characteristics of what they eat show more interest in healthy food practices, such as MedD.

The relationship between regular physical activity and adherence to MedD is consistent with the other relationships we have pointed to as indicators of healthy living. Alone, exercise does not necessarily predict healthy eating. Physical activity is the greatest benefit to a healthy life when the motivation to exercise is intrinsic rather than extrinsic [53], that is, exercising for personal enjoyment and satisfaction, as opposed to seeking an external benefit or reward [54]. Survey data from Padial, Viciana, and Palomares [27] suggest a case of extrinsically motivated exercise, when 77% of their sample reported nutritional deficiencies, although 86.6% exercised regularly.

4. Conclusions

The primary conclusion we derive from our results is that a significant number of people at the University of Almeria do not comply with the recommendations for healthy eating issued by competent authorities.

The second conclusion concerns student status at UAL. Of all the participant roles we tested, students are the least adherent to MedD. In our case study, academic education had little relevance to the level of MedD adherence. Even students of the Faculty of Health Sciences and the Faculty of Education, which offers degrees in Physical Education and Sports, did not show high adherence to MedD compared to other faculties.

As a third conclusion, the linear regression shows two personal variables—(1) Spanish women and (2) living with families and children—to have the greatest effect on the variability of MedD adherence. These two variables consistently predict high values for three critical indicators: healthy consumption habits, regular exercise, and a sustainable lifestyle (not wasting food and recycling).

Intervention Plan

Despite the detailed data on the Almeria University community's average level of MedD adherence, and due to the benefits that high MedD levels generate, we believe that intervention in food consumption is required in order to improve the health standards of the university community. We propose two major lines of work:

First, we must disseminate knowledge on healthy habits beyond the instruction currently received by students of Health Sciences and Physical Activity and Sports. Regardless of the role a person performs on the university campus, adequate knowledge of healthy eating and the implications of that knowledge for everyday life will facilitate an increase in MedD adherents and the transmission of adherence through their social relationships, both university, and family.

Second, we must intervene in the offerings of the many catering services on campus to encourage MedD-recommended food choices that utilize local products. As noted above, Almeria supplies the whole of Europe with fruit and vegetable products and has many fishing ports. Thus, instead of advertising unhealthy, ultra-processed foods, the university should publicize the benefits of MedD more widely.

This intervention began in an incipient way during the academic year 2022/2023 with the creation of a registered action protocol [55]. Its effects will be assessed in future studies.

Author Contributions: Study concept and design, M.M.H., Á.A.G. and J.C.C.O. Data acquisition, M.M.H., Á.A.G. and J.C.C.O. Analysis and interpretation of data, Á.A.G., M.M.H. and J.C.C.O. Preparation of manuscript, Á.A.G., M.M.H. and J.C.C.O. Critical revision of the manuscript for important intellectual content, Á.A.G., M.M.H. and J.C.C.O. All authors have read and agreed to the published version of the manuscript.

Funding: Funding was received from the Laboratory of Social and Cultural Anthropology (University of Almería).

Institutional Review Board Statement: The study was conducted according to the guidelines of the Declaration of Helsinki and Ley Orgánica de Protección de Datos y Garantía de Derechos Digitales (LOPDGDD 3/2018) that regulates the processing of data of both minors and adults.

Informed Consent Statement: Informed consent was obtained from all subjects involved in the study.

Data Availability Statement: Not applicable.

Conflicts of Interest: The authors declare no conflict of interest.

Ethical Considerations: This article is carried out within the framework of the UAL-ASASO Transfiere programme (2022–2023) and under which approval for data processing has been obtained through the bioethics committee, with reference code UALBIO2022/038.

References

1. Organización Mundial de la Salud. Enfermedades No Transmisibles. 2018. Available online: https://www.who.int/es/news-room/fact-sheets/detail/noncommunicable-diseases (accessed on 23 March 2023).
2. Jimeno-Martínez, A.; Maneschy, I.; Rupérez, A.I.; Moreno, L.A. Factores determinantes del comportamiento alimentario y su impacto sobre la ingesta y la obesidad en niños. *J. Behav. Feed.* **2021**, *1*, 60–71.
3. Dressl, N.L.; Balzaretti, M.L.; Barrosela, V.B.; Deluchi, D.; Rioja, M.; Torresani, E. Factores influyentes en la alimentación emocional y el riesgo de trastornos de la conducta alimentaria en mujeres adultas. *Rev. Nutr. Investig.* **2019**, 102–147.
4. Sozoranga, D.; León, D.; Mediavilla, C.; Palchisaca, Z. Comportamiento alimentario, actividad física e intención de práctica en estudiantes de bachillerato durante la pandemia. *Polo Conoc. Rev. Cient. Prof.* **2020**, *5*, 147–162.
5. Agencia Española de Seguridad Alimentaria. *Informe del Comité Científico de la Agencia Española de Seguridad Alimentaria y Nutrición Sobre Recomendaciones Dietéticas Saludables y Sostenibles Complementadas con Recomendaciones de Actividad Física Para la Población Española.*; Ministerio de Consumo: Madrid, Spain, 2022.
6. Keys, A. Coronary heart disease, serum cholesterol, and the diet. *Acta Med. Scand.* **1980**, *207*, 153–160. [CrossRef]
7. Serra, L.; Ribas, L.; García, R.; Pérez, C.; Peña, L.; Aranceta, J. Hábitos alimentarios y consumo de alimentos en la población infantil y juvenil española (1998–2000): Variables socioeconómicas y geográficas. *Med. Clín.* **2002**, *121*, 126–131.
8. Sánchez, M.; García, A.; Hidalgo, J.; García, M.Á.; Tarín, J.; Cano, A. Dieta mediterránea y salud: Una revisión sistemática de estudios epidemiológicos y ensayos de intervención. *Maturitas* **2020**, *136*, 25–37.
9. Romagnolo, D.; Selmin, O. Mediterranean diet and prevention of chronic diseases. *Nutr. Today* **2017**, *52*, 208. [CrossRef]
10. Sotos, M.; Mattei, J. Mediterranean diet and cardiometabolic diseases in racial/ethnic minority populations in the United States. *Nutrients* **2018**, *10*, 352. [CrossRef]
11. Agencia Española de Seguridad Alimentaria. *Informe del Comité Científico de la Agencia Española de Seguridad Alimentaria y Nutrición Sobre Recomendaciones Dietéticas Sostenibles y Recomendaciones de Actividad Física Para la Población*; Ministerio de Consumo: Madrid, Spain, 2022.
12. Caplliure, J.; Peralta, T.; Carrera, S.; Cuerda, M.; Drehmer, E.; López, M.; De la Rubia Ortí, J.E. Alternativa terapéutica de la dieta mediterránea cetogénica para mejorar la actividad mitocondrial en la Esclerosis Lateral Amiotrófica (ELA): Una Revisión Integral. *Cienc. Aliment. Nutr.* **2020**, *8*, 23–35.
13. Failde, J.M.; Ruiz, L.; Pérez, M.R.; Lameiras, M.; Rodríguez, Y. Evolución de la calidad de vida y comportamientos relacionados con la salud en estudiantes universitarios españoles. *Rev. Int. Planif. Gest. Salud* **2019**, *34*, 789–801.
14. Guzmán, M.; Lobo, M. Beneficios de la reducción del consumo de azúcares y aumento de la actividad física en adultos jóvenes con obesidad y la prevención de la diabetes. *Acta Acad.* **2020**, *67*, 185–194.
15. Trichopoulos, D. Diet and survival of elderly greeks-a link to the past. *Am. J. Clin. Nutr.* **1995**, *61*, S1346–S1350. [CrossRef] [PubMed]
16. Trichopoulou, A.; Bamia, C.; Trichopoulos, D. Anatomy of health effects of Mediterranean diet: Greek EPIC prospective cohort study. *Br. Med. J.* **2009**, *338*, b2337. [CrossRef] [PubMed]
17. Trichopoulou, A.; Costacou, T.; Bamia, C.; Trichopoulos, D. Adherence to a Mediterranean diet and survival in a Greek population. *N. Engl. J. Med.* **2003**, *348*, 2599–2608. [CrossRef]
18. Troncoso, C.; Amaya, J.P. Factores sociales en las conductas alimentarias de estudiantes universitarios. *Rev. Chil. Nutr.* **2009**, *36*, 1090–1097. [CrossRef]
19. Vilarnau, C.; Stracker, D.; Funtikov, A.; da Silva, R.; Estruch, R.; Bach-Faig, A. Worldwide adherence to Mediterranean Diet between 1960 and 2011. *Eur. J. Clin. Nutr.* **2019**, *72* (Suppl. S1), 83–91. [CrossRef]
20. Serra, L.; Castro, I.; Ruano, C. *La Dieta Mediterránea: Claves y Evolución en España*; Panorama Social: Madrid, Spain, 2014.
21. Vall, H.; Andrés, A.; Saldaña, C. El impacto de la pandemia por covid-19 y del confinamiento en las alteraciones alimentarias y el malestar emocional en adolescentes y jóvenes de España. *Behav. Psychol.* **2021**, *29*, 345–364. [CrossRef]
22. Bravo, S.; Castillo, A.; Izquierdo, D.; Rodas, P. Hábitos alimenticios, nocivos y rendimiento académico en estudiantes universitarios en tiempos de COVID-19. *Vive Rev. Salud* **2021**, *4*, 225–238.
23. Rojas, J.A. Alimentación emocional durante tiempos de COVID-19 en adultos jóvenes de 18 a 29 años. *Rev. Mex. Med. Forense Cienc. Salud* **2020**, *5*, 66–71.
24. Esparza, L.; Cruzado, A.; Dávila, M.; Díaz, Y.; La Cruz, D.; Ascoy, B.; Huamán, J. Modificaciones de la conducta alimentaria, actividad física y salud mental por la cuarentena COVID-19 en adultos jóvenes. *Rev. Med. Herediana* **2022**, *33*, 15–23. [CrossRef]
25. Instituto Nacional de Estadística. *Encuesta Nacional de Salud. Ministerio de Sanidad-Secretaría General de Salud Digital, Información e Innovación del Sistema Nacional de Salud*; INE: Madrid, Spain, 2022.
26. López, P.J.T.; Marcos, A.T.; Royo, J.M.P.; Carbayo, J.A.H.; Marcos, M.L.T.; Gil, J.F.L. Physical activity and its association with Mediterranean diet patterns among Spanish university students. *Nutr. Hosp. Organo Of. Soc. Esp. Nutr. Parenter. Enter.* **2022**, *39*, 603–609.

27. Padial, R.; Viciana, M.; Palomares, J. Adherencia a la dieta mediterránea, la actividad física y su relación con el IMC, en estudiantes universitarios del grado de primaria, mención de educación física, de Granada. *Educ. Sport Health Phys. Act.* **2018**, *2*, 30–49. [CrossRef]
28. Ministerio de Sanidad, Servicios Sociales e Igualdad. In Base de Datos Española de Composición de Alimentos. Available online: https://www.bedca.net/ (accessed on 23 March 2023).
29. Giménez, N. Estudio Nutricional de Población Mediterránea Situada en el Sureste Español y su Relación con Patologías Asociadas al Estado Nutricional. Ph.D. Thesis, Universidad de Murcia, Murcia, Spain, 2019.
30. Hodge, A.M.; Bassett, J.K.; Shivappa, N.; Hebert, J.R.; English, D.R.; Giles, G.G.; Severi, G. Dietary inflammatory index, Mediterranean diet score, and lung cancer: A prospective study. *Cancer Causes Control* **2016**, *27*, 907–917. [CrossRef] [PubMed]
31. García-Gabarra, A.; Castellà-Soley, M.; Calleja-Fernández, A. Ingestas de energía y nutrientes recomendadas en la Unión Europea: 2008–2016. *Nutr. Hosp.* **2017**, *34*, 490–498. [CrossRef] [PubMed]
32. Medina, F.X.; Aguilar, A.; Solé, J.M. Aspectos sociales y culturales sobre la obesidad: Reflexiones necesarias desde la salud pública. *Nutr. Clín. Diet. Hosp.* **2014**, *34*, 67–71.
33. Ruiz, E.; Ávila, J.M.; Valero, T.; Del Pozo, S.; Rodríguez, P.; Aranceta, J.; Varela, G. Ingesta, perfil y fuentes dietéticas de energía en la población española: Resultados del estudio ANIBES. *Nutrientes* **2015**, *7*, 4739–4762. [CrossRef]
34. Moncada, R.; Norte, A.; Zaragoza, A.; Fernández, J.; Davó, M. ¿Siguen patrones de dieta mediterránea los universitarios españoles? *Nutr. Hosp.* **2012**, *27*, 1952–1959.
35. Pastor, R.; Bibiloni, M.D.M.; Tur, J.A. Patrones de consumo de alimentos en estudiantes universitarios de Zamora. *Nutr. Hosp.* **2017**, *34*, 1424–1431.
36. Pérez, L.; Mingo, T.; Bayona, I.; Ferrer, M.; Márquez, E.; Ramírez, R.; Navas, C.; Navas, F. Calidad de la dieta en estudiantes universitarios con distinto perfil académico. *Nutr. Hosp.* **2015**, *31*, 2230–2239.
37. Redondo, M.P.; Mateo, B.; Carreño, L.; Marugán, J.M.; Fernández, M.; Camina, M. Ingesta dietética y adherencia a la dieta mediterránea en un grupo de estudiantes universitarios en función de la práctica deportiva. *Nutr. Hosp.* **2016**, *33*, 1172–1178. [CrossRef]
38. Sánchez, V.; Aguilar Martínez, A. Hábitos alimentarios y conductas relacionadas con la salud en una población universitaria. *Nutr. Hosp.* **2015**, *31*, 449–457.
39. Tárraga, A.; Panisello, J.M.; Carbayo, J.A.; López, J.F.; García, E.; Tárraga, P.J. Valoración de la adherencia a la dieta mediterránea en estudiantes universitarios de Ciencias de la Salud y su relación con el nivel de actividad física. *Nutr. Hosp.* **2021**, *38*, 814–820.
40. Sánchez, M.A.; Gutiérrez, A.; Rizo, M.; Cortés, E. Estudio longitudinal sobre la adherencia al patrón de Dieta Mediterránea en estudiantes de Ciencias de la salud. *Rev. Esp. Nutr. Hum. Diet.* **2018**, *22*, 4–13. [CrossRef] [PubMed]
41. Mieziene, B.; Emeljanovas, A.; Fatkulina, N.; Stukas, R. Dietary pattern and its correlates among Lithuanian young adults: Mediterranean diet approach. *Nutrients* **2020**, *12*, 2025. [CrossRef] [PubMed]
42. Santomauro, F.; Lorini, C.; Tanini, T.; Indiani, L.; Lastrucci, V.; Comodo, N.; Bonaccorsi, G. Adherence to Mediterranean diet in a sample of Tuscan adolescents. *Nutrition* **2014**, *30*, 1379–1383. [CrossRef]
43. Barrios, R.; Navarrete, E.; García, M.; González, S.; Valera, D.; Checa, J.; Giménez, G.; Vioque, J. Una menor adherencia a la dieta mediterránea se asocia a una peor salud auto-percibida en población universitaria. *Nutr. Hosp.* **2015**, *31*, 785–792.
44. Ramírez, R.; Márquez, E.M. Relación de la adherencia a la dieta mediterránea con el imc y la actividad física realizada en estudiantes universitarios. *Rev. Int. Deportes Colect.* **2016**, *26*, 36–43.
45. Benítez, A.; Sánchez, S.; Franco, L.; Bermejo, M.; Cubero, J. Adhesión a la dieta mediterránea en estudiantes de la Universidad de Extremadura: Un recurso en educación para la salud. *Rev. Fund. Educ. Méd.* **2016**, *19*, 287–289. [CrossRef]
46. Dernini, S.; Berry, E. Mediterranean diet: From a healthy diet to a sustainable dietary pattern. *Front. Nutr.* **2015**, *2*, 15. [CrossRef]
47. Alonso, R.; García, L.; Patino, M.C.; Sánchez, N.; Gómez, M.; Recio, J. Effectiveness of a multifactorial intervention in increasing adherence to the Mediterranean diet among patients with diabetes mellitus type 2: A controlled and randomized study (EMID study). *Nutrients* **2019**, *11*, 162. [CrossRef]
48. Talegawkar, S.A.; Bandinelli, S.; Bandeen-Roche, K.; Chen, P.; Milaneschi, Y.; Tanaka, T.; Semba, R.D.; Guralnik, J.M.; Ferrucci, L. A higher adherence to a Mediterranean-style diet is inversely associated with the development of frailty in community-dwelling elderly men and women. *J. Nutr.* **2012**, *142*, 2161–2166. [CrossRef] [PubMed]
49. Chumacero Moscoso, J.L. El ser y el Deber ser de la Mujer y del Hombre en el Cuidado Remunerado de Ancianos en Segovia. Master's Thesis, Universidad de Valladolid, Valladolid, Spain, 2018.
50. Martínez, L.M.M.; Araiza, A.; Uriarte, A.G.; Cólera, M.C.P. Género, espacio doméstico y socialización del cuidado: Algunas perspectivas de cambio. *Int. J. Dev. Educ. Psychol. Infad. Rev. Psicol.* **2011**, *5*, 181–186.
51. Abalde, N.; Pino, M. Familia, escuela y adherencia a la dieta mediterránea en infancia y adolescencia. *Rev. Estud. Investig. Psicol. Educ.* **2017**, *5*, 212–217.
52. Frías Armenta, M.; Barrios Gaxiola, M.I. Recursos que contribuyen al desarrollo positivo en jóvenes. *Escr. Psicol.* **2016**, *9*, 37–44. [CrossRef]
53. González, G.; Padial, R.; Espejo, E.; Chacón, R.; Puertas, P.; Pérez, A.J. Relación entre clima motivacional hacia el deporte y adherencia a la dieta mediterránea en estudiantes universitarios de educación física. *Int. J. Dev. Educ. Psychol.* **2017**, *4*, 285–295. [CrossRef]

54. Monserrat, M.; Arjona, Á.; Checa, J.C.; Salguero, D. Relationship between Negative Running Addiction and Eating Disorder Patterns in Runners. *Nutrients* **2021**, *13*, 4344. [CrossRef]
55. Checa, J.C.; Arjona, Á.; Rocamora, P.; Monserrat, M. Protocolo de Actuación Programa ASASO-UAL. Inscrito en el Registro General de la Propiedad Intelectual el 4/3/2022 con Número de Asiento Registral 04/2022/3684. 2022. Available online: http://hdl.handle.net/10835/13980 (accessed on 23 March 2023).

nutrients

MDPI

Article

Osteoporosis Risk in Hemodialysis Patients: The Roles of Gender, Comorbidities, Biochemical Parameters, Health and Diet Literacy

Lan T. H. Le [1,2,3,†], Loan T. Dang [4,5,†], Tsae-Jyy Wang [4], Tuyen G. Do [6], Dung H. Nguyen [6], Trung A. Hoang [6], Minh D. Pham [7,8], Binh N. Do [9,10], Hoang C. Nguyen [3,11], Tu T. Tran [12,13], Linh V. Pham [14,15], Lien T. H. Nguyen [14], Hoi T. Nguyen [16], Nga T. Trieu [17], Thinh V. Do [18], Manh V. Trinh [19], Tung H. Ha [20], Dung T. Phan [21,22], Shwu-Huey Yang [23,24,25], Ngoc N. M. Le [26], Kien T. Nguyen [27] and Tuyen Van Duong [12,23,*]

1 Training and Direction of Healthcare Activity Center, Thai Nguyen National Hospital, Thai Nguyen City 241-24, Vietnam
2 Biochemistry Department, Thai Nguyen National Hospital, Thai Nguyen City 241-24, Vietnam
3 Director Office, Thai Nguyen National Hospital, Thai Nguyen City 241-24, Vietnam
4 School of Nursing, National Taipei University of Nursing and Health Sciences, Taipei 112-19, Taiwan
5 Faculty of Nursing and Midwifery, Hanoi Medical University, Hanoi 115-20, Vietnam
6 Hemodialysis Department, Nephro-Urology-Dialysis Center, Bach Mai Hospital, Hanoi 115-19, Vietnam
7 Department of Nutrition, Military Hospital 103, Hanoi 121-08, Vietnam
8 Department of Nutrition, Vietnam Military Medical University, Hanoi 121-08, Vietnam
9 Department of Military Science, Vietnam Military Medical University, Hanoi 121-08, Vietnam
10 Department of Infectious Diseases, Vietnam Military Medical University, Hanoi 121-08, Vietnam
11 President Office, Thai Nguyen University of Medicine and Pharmacy, Thai Nguyen City 241-17, Vietnam
12 International Ph.D. Program in Medicine, College of Medicine, Taipei Medical University, Taipei 110-31, Taiwan
13 Department of Internal Medicine, Thai Nguyen University of Medicine and Pharmacy, Thai Nguyen 241-17, Vietnam
14 Department of Pulmonary & Cardiovascular Diseases, Hai Phong University of Medicine and Pharmacy Hospital, Hai Phong 042-12, Vietnam
15 President Office, Hai Phong University of Medicine and Pharmacy, Hai Phong 042-12, Vietnam
16 Director Office, Hai Phong International Hospital, Hai Phong 047-08, Vietnam
17 Hemodialysis Division, Hai Phong International Hospital, Hai Phong 047-08, Vietnam
18 Director Office, Bai Chay Hospital, Ha Long 011-21, Vietnam
19 Director Office, Quang Ninh General Hospital, Ha Long 011-08, Vietnam
20 Director Office, General Hospital of Agricultural, Hanoi 125-16, Vietnam
21 Faculty of Nursing, Hanoi University of Business and Technology, Hanoi 116-22, Vietnam
22 Nursing Office, Thien An Obstetrics and Gynecology Hospital, Hanoi 112-06, Vietnam
23 School of Nutrition and Health Sciences, Taipei Medical University, Taipei 110-31, Taiwan
24 Nutrition Research Center, Taipei Medical University Hospital, Taipei 110–31, Taiwan
25 Research Center of Geriatric Nutrition, Taipei Medical University, Taipei 110–31, Taiwan
26 College of Medicine, Hanoi Medical University, Hanoi 115-20, Vietnam
27 Department of Health Promotion, Faculty of Social and Behavioral Sciences, Hanoi University of Public Health, Hanoi 119-10, Vietnam
* Correspondence: tvduong@tmu.edu.tw; Tel.: +886-2-2736-1661 (ext. 6545)
† These authors contributed equally to this work.

Abstract: Osteoporosis is a common bone health disorder in hemodialysis patients that is linked with a higher morbidity and mortality rate. While previous studies have explored the associated factors of osteoporosis, there is a lack of studies investigating the impacts of health literacy (HL) and digital healthy diet literacy (DDL) on osteoporosis. Therefore, we aimed to investigate the associations of HL, DDL, and other factors with osteoporosis among hemodialysis patients. From July 2020 to March 2021, a cross-sectional study was conducted on 675 hemodialysis patients in eight hospitals in Vietnam. The data were collected by using the osteoporosis self-assessment tool for Asians (OSTA) and the 12-item short form of the health literacy questionnaire (HLS-SF12) on digital healthy diet literacy (DDL) and hemodialysis dietary knowledge (HDK). In addition, we also collected information about the socio-demographics, the clinical parameters, the biochemical parameters, and physical activity. Unadjusted and adjusted multinomial logistic regression models were utilized in order to investigate the associations. The proportion of patients at low, medium, and high levels of osteoporosis risk was 39.6%, 40.6%, and 19.8%, respectively. In the adjusted models, women had a higher likelihood of osteoporosis risk than men (odds ratio, OR, 3.46; 95% confidence interval, 95% CI, 1.86, 6.44; $p < 0.001$; and OR, 6.86; 95% CI, 2.96, 15.88; $p < 0.001$). The patients with rheumatoid arthritis (OR, 4.37; 95% CI, 1.67, 11.52; $p = 0.003$) and stomach ulcers (OR, 1.95; 95% CI, 1.01, 3.77; $p = 0.048$) were more likely to have a higher likelihood of osteoporosis risk than those without. The patients who had a higher waist circumference (WC), HL, and DDL were less likely to have a medium level of osteoporosis risk (OR, 0.95; 95% CI, 0.92, 0.98; $p = 0.004$; OR, 0.92; 95% CI, 0.88, 0.96; $p < 0.001$; OR, 0.96; 95% CI, 0.93, 0.99; $p = 0.017$, respectively) and a high level of osteoporosis risk (OR, 0.93; 95% CI, 0.89, 0.97; $p = 0.001$; OR, 0.89; 95% CI, 0.84, 0.94; $p < 0.001$; OR, 0.95; 95% CI, 0.91, 0.99; $p = 0.008$, respectively) compared with a low level of osteoporosis risk and to those with a lower WC, HL, and DDL. In addition, higher levels of hemoglobin (Hb) (OR, 0.79; 95% CI, 0.66, 0.95; $p = 0.014$), hematocrit (Hct) (OR, 0.95; 95% CI, 0.92, 0.99; $p = 0.041$), albumin (OR, 0.91; 95% CI, 0.83, 0.99; $p = 0.030$), and education (OR, 0.37; 95% CI, 0.16, 0.88; $p = 0.025$) were associated with a lower likelihood of a high level of osteoporosis risk. In conclusion, osteoporosis risk is highly prevalent in hemodialysis patients. Improved HL, DDL, education, WC, albumin, Hb, and Hct levels should be considered in preventing hemodialysis patients from developing osteoporosis.

Keywords: hemodialysis; osteoporosis; fracture; health literacy; digital healthy diet literacy; comorbidities; biochemical parameters; detection; prevention; Vietnam

1. Introduction

End-stage renal disease is a global health crisis [1,2]. The worldwide use of renal replacement therapies has increased remarkably from 2618 million people in 2010 to an estimated 5439 million people by 2030 [1]. Among the treatment modalities, hemodialysis is the most common in most countries, including Vietnam [2,3].

Osteoporosis is "a skeletal condition characterized by decreased density (mass/volume) of normally mineralized bone", which leads to a high risk of fracture [4]. Osteoporosis is observed in a large number of hemodialysis patients, ranging from 23% to 41% [5–7]. The consequences of osteoporosis, such as the increased risk of fracture and the greater morbidity and mortality rate, have been documented in the literature [8,9]. Therefore, osteoporosis should be taken into account in the management of hemodialysis patients in order to reduce the burdens on the healthcare system and patients.

There are many factors that may contribute to an increased osteoporosis risk in chronic kidney patients, including abnormal biochemical markers (e.g., calcium, phosphorus, vitamin D, and parathyroid hormone), inflammatory cytokines status, sarcopenia, corticoid use, and lifestyle [10–13]. Factors that are associated with osteoporosis in pre-dialysis or hemodialysis patients have been found in previous studies, e.g., being female, being of an older age, and having a low body mass index [7,14,15]. Abdominal obesity was found to be a preventable factor for osteoporosis risk in hemodialysis patients [16].

Health literacy (HL) and digital healthy diet literacy (DDL) are defined as the individual's capacity to find, understand, appraise, and apply the information that is related to health and digital-healthy-diet-related information in order to prevent disease, to improve healthy eating behavior, and to promote health outcomes [17,18]. The benefits of adequate health literacy in hemodialysis patients have been reported in prior studies, such as improved fluid management and psychological health [19,20]. However, there is limited information about the impacts of health literacy and digital healthy diet literacy on osteoporosis risk in hemodialysis patients. Meanwhile, insufficient health literacy has been associated with a lower adoption rate of osteoporosis-preventive behaviors [21], as well as a higher non-adherence to osteoporosis treatment [22].

Therefore, we conducted a multi-center study in order to explore the associated factors of osteoporosis in hemodialysis patients, where the roles of gender, comorbidities, biochemical parameters, HL, and DDL were emphasized. We hypothesized that the patients with higher HL and DDL, and greater levels in some biochemical components, had a lower likelihood of osteoporosis, whereas being female and living with comorbidities had an increased likelihood of osteoporosis.

2. Materials and Methods

2.1. Study Design and Sample

A cross-sectional study was conducted from July 2020 to March 2021. A total of 1048 eligible participants who were being treated at hemodialysis centers from eight hospitals in Vietnam were recruited, including Bai Chay Hospital (n = 81), Quang Ninh General Hospital (n = 103), Hai Phong International Hospital (n = 43), Hai Phong University of Medicine and Pharmacy Hospital (n = 82), Bach Mai Hospital (n = 251), Military Hospital 103 (n = 147), General Hospital of Agricultural(n = 171), and National Thai Nguyen Hospital (n = 170). A sample of 675 participants (who were aged 45 years or older, had received hemodialysis treatment for at least three months, and were able to communicate in Vietnamese) was analyzed.

2.2. Measurements

2.2.1. The Risk of Osteoporosis

The osteoporosis self-assessment tool for Asians (OSTA) was used to evaluate the risk of osteoporosis. Koh et al. (2001) developed OSTA to screen the fracture risk among post-menopausal women in Asia. This self-assessment tool was not only applied to women, but also to men at risk of osteoporosis [23]. The OSTA score was calculated using Formula (1). Our present study used the dry weight of the participants to calculate the OSTA score.

$$\text{OSTA score} = [\text{weight (kg)} - \text{age (year)}] \times 0.2 \quad (1)$$

The risk of osteoporosis was classified into three groups, in which a score > -1 presents a low risk, a score between -4 and -1 presents a medium risk, and a score < -4 presents a high risk [24].

The OSTA has been reported to be an acceptable tool in detecting the fracture risk and osteoporosis risk in hemodialysis patients [25]. It has also been tested in the Vietnamese population and has shown high sensitivity and specificity, at 74.6% and 81.4%, respectively [26].

2.2.2. Socio-Demographics

The socio-demographic information was collected, including the age (year), gender (men vs. women), marital status (living with/without partner), educational status (illiterate or elementary, junior high school, and senior high school or above), occupation (working vs. not working), social status (low vs. medium or high), ability to pay for medication (very or fairly difficult vs. very or fairly easy), dry weight (kg), and hemodialysis vintage (years).

2.2.3. Clinical Parameters

The clinical parameters were assessed, including comorbid conditions such as rheumatoid arthritis, stomach ulcers, and suspected COVID-19 symptoms (S-COVID19-S), waist circumference after dialysis (cm), and diuretic usage. The participants were screened and categorized as having S-COVID-19-S if they experienced any of the following symptoms: fever, cough, fatigue, dyspnea, myalgia, sputum production/expectoration, sore throat, running nose, confusion, headache, chest pain, rhinorrhea, diarrhea, and/or nausea/vomiting [27].

2.2.4. Biochemical Parameters

The laboratory indicators were collected using chart review, including Hb (g/dL); mean corpuscular volume, MCV (fL); Hct (%); blood cells (white blood cells, $10^3/\mu L$; red blood cells, $10^6/\mu L$; platelet, $10^3/\mu L$); albumin (mg/dL); serum electrolytes (K^+, mEq/L; Na^+ and Cl^-, mmol/L); phosphates (mg/dL); and parathyroid hormone (pg/mL).

2.2.5. Physical Activities

The level of physical activity was measured using the international physical activity questionnaire, short version [28]. The tool was validated and used in Vietnam [20,29]. The patients rated their time spent on four daily activities, including sitting, walking, moderate, and vigorous physical activities throughout the last seven days. The overall physical activity score was calculated as per the instructions from previous studies [20,28].

2.2.6. Health Literacy, Digital Healthy Diet Literacy, and Hemodialysis Diet Knowledge

The 12-item short form of the health literacy questionnaire (HLS-SF12) [30,31] and the digital healthy diet literacy (DDL-4) [18] were used to assess the HL and DDL of the participants. These scales have been validated and widely used in the Vietnamese population [18,30,32,33]. The participants chose one of four options to describe their difficulty for each question, in which, "1" was "very difficult" "2" was "fairly difficult", "3" was "fairly easy", and "4" was "very easy". The HL and DDL indices were calculated using Formula (2). The higher index scores present the better HL or DDL levels [18,34].

$$\text{Index} = (\text{Mean} - 1) \times (50/3) \tag{2}$$

where *Index* is the specific index calculated, *Mean* is the mean of all participating items for each individual, 1 is the minimal possible value of the mean (leading to a minimum value of the index of 0), 3 is the range of the mean, and 50 is the chosen maximum value.

In addition, we used the hemodialysis dietary knowledge (HDK) scale to investigate the participants' knowledge about the hemodialysis diet. This scale contains ten questions about protein, potassium, phosphorus, sodium, and water [35]. There are three possible options, including "correct," "incorrect," and "not sure". The correct answer was categorized as "correct", while incorrect or "not sure" answers were categorized as "incorrect". The possible HDK score varies from 0 to 10, in which a higher score indicates better knowledge. The psychometric testing of HDK was conducted in a previous study [20].

2.3. Data Collection Procedure

The research assistants, including doctors, nurses, and medical students, collected the data after receiving a 4-h training session by two senior researchers at each hospital. Safety guidance for the prevention and control of COVID-19 was also provided during the training, including wearing masks, washing hands, and maintaining physical distance [36].

Participation in this study was completely voluntary. After receiving the consent forms, face-to-face interviews were conducted on patients at the hemodialysis departments. It took about 20–30 min to complete the questionnaire. Then, the research assistants collected information related to the clinical and biochemical parameters from medical records. Finally, all of the data were coded, cleaned, and analyzed confidentially by the researchers.

2.4. Data Analysis

Frequency and percentage were used for a categorical variable, while mean and standard deviation were used for a continuous variable using the chi-square test and one-way ANOVA appropriately. For the non-normal distributed variables, median and interquartile range were reported using the Kruskal–Wallis test. The unadjusted and adjusted models were performed by multinomial logistic regression to identify the associated factors of osteoporosis risks (using the low risk group as the reference). Only the factors with $p < 0.20$ in the unadjusted model were selected into the adjusted model [37]. In the adjusted model, each factor in each subgroup was adjusted by other factors in other subgroups. The correlations among the independent variables were checked prior to running the multinomial logistic regression to determine if these variables were highly correlated. The Spearman correlation coefficients of these variables that were less than 0.3 were accepted to be added to the adjusted model (Supplementary Table S1). All statistical analyses were performed using IBM SPSS Version 26.0 (IBM Corp., Armonk, NY, USA). Statistical significance was established at $p < 0.05$.

3. Results

3.1. Participants' Socio-Demographics

The participants' characteristics are described in Table 1. Of the 675 patients, 337 (50.1%) were male and 336 (49.9%) were female, with a mean age of 61.1 ± 9.6. Overall, the prevalence of osteoporosis risks at low, medium, and high levels were 39.6%, 40.6%, and 19.8%, respectively. The prevalence of low, medium, and high risks of osteoporosis was significantly different in some variables in the groups of socio-demographics (gender, education level, marital status, and medication payment ability); the clinical parameters (rheumatoid arthritis, waist circumference, and diuretic usage); the biochemical parameters (level of serum albumin); and the health literacy and digital health diet literacy ($p < 0.05$).

Table 1. Patients' characteristics and OSTA (n = 675).

Variables	Total n (%)	OSTA			*p*
		Low (n;% = 267; 39.6)	**Medium (n;% = 274; 40.6)**	**High (n;% = 134; 19.8)**	
Socio-demographics					
Gender					<0.001 [a]
Male	337 (50.1)	176 (65.9)	119 (43.6)	42 (31.6)	
Female	336 (49.9)	91 (34.1)	154 (56.4)	91 (68.4)	
Education					0.001 [a]
Illiterate or elementary	316 (50.5)	101 (41.4)	142 (55.7)	73 (57.5)	
Junior high school	182 (29.1)	91 (31.3)	67 (26.3)	24 (18.9)	
Senior high school or above	128(20.4)	52 (21.3)	46 (18.0)	30 (23.6)	
Working status					0.660 [a]
Not working	249 (36.9)	93 (34.8)	104 (38.0)	52.0 (38.8)	
Working	426 (63.1)	174 (65.2)	170 (62.0)	82 (61.2)	
Marital status					0.009 [a]
Without partner	52 (7.8)	13 (4.9)	21 (7.8)	18 (13.6)	
With partner	616 (92.2)	253 (95.1)	249 (92.2)	114 (86.4)	
Social status					0.318 [a]
Low	198 (29.3)	70 (26.2)	88 (32.1)	40 (29.9)	
Middle and high	477 (70.7)	197 (73.8)	186 (67.9)	94 (70.1)	
Medication payment ability					0.035 [a]
Very or fairly difficult	521 (782)	219 (82.3)	209 (77.7)	93 (71.0)	
Very or fairly easy	145 (21.8)	47 (17.7)	60 (22.3)	38 (29.0)	
Hemodialysis vintage, years (Median, IQR)	4.4 (2.2, 7.9)	4.4 (2.4, 7.9)	4.4 (2.4, 8.2)	4.2 (2.0, 7.9)	0.966 [b]

Table 1. *Cont.*

Variables	Total n (%)	OSTA			p
		Low (n;% = 267; 39.6)	Medium (n;% = 274; 40.6)	High (n;% = 134; 19.8)	
Clinical Parameters					
S-COVID-19-S					0.057 [a]
Without S-COVID-19-S	204 (30.2)	94 (35.2)	77 (28.1)	33 (24.6)	
With S-COVID-19-S	471 (69.8)	173 (64.8)	197 (71.9)	101 (74.4)	
Rheumatoid arthritis					<0.001 [a]
No	606 (89.8)	251 (94.0)	248 (90.5)	107 (79.9)	
Yes	69 (10.2)	16 (6.0)	26 (9.5)	27 (20.1)	
Stomach ulcers					0.068 [a]
No	538 (79.7)	224 (83.9)	208 (75.9)	106 (79.1)	
Yes	137 (20.3)	43 (16.1)	66 (24.1)	28 (20.9)	
Diuretic usage					0.002 [a]
No	351 (73.1)	156 (81.3)	135 (69.9)	60 (63.2)	
Yes	129 (26.9)	36 (18.8)	58 (30.1)	35 (36.8)	
HBsAg					0.853 [a]
Negative	425 (91.6)	164 (91.6)	170 (90.9)	91 (92.9)	
Positive	39 (8.4)	15 (8.4)	17 (9.1)	7 (7.1)	
HCV					0.678 [a]
Negative	330 (71.1)	127 (70.9)	130 (69.5)	73 (74.5)	
Positive	134 (28.9)	52 (29.1)	57 (30.5)	25 (25.5)	
WC, cm (Mean ± SD)	76.9 ± 9.9	78.9 ± 9.7	75.7 ± 9.8	75.5 ±10.4	0.001 [c]
Biochemical parameters					
Hb, g/dL (Median, IQR)	9.7 (8.4, 11.1)	9.8 (8.6, 11.1)	9.8 (8.3, 11.3)	9.4 (7.9, 10.7)	0.064 [b]
WBC, $10^3/\mu L$ (Median, IQR)	5.9 (4.5, 7.3)	5.8 (4.5, 7.0)	6.0 (4.5, 7.5)	6.0 (4.6, 7.4)	0.606 [b]
RBC, $10^6/\mu L$ (Median, IQR)	3.3 (2.7, 3.7)	3.3 (2.8, 3.8)	3.3 (2.7, 3.8)	3.1 (2.7, 3.7)	0.593 [b]
MCV, fL (Median, IQR)	90.0 (83.0, 94.6)	89.7 (83.4, 94.2)	89.9 (80.7, 94.1)	91.6 (85.3, 95.9)	0.099 [b]
Hct, % (Mean ± SD)	30.0 ± 5.8	30.1 ± 5.3	30.5 ± 6.3	28.9 ± 5.7	0.095 [c]
PLT, $10^3/\mu L$ (Median, IQR)	205.0 (163.0, 245.0)	197.0 (163.0, 236.0)	206.0 (168.0, 252.0)	208.0 (157.0, 251.0)	0.200 [b]
PO_4, mg/dL (Median, IQR)	1.8 (1.4, 2.6)	1.8 (1.4, 2.4)	1.7 (1.4, 2.8)	2.0 (1.3, 3.4)	0.800 [b]
PTH, pg/mL (Median, IQR)	23.9 (16.4, 45.8)	23.4 (16.5, 43.5)	25.2 (14.1, 46.5)	25.2 (19.1, 51.0)	0.568 [b]
K^+, mEq/L (Mean ± SD)	4.2 ± 0.9	4.2 ± 0.9	4.3 ± 0.9	4.2 ± 0.8	0.817 [c]
Na^+, mmol/L (Mean ± SD)	135.9 ± 4.7	136.3 ± 3.1	135.7 ± 5.3	135.9 ± 5.9	0.518 [c]
Cl^-, mmol/L (Mean ± SD)	97.8 ± 5.1	97.3 ± 4.4	97.9 ± 5.9	98.5 ± 4.7	0.193 [c]
Albumin, mg/dL (Mean ± SD)	38.7 ± 5.6	39.3 ± 6.3	38.7 ± 4.9	37.3 ± 5.6	0.047 [c]
Physical activity, MET-min/wk					0.895 [a]
Tertile 1 (MET ≤ 180)	168 (33.5)	67 (34.5)	68 (33.0)	33 (32.4)	
Tertile 2 (180 < MET ≤ 723)	164 (32.7)	59 (30.4)	72 (35.0)	33 (32.4)	
Tertile 3 (MET > 723)	170 (33.9)	68 (35.1)	66 (32.0)	36 (35.3)	

Table 1. *Cont.*

Variables	Total n (%)	OSTA			*p*
		Low (n;% = 267; 39.6)	Medium (n;% = 274; 40.6)	High (n;% = 134; 19.8)	
Health/diet literacy and diet knowledge					
HL index (Mean ± SD)	25.2 ± 9.2	25.6 ± 8.6	22.9 ± 9.3	22.2 ± 9.3	<0.001 [c]
DDL index (Mean ± SD)	24.1 ± 11.4	25.1 ± 11.1	21.2 ± 11.3	20.6 ± 1.7	<0.001 [c]
HDK (Mean ± SD)	5.4 ± 2.5	5.2 ± 2.5	5.3 ± 2.4	5.3 ± 2.6	0.788 [c]

Abbreviation: SD, standard deviation; IQR, interquartile range; S-COVID-19-S, suspected COVID-19 symptoms; HBsAg, hepatitis B surface antigen; HCV, hepatitis C virus; WC, waist circumference; Hb, hemoglobin; WBC, white blood cell; RBC, red blood cell; MCV, mean corpuscular volume; Hct, hematocrit; PLT, platelet count; PO4, phosphates; PTH, parathyroid hormone; K^+, kali; Na^+, natri; Cl^-, clo; MET-min/wk, metabolic equivalent task scored in minutes per week; HL, health literacy; DDL, digital health diet literacy; HDK, hemodialysis dietary knowledge; OSTA, osteoporosis self-assessment tool for Asians. [a] Result of the chi-square test; [b] Result of Kruskal–Wallis test; [c] Result of one-way ANOVA.

3.2. Associated Factors of Osteoporosis

Table 2 shows the results of the unadjusted and the adjusted multinomial logistic regression models. In the adjusted model, a medium osteoporosis risk (OR, 3.46; 95% CI, 1.86, 6.44; $p < 0.001$) and a high osteoporosis risk (OR, 6.86; 95% CI, 2.96, 15.88; $p < 0.001$) were more likely in the female participants. The participants who were at a high risk of osteoporosis were more likely to have rheumatoid arthritis (OR, 4.37; 95% CI, 1.67, 11.52; $p = 0.003$), while those at a medium risk of osteoporosis were more likely to have stomach ulcers (OR, 1.95; 95% CI, 1.01, 3.77; $p = 0.048$). The odds of a medium osteoporosis risk decreased by 5%, 8%, and 4% for each increment by one unit in waist circumference (OR, 0.95; 95% CI, 0.92, 0.98; $p = 0.004$), HL (OR, 0.92; 95% CI, 0.88, 0.96; $p < 0.001$), and DDL (OR, 0.96; 95% CI, 0.93, 0.99; $p = 0.017$), respectively. The odds of a high osteoporosis risk declined by 7%, 21%, 5%, 9%, 11%, and 5% for each increment by one unit in waist circumference (OR, 0.93; 95% CI, 0.89, 0.97; $p = 0.001$), Hb level (OR, 0.79; 95% CI, 0.66, 0.95; $p = 0.014$), Hct (OR, 0.95; 95% CI, 0.92, 0.99; $p = 0.041$), albumin level (OR, 0.91; 95% CI, 0.83, 0.99; $p = 0.030$), HL (OR, 0.89; 95% CI, 0.84, 0.94; $p < 0.001$), and DDL (OR, 0.95; 95% CI, 0.91, 0.99; $p = 0.008$), respectively. The patients with a junior high school level of education had a lower likelihood of having osteoporosis risk compared to those who were illiterate or at the elementary level of education (OR, 0.37; 95% CI, 0.16, 0.88; $p = 0.025$).

Table 2. Associated factors of osteoporosis via unadjusted and adjusted multinominal logistic regression analysis.

Associated Factors	Medium Risk of Osteoporosis *				High Risk of Osteoporosis *			
	Unadjusted Model		Adjusted Model		Unadjusted Model		Adjusted Model	
	OR (95% CI)	*p*	OR (95% CI)	*p*	OR (95% CI)	*p*	OR (95% CI)	*p*
Socio-demographics								
Gender			1.00					
Male	1.00				1.00		1.00	
Female	2.50 (1.77, 3.55)	<0.001	3.46 (1.86, 6.44)	<0.001 [a]	4.19 (2.69, 6.54)	<0.001	6.86 (2.96, 15.88)	<0.001 [a]
Education								
Illiterate or elementary	1.00		1.00		1.00		1.00	
Junior high school	0.52 (0.35, 0.79)	0.002	0.63 (0.33, 1.20)	0.158 [a]	0.37 (0.21, 0.63)	<0.001	0.37 (0.16, 0.88)	0.025 [a]
Senior high school or above	0.63 (0.39, 1.01)	0.054	1.02 (0.41, 2.53)	0.963 [a]	0.80 (0.47, 1.37)	0.414	0.82 (0.27, 2.53)	0.731 [a]

Table 2. *Cont.*

Associated Factors	Medium Risk of Osteoporosis *				High Risk of Osteoporosis *			
	Unadjusted Model		Adjusted Model		Unadjusted Model		Adjusted Model	
	OR (95% CI)	p	OR (95% CI)	p	OR (95% CI)	p	OR (95% CI)	p
Working status								
Not working	1.00				1.00			
Working	0.87 (0.62, 1.24)	0.450			0.84 (0.55, 1.29)	0.435		
Marital status								
Without partner	1.00				1.00		1.00	
With partner	0.61 (0.30, 1.24)	0.173	0.82 (0.09, 6.97)	0.817 [a]	0.33 (0.15, 0.69)	0.003	0.60 (0.06, 6.46)	0.674 [a]
Social status								
Low	1.00		1.00		1.00		1.00	
Middle and high	0.75 (0.52, 0.09)	0.132	1.15 (0.60, 2.23)	0.673 [a]	0.84 (0.53, 1.32)	0.442	1.07 (0.46, 2.50)	0.874 [a]
Medication payment ability								
Very or fairly difficult	1.00		1.00		1.00		1.00	
Very or fairly easy	1.34 (0.87, 2.05)	0.181	1.63 (0.69, 3.84)	0.265 [a]	1.90 (1.16, 3.11)	0.010	0.98 (0.32, 2.97)	0.968 [a]
Hemodialysis vintage, years	1.01 (0.97, 1.05)	0.620			0.99 (0.94, 1.04)	0.609		
Clinical parameters								
S-COVID-19-S								
Without S-COVID-19-S	1.00		1.00		1.00		1.00	
With S-COVID-19-S	1.39 (0.97, 2.00)	0.076	1.18 (0.62, 2.24)	0.620 [b]	1.66 (1.04, 2.65)	0.033	2.37 (0.93, 6.07)	0.071 [b]
Rheumatoid arthritis								
No	1.00		1.00		1.00		1.00	
Yes	1.65 (0.86, 3.14)	0.132	0.92 (0.37, 2.33)	0.865 [b]	3.96 (2.05, 7.65)	<0.001	4.37 (1.67, 11.52)	0.003 [b]
Stomach ulcers								
No	1.00		1.00		1.00		1.00	
Yes	1.65 (1.08, 2.54)	0.021	1.95 (1.01, 3.77)	0.048 [b]	1.38 (0.81, 2.34)	0.237	1.53 (0.66, 3.54)	0.322 [b]
Diuretic usage								
No	1.00		1.00		1.00		1.00	
Yes	1.86 (1.16, 2.99)	0.010	1.22 (0.63, 2.34)	0.562 [b]	2.53 (1.46, 4.39)	0.001	2.19 (0.99, 4.86)	0.053 [b]
HBsAg								
Negative	1.00				1.00			
Positive	1.09 (0.53, 2.26)	0.810			0.84 (0.33, 2.14)	0.716		
HCV								
Negative	1.00				1.00			
Positive	1.07 (0.68, 1.68)	0.765			0.84 (0.48, 1.46)	0.530		
WC	0.97 (0.95, 0.99)	0.001	0.95 (0.92, 0.98)	0.004 [b]	0.97 (0.94, 0.99)	0.008	0.93 (0.89, 0.97)	0.001 [b]
Biochemical parameters								
Hb	0.99 (0.87, 1.09)	0.779	0.98 (0.86, 1.13)	0.802 [c]	0.85 (0.75, 0.97)	0.017	0.79 (0.66, 0.95)	0.014 [c]
WBC	1.05 (0.97, 1.14)	0.248			1.06 (0.96, 1.18)	0.266		
RBC	1.07 (0.85, 1.35)	0.569			0.89 (0.66, 1,21)	0.465		
MCV	0.99 (0.98, 1.01)	0.814	0.99 (0.97, 1.01)	0.411 [c]	1.02 (0.99, 1.04)	0.124	1.01 (0.98, 1.04)	0.549 [c]
Hct	1.01 (0.98, 1.05)	0.592	1.01 (0.97, 1.06)	0.679 [c]	0.96 (0.92, 1.01)	0.089	0.95 (0.92, 0.99)	0.041 [c]
PLT	1.01 (0.99, 1.01)	0.221			1.01 (0.99, 1.01)	0.441		
PO_4	1.08 (0.89, 1.32)	0.435			1.06 (0.84, 1.35)	0.610		
PTH	1.01 (0.98, 1.02)	0.876			1.01 (0.99, 1.03)	0.311		

Table 2. *Cont.*

Associated Factors	Medium Risk of Osteoporosis *				High Risk of Osteoporosis *			
	Unadjusted Model		Adjusted Model		Unadjusted Model		Adjusted Model	
	OR (95% CI)	*p*	OR (95% CI)	*p*	OR (95% CI)	*p*	OR (95% CI)	*p*
K^+	1.09 (0.84, 1.40)	0.524			1.05 (0.77, 1.43)	0.768		
Na^+	0.97 (0.92, 1.02)	0.257			0.98 (0.92, 1.04)	0.506		
Cl^-	1.03 (0.98, 1.08)	0.200	1.02 (0.96, 1.07)	0.538 [c]	1.05 (0.99, 1.11)	0.083	1.02 (0.96, 1.10)	0.503 [c]
Albumin	0.98 (0.96, 1.02)	0.395	0.98 (0.91, 1.05)	0.286 [c]	0.93 (0.88, 0.98)	0.012	0.91 (0.83, 0.99)	0.030 [c]
Physical activity								
Tertile 1 (MET ≤ 180)	1.00				1.00			
Tertile 2 (180 < MET ≤ 723)	1.20 (0.74, 1.95)	0.454			1.14 (0.63, 2.06)	0.676		
Tertile 3 (MET > 723)	0.96 (0.59, 1.54)	0.855			1.08 (0.60, 1.92)	0.807		
Health/diet literacy and diet knowledge								
HL index	0.97 (0.95, 0.99)	0.001	0.92 (0.88, 0.96)	<0.001 [d]	0.96 (0.94, 0.98)	0.001	0.89 (0.84, 0.94)	<0.001 [c]
DDL index	0.97 (0.95, 0.98)	<0.001	0.96 (0.93, 0.99)	0.017 [d]	0.97 (0.95, 0.98)	<0.001	0.95 (0.91, 0.99)	0.008 [c]
HDK	1.02 (0.95, 1.09)	0.668			1.03 (0.95, 1.12)	0.502		

Abbreviation: OR, odds ratio; CI, confidence interval; SD, standard deviation; S-COVID-19-S, suspected COVID-19 symptoms; HBsAg, hepatitis B surface antigen; HCV, hepatitis C virus; WC, waist circumference; Hb, hemoglobin; WBC, white blood cell; RBC, red blood cell; MCV, mean corpuscular volume; Hct, hematocrit; PLT, platelet count; PO_4, phosphates; PTH, parathyroid hormone; K^+, kali; Na^+, natri; Cl^-, clo; HL, health literacy; DDL, digital health diet literacy; HDK, hemodialysis dietary knowledge; OSTA, osteoporosis self-assessment tool for Asians. * Low risk of osteoporosis is the reference group. [a] the adjusted multinominal logistic regression, which adjusted for variables ($p < 0.2$) in the groups of clinical parameters, biochemical parameters, health/diet literacy and diet knowledge; [b] the adjusted multinominal logistic regression, which adjusted for variables ($p < 0.2$) in the groups of socio-demographics, biochemical parameters, health/diet literacy and diet knowledge; [c] the adjusted multinominal logistic regression, which adjusted for variables ($p < 0.2$) in the groups of socio-demographics, clinical parameters, health/diet literacy and diet knowledge; [d] the adjusted multinominal logistic regression, which adjusted for variables ($p < 0.2$) in the groups of socio-demographics, clinical parameters, and biochemical parameters.

4. Discussion

Using a self-assessment tool, more than 60% of our hemodialysis patients presented a medium and high level of osteoporosis risk. The high prevalence of osteoporosis in hemodialysis patients has been reported in previous studies that used different diagnostic methods, such as an ultrasound bone densitometry [38], a bone density scan [5,6], and a bone histomorphometry [39]. The OSTA has been suggested for early osteoporosis detection in the healthy population [26] or in individuals with type 2 diabetes mellitus [40]. It is also capable of distinguishing the fracture status in hemodialysis patients [25]. This screening tool may help physicians to prioritize the high-risk patients for further diagnosis and for specific strategies to manage those patients.

In this study, we found that higher HL, DDL, and waist circumference, and higher levels of Hb, Hct, albumin, and education, protected our participants from osteoporosis risk, while being female and having comorbid diseases were associated with a higher likelihood of having bone health disorder.

The most important finding in this study is that higher HL and DDL were associated with a lower likelihood of osteoporosis risk in patients who were undergoing hemodialysis. Similarly, our patients with a higher education level had lower odds of osteoporosis, which is in line with another study's findings [41]. In fact, the promotion of healthy habits, a balanced nutrient intake, and regular exercise is highly recommended in order to reduce the risk of osteoporosis [42,43]. People with higher HL and DDL scores tend to have better eating behaviors [18,44]. However, the level of HL among hemodialysis patient was insufficient [45]. Nowadays, numerous resources, such as the Internet, media, books, etc., can provide hemodialysis patients with information about healthy eating; however, not all of these methods are qualified. Thus, particular attention should be given to such interventions in order to improve patients' health and healthy diet literacy. For example, these patients should be educated and suggested formal websites in order to help them with adequate literacy about the hemodialysis diet.

Another important finding in the present study is that the waist circumference protected our participants from the risk of osteoporosis. This finding is congruent with a previous study that supported a lower risk of osteoporosis in hemodialysis patients with abdominal obesity [16]. A higher waist circumference reflects abdominal obesity, which may increase bone density by stimulating bone growth and improving the bones' weight tolerance [46]. However, other studies have reported that people with a higher waist circumference/abdominal obesity have a higher risk of osteoporosis/fractures or a worse bone mineral density [47–49]. The inconsistency between these results may be due to the difference between the studies in the measuring methods, the fracture sites, the covariates, and the waist circumference classification. Thus, further studies assessing the relationship between waist circumference and osteoporosis risk among hemodialysis patients are needed.

Remarkably, in this study, higher serum albumin was significantly associated with lower odds of osteoporosis risk. In line with our findings, another study on rheumatoid arthritis patients during the postmenopausal stage revealed that the serum albumin concentrations were lower in the osteoporosis group than in the non-osteoporosis group [50]. Likewise, hypoalbuminemia was associated with a higher risk of osteoporosis and future fractures [51,52]. A possible explanation for this association is that low levels of serum albumin may directly activate osteoclasts and inhibit osteogenesis through its link with the nuclear factor-κB [53]. Moreover, our study found that higher Hb and Hct levels were protective factors against osteoporosis. This concurs with other studies [54–56]. In fact, lower levels of Hb and Hct reflect an anemia status, which increases osteoclast activity [55]. Hence, in clinical practice, health care providers should be aware of the correction between albumin, Hb, and Hct levels in order to protect against osteoporosis in hemodialysis patients.

Inversely, being female was associated with an increased level of osteoporosis risk in our participants. It has been indicated consistently in the literature that women have a higher risk of osteoporosis than men [7,57]. Bone loss may be due to a deficiency in estrogen, which is highly prevalent in menopausal women [58]. However, other studies have found that decreased estrogen levels play a major role in osteoporosis development for both sexes [59,60]. Therefore, although female patients receive more attention in early osteoporosis detection, osteoporosis in men should also be taken into account.

Our findings have also indicated that hemodialysis patients who have comorbid diseases tend to have a higher level of osteoporosis risk. Patients who are diagnosed with rheumatoid arthritis have a higher risk of osteoporosis, which is possibly due to their inflammation status, cytokine release, and autoantibody production [61]. Meanwhile, persistent inflammation in chronic kidney disease is obviously present [62]. Notably, having stomach ulcers was another risk factor of osteoporosis in our participants. This finding is consistent with the findings from previous studies [63,64]. A possible explanation for this association is that patients with peptic ulcers are usually treated with omeprazole, which has a negative association with the risk of vertebral fractures [65]. Therefore, early diagnosis and the establishment and implementation of appropriate alternative treatments for hemodialysis patients with other diseases could reduce osteoporosis risk.

This study has some limitations. Firstly, the causality of the protective factors on osteoporosis was not able to be confirmed in a cross-sectional study design. Further experimental studies are suggested in order to examine the effects of the biochemical components and health and diet literacy on osteoporosis in hemodialysis patients. Secondly, the biochemical parameters (e.g., vitamin D, calcium, and liver enzymes) that may contribute to osteoporosis have not been investigated in this study due to insufficient data. Thirdly, the OSTA score was intended to reflect the osteoporosis risk or the fracture risk instead of confirmed osteoporosis status. Therefore, the results should be interpreted with caution. The use of a combination of osteoporosis diagnosis methods (e.g., using bone biopsy or biochemical parameters) is suggested in future research and clinical practice. Despite the limitations, OSTA may be an acceptable solution in detecting the osteoporosis risk in some contexts, particularly those regarding issues such as the trained technicians required, high cost, and instrument availability.

5. Conclusions

In this study, we have found that female patients and those with comorbid conditions were more likely to have osteoporosis/fracture risk. Meanwhile, patients with higher health and diet literacy, education, waist circumference, and greater levels of some biochemical components (albumin, Hb, and Hct) had a lower likelihood of osteoporosis risk. The results suggest that these protective factors should be a consideration in future interventions in order to prevent osteoporosis/fracture risk in hemodialysis patients.

Supplementary Materials: The following supporting information can be downloaded at: https://www.mdpi.com/article/10.3390/nu14235122/s1, Table S1: The correlations between independent variables.

Author Contributions: Conceptualization, L.T.H.L., L.T.D., T.-J.W., T.G.D., D.H.N., T.A.H., M.D.P., B.N.D., H.C.N., T.T.T., L.V.P., L.T.H.N., H.T.N., N.T.T., T.V.D. (Thinh V. Do), M.V.T., T.H.H., D.T.P., S.-H.Y., N.N.M.L., K.T.N. and T.V.D. (Tuyen V. Duong); Data curation, L.T.H.L., T.G.D., M.D.P., H.C.N., L.V.P., H.T.N., T.V.D. (Thinh V. Do), M.V.T. and T.H.H.; Formal analysis, L.T.H.L. and L.T.D.; Funding acquisition, T.V.D. (Tuyen V. Duong); Investigation, L.T.H.L., L.T.D., T.-J.W., T.G.D., D.H.N., T.A.H., M.D.P., B.N.D., H.C.N., T.T.T., L.V.P., L.T.H.N., H.T.N., N.T.T., T.V.D. (Thinh V. Do), M.V.T., T.H.H., D.T.P., S.-H.Y., N.N.M.L., K.T.N. and T.V.D. (Tuyen V. Duong); Methodology, L.T.H.L., L.T.D., T.-J.W., T.G.D., D.H.N., T.A.H., M.D.P., B.N.D., H.C.N., T.T.T., L.V.P., L.T.H.N., H.T.N., N.T.T., T.V.D. (Thinh V. Do), M.V.T., T.H.H., D.T.P., S.-H.Y., N.N.M.L., K.T.N. and T.V.D. (Tuyen V. Duong); Project administration, L.T.H.L., L.T.D. and T.V.D. (Tuyen V. Duong); Resources, T.G.D., M.D.P., H.C.N., L.V.P., H.T.N., T.V.D. (Thinh V. Do), M.V.T., T.H.H. and T.V.D. (Tuyen V. Duong); Software, L.T.H.L., L.T.D. and T.V.D. (Tuyen V. Duong); Supervision, T.V.D. (Tuyen V. Duong); Validation, L.T.H.L., L.T.D., T.-J.W., T.G.D., D.H.N., T.A.H., M.D.P., B.N.D., H.C.N., T.T.T., L.V.P., L.T.H.N., H.T.N., N.T.T., T.V.D. (Thinh V. Do), M.V.T., T.H.H., D.T.P., S.-H.Y., N.N.M.L., K.T.N. and T.V.D. (Tuyen V. Duong); Visualization, L.T.H.L. and L.T.D.; Writing—original draft, L.T.H.L., L.T.D. and T.V.D. (Tuyen V. Duong); Writing—review and editing, L.T.H.L., L.T.D., T.-J.W., T.G.D., D.H.N., T.A.H., M.D.P., B.N.D., H.C.N., T.T.T., L.V.P., L.T.H.N., H.T.N., N.T.T., T.V.D. (Thinh V. Do), M.V.T., T.H.H., D.T.P., S.-H.Y., N.N.M.L., K.T.N. and T.V.D. (Tuyen V. Duong). All authors have read and agreed to the published version of the manuscript.

Funding: This study was supported by Military Hospital 103, Thai Nguyen National Hospital, and Taipei Medical University and the National Science and Technology Council, Taiwan (MOST 111-2410-H-038-008-MY2).

Institutional Review Board Statement: This study was conducted in accordance with the Declaration of Helsinki and approved by the Institutional Review Board of Hanoi University of Public Health in Vietnam (IRB No. 225/2020/YTCC-HD3).

Informed Consent Statement: Informed consent was obtained from all subjects involved in this study.

Data Availability Statement: Data will be available upon reasonable request to the corresponding author.

Acknowledgments: The authors would like to thank all of the healthcare providers and patients who participated in this study from Bach Mai Hospital, Military Hospital 103, General Hospital of Agricultural, National Thai Nguyen Hospital, Hai Phong University of Medicine and Pharmacy Hospital, Hai Phong International Hospital, Quang Ninh General Hospital, and Bai Chay Hospital.

Conflicts of Interest: The authors declare no conflict of interest. The funders had no role in the design of this study; in the collection, analyses, or interpretation of data; in the writing of the manuscript, or in the decision to publish the results.

References

1. Liyanage, T.; Ninomiya, T.; Jha, V.; Neal, B.; Patrice, H.M.; Okpechi, I.; Zhao, M.H.; Lv, J.; Garg, A.X.; Knight, J.; et al. Worldwide access to treatment for end-stage kidney disease: A systematic review. *Lancet* **2015**, *385*, 1975–1982. [CrossRef] [PubMed]
2. Thurlow, J.S.; Joshi, M.; Yan, G.; Norris, K.C.; Agodoa, L.Y.; Yuan, C.M.; Nee, R. Global Epidemiology of End-Stage Kidney Disease and Disparities in Kidney Replacement Therapy. *Am. J. Nephrol.* **2021**, *52*, 98–107. [CrossRef] [PubMed]
3. Bhargava, V.; Jasuja, S.; Tang, S.C.; Bhalla, A.K.; Sagar, G.; Jha, V.; Ramachandran, R.; Sahay, M.; Alexander, S.; Vachharajani, T.; et al. Peritoneal dialysis: Status report in South and South East Asia. *Nephrology* **2021**, *26*, 898–906. [CrossRef] [PubMed]
4. Glaser, D.L.; Kaplan, F.S. Osteoporosis. Definition and clinical presentation. *Spine* **1997**, *22*, 12s–16s. [CrossRef]
5. Slouma, M.; Sahli, H.; Bahlous, A.; Laadhar, L.; Smaoui, W.; Rekik, S.; Gharsallah, I.; Sallami, M.; Moussa, F.B.; Elleuch, M.; et al. Mineral bone disorder and osteoporosis in hemodialysis patients. *Adv. Rheumatol.* **2020**, *60*, 15. [CrossRef]
6. Hashimoto, H.; Shikuma, S.; Mandai, S.; Adachi, S.; Uchida, S. Calcium-based phosphate binder use is associated with lower risk of osteoporosis in hemodialysis patients. *Sci. Rep.* **2021**, *11*, 1648. [CrossRef]
7. Karatas, A.; Erdem, E.; Arıcı, Y.K.; Canakci, E.; Turkmen, E.; Turker, N.T. The frequency of osteoporosis in patients with predialysis chronic renal failure and the factors affecting the development of osteoporosis. *Niger. J. Clin. Pract.* **2022**, *25*, 137–143. [CrossRef]
8. Yenchek, R.H.; Ix, J.H.; Shlipak, M.G.; Bauer, D.C.; Rianon, N.J.; Kritchevsky, S.B.; Harris, T.B.; Newman, A.B.; Cauley, J.A.; Fried, L.F. Bone mineral density and fracture risk in older individuals with CKD. *Clin. J. Am. Soc. Nephrol.* **2012**, *7*, 1130–1136. [CrossRef]
9. Lin, Z.Z.; Wang, J.J.; Chung, C.R.; Huang, P.C.; Su, B.A.; Cheng, K.C.; Chio, C.C.; Chien, C.C. Epidemiology and mortality of hip fracture among patients on dialysis: Taiwan National Cohort Study. *Bone* **2014**, *64*, 235–239. [CrossRef]
10. Hsu, C.Y.; Chen, L.R.; Chen, K.H. Osteoporosis in Patients with Chronic Kidney Diseases: A Systemic Review. *Int. J. Mol. Sci.* **2020**, *21*, 6846. [CrossRef]
11. Tasnim, N.; Dutta, P.; Nayeem, J.; Masud, P.; Ferdousi, A.; Ghosh, A.S.; Hossain, M.; Rajia, S.; Kubra, K.T.; Sakibuzzaman, M.; et al. Osteoporosis, an Inevitable Circumstance of Chronic Kidney Disease: A Systematic Review. *Cureus* **2021**, *13*, e18488. [CrossRef] [PubMed]
12. Panuccio, V.; Enia, G.; Tripepi, R.; Aliotta, R.; Mallamaci, F.; Tripepi, G.; Zoccali, C. Pro-inflammatory cytokines and bone fractures in CKD patients. An exploratory single centre study. *BMC Nephrol.* **2012**, *13*, 134. [CrossRef] [PubMed]
13. Rashid, A.; Chaudhary Hauge, S.; Suetta, C.; Hansen, D. Sarcopenia and risk of osteoporosis, falls and bone fractures in patients with chronic kidney disease: A systematic review. *PLoS ONE* **2022**, *17*, e0262572. [CrossRef] [PubMed]
14. Najar, M.S.; Mir, M.M.; Muzamil, M. Prevalence of osteoporosis in patients with chronic kidney disease (stages 3–5) in comparison with age- and sex-matched controls: A study from Kashmir Valley Tertiary Care Center. *Saudi J. Kidney Dis. Transplant.* **2017**, *28*, 538–544. [CrossRef]
15. Mahzari, M.M.; Alibrahim, A.R.; Alghamdi, N.A.; Alsadhan, M.A.; Almoamary, S.M.; Masuadi, E.M.; Al Shahrani, A.S. Prevalence and Risk Factors of Osteoporosis in Saudi End-Stage Renal Disease Patients on Hemodialysis. *Saudi J. Med. Med. Sci.* **2022**, *10*, 259–265. [CrossRef]
16. Wung, C.H.; Chung, C.Y.; Wu, P.Y.; Huang, J.C.; Tsai, Y.C.; Chen, S.C.; Chiu, Y.W.; Chang, J.M. Associations between Metabolic Syndrome and Obesity-Related Indices and Bone Mineral Density T-Score in Hemodialysis Patients. *J. Pers. Med.* **2021**, *11*, 775. [CrossRef]
17. Sørensen, K.; Van den Broucke, S.; Fullam, J.; Doyle, G.; Pelikan, J.; Slonska, Z.; Brand, H. Health literacy and public health: A systematic review and integration of definitions and models. *BMC Public Health* **2012**, *12*, 80. [CrossRef]
18. Duong, T.V.; Pham, K.M.; Do, B.N.; Kim, G.B.; Dam, H.T.B.; Le, V.T.; Nguyen, T.T.P.; Nguyen, H.T.; Nguyen, T.T.; Le, T.T.; et al. Digital Healthy Diet Literacy and Self-Perceived Eating Behavior Change during COVID-19 Pandemic among Undergraduate Nursing and Medical Students: A Rapid Online Survey. *Int. J. Environ. Res. Public Health* **2020**, *17*, 7185. [CrossRef]
19. Chen, C.; Zheng, J.; Driessnack, M.; Liu, X.; Liu, J.; Liu, K.; Peng, J.; You, L. Health literacy as predictors of fluid management in people receiving hemodialysis in China: A structural equation modeling analysis. *Patient Educ. Couns.* **2021**, *104*, 1159–1167. [CrossRef]
20. Dang, L.T.; Luong, T.C.; Nguyen, D.H.; Hoang, T.A.; Nguyen, H.T.; Nguyen, H.C.; Duong, T.H.; Tran, T.T.; Pham, L.V.; Ngo, T.V.; et al. The Associations of Suspected COVID-19 Symptoms with Anxiety and Depression as Modified by Hemodialysis Dietary Knowledge: A Multi-Dialysis Center Study. *Nutrients* **2022**, *14*, 2364. [CrossRef]
21. Panahi, R.; Yekefallah, L.; Shafaei, M.; Dehghankar, L.; Anbari, M.; Hosseini, N.; Hasannia, E. Effect of health literacy among students on the adoption of osteoporosis-preventive behaviors in Iran. *J. Educ. Health Promot.* **2020**, *9*, 191. [CrossRef] [PubMed]
22. Roh, Y.H.; Koh, Y.D.; Noh, J.H.; Gong, H.S.; Baek, G.H. Effect of health literacy on adherence to osteoporosis treatment among patients with distal radius fracture. *Arch. Osteoporos* **2017**, *12*, 42. [CrossRef] [PubMed]
23. Kung, A.W.; Ho, A.Y.; Ross, P.D.; Reginster, J.Y. Development of a clinical assessment tool in identifying Asian men with low bone mineral density and comparison of its usefulness to quantitative bone ultrasound. *Osteoporos Int.* **2005**, *16*, 849–855. [CrossRef] [PubMed]
24. Koh, L.K.; Sedrine, W.B.; Torralba, T.P.; Kung, A.; Fujiwara, S.; Chan, S.P.; Huang, Q.R.; Rajatanavin, R.; Tsai, K.S.; Park, H.M.; et al. A simple tool to identify asian women at increased risk of osteoporosis. *Osteoporos Int.* **2001**, *12*, 699–705. [CrossRef] [PubMed]
25. Chang, A.J.; Ying, Q.; Chen, X.N.; Wang, W.M.; Chen, N. Evaluation of three risk assessment tools in discriminating fracture status among Chinese patients undergoing hemodialysis. *Osteoporos Int.* **2016**, *27*, 3599–3606. [CrossRef]

26. Bui, M.H.; Dao, P.T.; Khuong, Q.L.; Le, P.A.; Nguyen, T.T.; Hoang, G.D.; Le, T.H.; Pham, H.T.; Hoang, H.T.; Le, Q.C.; et al. Evaluation of community-based screening tools for the early screening of osteoporosis in postmenopausal Vietnamese women. *PLoS ONE* **2022**, *17*, e0266452. [CrossRef]
27. BMJ Best Practice. Coronavirus Disease 2019 (COVID-19), History and Exam. 2020. Available online: https://bestpractice.bmj.com/topics/en-gb/3000201/history-exam (accessed on 19 May 2021).
28. Craig, C.L.; Marshall, A.L.; Sjöström, M.; Bauman, A.E.; Booth, M.L.; Ainsworth, B.E.; Pratt, M.; Ekelund, U.; Yngve, A.; Sallis, J.F.; et al. International physical activity questionnaire: 12-country reliability and validity. *Med. Sci. Sport. Exerc.* **2003**, *35*, 1381–1395. [CrossRef]
29. Pham, T.; Bui, L.; Nguyen, A.; Nguyen, B.; Tran, P.; Vu, P.; Dang, L. The prevalence of depression and associated risk factors among medical students: An untold story in Vietnam. *PLoS ONE* **2019**, *14*, e0221432. [CrossRef]
30. Duong, T.V.; Aringazina, A.; Kayupova, G.; Nurjanah; Pham, T.V.; Pham, K.M.; Truong, T.Q.; Nguyen, K.T.; Oo, W.M.; Su, T.T.; et al. Development and Validation of a New Short-Form Health Literacy Instrument (HLS-SF12) for the General Public in Six Asian Countries. *Health Lit. Res. Pract.* **2019**, *3*, e91–e102. [CrossRef]
31. Duong, T.V.; Chang, P.W.; Yang, S.-H.; Chen, M.-C.; Chao, W.-T.; Chen, T.; Chiao, P.; Huang, H.-L. A new comprehensive short-form health literacy survey tool for patients in general. *Asian Nurs. Res. (Korean Soc. Nurs. Sci.)* **2017**, *11*, 30–35. [CrossRef]
32. Duong, T.V.; Nguyen, T.T.P.; Pham, K.M.; Nguyen, K.T.; Giap, M.H.; Tran, T.D.X.; Nguyen, C.X.; Yang, S.-H.; Su, C.-T. Validation of the short-form health literacy questionnaire (HLS-SF12) and its determinants among people living in rural areas in Vietnam. *Int. J. Environ. Res. Public Health* **2019**, *16*, 3346. [CrossRef] [PubMed]
33. Ho, H.V.; Hoang, G.T.; Pham, V.T.; Duong, T.V.; Pham, K.M. Factors associated with health literacy among the elderly people in Vietnam. *Biomed. Res. Int.* **2020**, *2020*, 3490635. [CrossRef]
34. HLS-EU Consortium. Comparative Report of Health literacy in Eight EU Member States. The European Health Literacy Project 2009–2012. 2012. Available online: https://www.healthliteracyeurope (accessed on 19 May 2021).
35. Ryu, H.; Jeon, H.J.; Sun, H.-K.; Han, K.H.; Whang, C.G.; Han, S.Y. Repeated education improves diet compliance in maintenance Hemodialysis Patients. *Int. J. Urol. Nephrol.* **2014**, *2*, 63–68.
36. WHO. Coronavirus Disease (COVID-19) Technical Guidance: Infection Prevention and Control/Wash. Available online: https://www.who.int/emergencies/diseases/novel-coronavirus-2019/technical-guidance/infection-prevention-and-control (accessed on 20 May 2020).
37. Maldonado, G.; Greenland, S. Simulation study of confounder-selection strategies. *Am. J. Epidemiol.* **1993**, *138*, 923–936. [CrossRef]
38. Kuo, L.-L.; Tsai, W.-H.; Yu, C.-M.; Yang, C.-C. Risk Factors for Osteoporosis among Hemodialysis Patients. *Taipei City Med. J.* **2012**, *9*, 234–243. [CrossRef]
39. Barreto, F.C.; Barreto, D.V.; Moyses, R.M.; Neves, C.L.; Jorgetti, V.; Draibe, S.A.; Canziani, M.E.; Carvalho, A.B. Osteoporosis in hemodialysis patients revisited by bone histomorphometry: A new insight into an old problem. *Kidney Int.* **2006**, *69*, 1852–1857. [CrossRef]
40. Tang, J.L.; Pan, B.B.; Shu, Y.; Gu, Y.F.; Liu, S. Evaluation of two tools for the early screening of osteoporosis in postmenopausal Chinese women with type 2 diabetes mellitus. *J. Int. Med. Res.* **2020**, *48*, 300060520903889. [CrossRef]
41. Maddah, M.; Sharami, S.H.; Karandish, M. Educational difference in the prevalence of osteoporosis in postmenopausal women: A study in northern Iran. *BMC Public Health* **2011**, *11*, 845. [CrossRef]
42. Muñoz-Garach, A.; García-Fontana, B.; Muñoz-Torres, M. Nutrients and Dietary Patterns Related to Osteoporosis. *Nutrients* **2020**, *12*, 1986. [CrossRef]
43. Baccaro, L.F.; Conde, D.M.; Costa-Paiva, L.; Pinto-Neto, A.M. The epidemiology and management of postmenopausal osteoporosis: A viewpoint from Brazil. *Clin. Interv. Aging* **2015**, *10*, 583–591. [CrossRef]
44. Do, B.N.; Nguyen, P.A.; Pham, K.M.; Nguyen, H.C.; Nguyen, M.H.; Tran, C.Q.; Nguyen, T.T.P.; Tran, T.V.; Pham, L.V.; Tran, K.V.; et al. Determinants of Health Literacy and Its Associations With Health-Related Behaviors, Depression Among the Older People With and Without Suspected COVID-19 Symptoms: A Multi-Institutional Study. *Front. Public Health* **2020**, *8*, 581746. [CrossRef] [PubMed]
45. Khamis, S.; Emara, M.; Elnashar, M.; Khalil, M.; Kasemy, Z. Development of Health Literacy for Regular Hemodialysis Patients in Menoufia Governorate: A Cross-Sectional Study. *Open J. Nephrol.* **2021**, *11*, 199–216. [CrossRef]
46. Reid, I.R. Fat and bone. *Arch. Biochem. Biophys.* **2010**, *503*, 20–27. [CrossRef]
47. Park, G.R.; Kim, H.S.; Kim, Y.T.; Chung, H.J.; Ha, S.J.; Kim, D.W.; Kang, D.R.; Kim, J.Y.; Lee, M.Y.; Lee, J.Y. Waist circumference and the risk of lumbar and femur fractures: A nationwide population-based cohort study. *Eur. Rev. Med. Pharmacol. Sci.* **2021**, *25*, 1198–1205. [CrossRef] [PubMed]
48. Ofir, O.; Buch, A.; Rouach, V.; Goldsmith, R.; Stern, N.; Monsonego-Ornan, E. Association between abdominal obesity and fragility fractures among elderly Israeli women. *Aging Clin. Exp. Res.* **2020**, *32*, 1459–1467. [CrossRef]
49. Hua, Y.; Fang, J.; Yao, X.; Zhu, Z. Can waist circumference be a predictor of bone mineral density independent of BMI in middle-aged adults? *Endocr. Connect.* **2021**, *10*, 1307–1314. [CrossRef]
50. Nagayama, Y.; Ebina, K.; Tsuboi, H.; Hirao, M.; Hashimoto, J.; Yoshikawa, H.; Okada, S.; Nakata, K. Low serum albumin concentration is associated with increased risk of osteoporosis in postmenopausal patients with rheumatoid arthritis. *J. Orthop. Sci.* **2021**, *27*, 1283–1290. [CrossRef]

51. Kunutsor, S.K.; Voutilainen, A.; Whitehouse, M.R.; Seidu, S.; Kauhanen, J.; Blom, A.W.; Laukkanen, J.A. Serum Albumin and Future Risk of Hip, Humeral, and Wrist Fractures in Caucasian Men: New Findings from a Prospective Cohort Study. *Med. Princ. Pract.* **2019**, *28*, 401–409. [CrossRef]
52. Afshinnia, F.; Wong, K.K.; Sundaram, B.; Ackermann, R.J.; Pennathur, S. Hypoalbuminemia and Osteoporosis: Reappraisal of a Controversy. *J. Clin. Endocrinol. Metab.* **2016**, *101*, 167–175. [CrossRef]
53. Abu-Amer, Y. NF-κB signaling and bone resorption. *Osteoporos Int.* **2013**, *24*, 2377–2386. [CrossRef]
54. Xiu, S.; Mu, Z.; Sun, L.; Zhao, L.; Fu, J. Hemoglobin level and osteoporosis in Chinese elders with type 2 diabetes mellitus. *Nutr. Diabetes* **2022**, *12*, 19. [CrossRef]
55. Kim, S.Y.; Yoo, D.M.; Min, C.; Choi, H.G. Association between Osteoporosis and Low Hemoglobin Levels: A Nested Case-Control Study Using a National Health Screening Cohort. *Int. J. Environ. Res. Public Health* **2021**, *18*, 8598. [CrossRef] [PubMed]
56. Yoo, J.; Lee, B.J. Anthropometric, biochemical, and nutritional risk factors for osteoporosis in Korean adults based on a large cross-sectional study. *PLoS ONE* **2021**, *16*, e0261361. [CrossRef] [PubMed]
57. Alswat, K.A. Gender Disparities in Osteoporosis. *J. Clin. Med. Res.* **2017**, *9*, 382–387. [CrossRef] [PubMed]
58. Klein-Nulend, J.; van Oers, R.F.; Bakker, A.D.; Bacabac, R.G. Bone cell mechanosensitivity, estrogen deficiency, and osteoporosis. *J. Biomech* **2015**, *48*, 855–865. [CrossRef] [PubMed]
59. Gennari, L.; Khosla, S.; Bilezikian, J.P. Estrogen and fracture risk in men. *J. Bone Miner. Res.* **2008**, *23*, 1548–1551. [CrossRef]
60. Atroshi, I.; Ahlander, F.; Billsten, M.; Ahlborg, H.G.; Mellström, D.; Ohlsson, C.; Ljunggren, O.; Karlsson, M.K. Low calcaneal bone mineral density and the risk of distal forearm fracture in women and men: A population-based case-control study. *Bone* **2009**, *45*, 789–793. [CrossRef]
61. Adami, G.; Fassio, A.; Rossini, M.; Caimmi, C.; Giollo, A.; Orsolini, G.; Viapiana, O.; Gatti, D. Osteoporosis in Rheumatic Diseases. *Int. J. Mol. Sci.* **2019**, *20*, 5867. [CrossRef]
62. Akchurin, O.M.; Kaskel, F. Update on inflammation in chronic kidney disease. *Blood Purif.* **2015**, *39*, 84–92. [CrossRef]
63. Yoon, P.H.; An, S.J.; Jeong, S.H.; Yang, Y.J.; Hong, Y.P. Association between Peptic Ulcer Disease and Osteoporosis: The Population-Based Longitudinal Cohort Study in Korea. *Int. J. Environ. Res. Public Health* **2019**, *16*, 2777. [CrossRef]
64. Wu, C.H.; Tung, Y.C.; Chai, C.Y.; Lu, Y.Y.; Su, Y.F.; Tsai, T.H.; Kuo, K.L.; Lin, C.L. Increased Risk of Osteoporosis in Patients With Peptic Ulcer Disease: A Nationwide Population-Based Study. *Medicine* **2016**, *95*, e3309. [CrossRef] [PubMed]
65. Roux, C.; Briot, K.; Gossec, L.; Kolta, S.; Blenk, T.; Felsenberg, D.; Reid, D.M.; Eastell, R.; Glüer, C.C. Increase in vertebral fracture risk in postmenopausal women using omeprazole. *Calcif. Tissue Int.* **2009**, *84*, 13–19. [CrossRef] [PubMed]

nutrients

MDPI

Article

Inpatient Rehabilitation during Intensive Refeeding in Severe Anorexia Nervosa

Marc Dauty [1,2,3,4], Pierre Menu [1,2,3,4], Baptiste Jolly [1], Sylvain Lambert [5], Bruno Rocher [5], Maëlle Le Bras [6], Adam Jirka [7], Pascale Guillot [8], Stéphane Pretagut [2,3] and Alban Fouasson-Chailloux [1,2,3,4,*]

1 Service de Médecine Physique et Réadaptation Locomotrice et Respiratoire, CHU Nantes, Nantes Université, 44093 Nantes, France; marc.dauty@chu-nantes.fr (M.D.); pierre.menu@chu-nantes.fr (P.M.); baptiste.jolly@chu-nantes.fr (B.J.)
2 Service de Médecine du Sport, CHU Nantes, Nantes Université, 44093 Nantes, France; stephane.pretagut@chu-nantes.fr
3 IRMS, Institut Régional de Médecine du Sport, 44093 Nantes, France
4 Inserm UMR 1229, Regenerative Medicine and Skeleton, RMeS, Nantes Université, ONIRIS, 44042 Nantes, France
5 Psychiatrie et Santé Mentale, UIC 18, CHU Nantes, Nantes Université, 44000 Nantes, France; sylvain.lambert@chu-nantes.fr (S.L.); bruno.rocher@chu-nantes.fr (B.R.)
6 Service d'Endocrinologie, Diabétologie et Nutrition, Institut du Thorax, CHU Nantes, Nantes Université, 44000 Nantes, France; maelle.lebras@chu-nantes.fr
7 Equipe Transversale D'assistance Nutritionnelle, CHU Nantes, Nantes Université, 44000 Nantes, France; adam.jirka@chu-nantes.fr
8 Service de Rhumatologie, CHU Nantes, Nantes Université, 44000 Nantes, France; pascale.guillot@chu-nantes.fr
* Correspondence: alban.fouassonchailloux@chu-nantes.fr

Abstract: Severe forms of anorexia nervosa are responsible for weight loss and life-threatening consequences. Refeeding represents a real psychiatric and somatic challenge. Physical activities are usually not recommended during intensive refeeding in order to avoid energy expenditure. This study assessed the interest in an early return to controlled physical activities, during a hospitalization in a Physical Medicine and Rehabilitation (PMR) department, including continuous nasogastric refeeding and psychiatric care. A total of 37 subjects aged 32 ± 11 years old performed inpatient physical activities during nasogastric refeeding initiated after intensive care. The physical activity program was adapted according to the hyperactivity of the patients. Evaluation parameters were weight, body mass index (BMI), body composition (fat, lean, and bone masses), and function (strength, balance, walking, ventilation). Patient satisfaction, re-hospitalizations, and physical activities continuation were assessed at 12 months of follow-up. Weight, BMI, and body fat increased significantly (+2.7 ± 1.7 kg; +1.0 ± 0.6 kg/m^2; +1.7 ± 2.5 kg, respectively). Muscle strength increased even if the lean mass did not. Walking distance, balance, and respiratory function were significantly improved. Weight and fat mass gains did not differ according to the presence or absence of hyperactivity. At 12 months, 46% of the patients continued to be physically active, but 21% of the patients had been re-hospitalized. The early return to controlled physical activities in PMR hospitalization does not compromise the efficiency of intensive refeeding in severe anorexia nervosa patients.

Keywords: anorexia nervosa; body mass index; physical activities; muscle strength; hyperactivity

1. Introduction

Anorexia nervosa is a psychiatric illness that mainly affects young women aged 15 to 19, with an incidence between 4.2 and 8.3/100,000/year [1,2]. The disease evolution is variable, from recovery to chronic forms with the possibility of death due to ionic disorders, infection, or suicide (0.5% a year) [3–5]. Patients with serious forms of malnutrition are hospitalized for continuous nasogastric refeeding because of severe somatic conditions requiring a multidisciplinary management [6–10]. Weight loss is often associated with a loss of strength and an increase in daily-life dependency [11,12]. The management has several objectives, with the increase in weight and Body Mass Index (BMI) as benchmarks, reflecting the clinical improvement of the patient [8,11]. For severe forms of anorexia nervosa, a period of continuous nasogastric refeeding carried out in intensive care is usually necessary in order to correct ionic and energy imbalances [13]. Then, returning home can be considered, but there are risks of recurrence [8]. Alternatives to hospitalization most often require oral nutrition to be restarted [8]. Hospitalization in the Physical Medicine and Rehabilitation (PMR) department has the ability to offer physiotherapy care and adapted physical activities to help the patient recover strength and autonomy (e.g., walking, sit-to-stand without assistance) while continuing intensive refeeding [14]. The practice of physical activities was first proposed in 1970 by Blinder et al. [15]. A weight gain of 3.9 pounds per week (+1.75 kg) was obtained in patients during a stay of 6 weeks, which included the practice of resistance exercises. Since then, different meta-analyses have shown that muscle strength and function were improved without negative effects on anthropometric measurements (body weight and BMI) in the case of calorie intake adjustment [16–18]. The practice of physical activities could also improve body perception, eating disorder symptoms, mood, and quality of life [14,17,19,20]. However, controlling physical activities is essential because of the malnourished state of the subjects, who may also present hyperactivity [21]. This hyperactivity can be intentional so as to lose weight and control body weight, or unintentional but due to obsession compulsions, which poses the problem of the dependence on physical activity, accompanied by an anxious state or even depression if these activities are no longer practiced [22,23]. Conversely, physical activity can be used to reduce anxiety [24]. Hyperactivity is present in 30 to 75% of the anorexic subjects and is responsible for difficulties in refeeding, risk of drop-out during treatment and recurrences [25]. Therefore exercise has been considered a behavior problem and is usually forbidden during refeeding. The goal of PMR hospitalization is, therefore, to continue nasogastric refeeding and psychiatric care while performing controlled and adapted physical activities.

The main objective of this study was to assess if this original treatment, performed during intensive nasogastric refeeding, improved muscle strength and patients' autonomy. The secondary objectives were to compare the results depending on the presence or absence of hyperactivity and to know if physical activities were safe, and then, if safe, continue them over a 12-month period.

2. Materials and Methods

2.1. Population

We included patients from 2015 to 2020 addressed for hospitalization in the PMR department. Subjects had to present anorexia nervosa. They were hospitalized following a stay in intensive care for refeeding. The diagnosis of anorexia nervosa was made by a psychiatrist specializing in eating disorders according to the DSM-V classification of the American Psychiatric Association [26].

Before entering PMR hospitalization, any ionic disorder and hepatic cytolysis had been corrected during the hospital stay in intensive care. In addition, the patients had to give their consent to perform physical exercises during refeeding after consulting the psychiatrist. A three-partite contract (Patient, PMR Physician, and Psychiatrist) for a renewable period of 4 weeks was signed at the entry into the PMR inpatient care. Patients who presented a weight loss unrelated to anorexia nervosa or a psychiatric condition contraindicating PMR care were not included. Patients with vestibular and cerebellar disorders, polyneuropathy, or musculoskeletal traumatism, as well as asthmatic respiratory disease or smokers, were excluded.

All the patients gave written consent to participate in the study. The local ethics committee (Comité Nantais d'Ethique en Médecine du Sport) approved the protocol under the number of registration CNEMS-2022-001. The study was also declared to the Research

Department of the University Hospital. The study was in accordance with the declaration of Helsinki [20].

2.2. Contracted Support for PMR Management

The objectives of the PMR care were (1) to continue the weight gain of more than 500 g a week with weighing carried out twice a week, (2) to stop the nasogastric tube feeding gradually (intake at the entry of PMR >1500 Kcal/day) according to a reduction of 250 Kcal per week if the weekly objective of weight gain was reached. On discharge, oral feeding should be exclusive, and (3) to perform controlled physical activities to improve strength, balance, respiratory function, and walking autonomy. Cardiac contraindications were previously assessed: hypotension <80/50 mmHg, bradycardia <50 beats/min, arrhythmia, QRS abnormalities [27].

2.3. Program of Physical Activities

The exercise program was developed based on the results of Ng et al. and Moola et al. in 2013 [16,17]. This program was monitored 3 times a week by a PMR physician and controlled by a physiotherapist and a sports instructor. The first week was devoted to the somatic evaluation, which allowed the initiation of physical activities for 1 h a day and to determine whether the patient presented signs of hyperactivity or not. Due to multiple definitions of hyperactivity in anorexia nervosa [25], the diagnosis of hyperactivity was made if the subject attempted to perform exercises in addition to the controlled exercise requested.

During the following weeks, 1-h sessions were performed twice a day, 5 days out of 7, with a 10-min warm-up and a 10-min cool-down. The morning was dedicated to muscle stretching exercises of the upper and lower limbs, postural maintenance of the trunk (started by 15 s of maintenance targeting stiffness and gradually increased to 30 s × 2 sets), balance (monopodal support: eyes open then closed, for 10 s), and relaxation including breath control with thoracic expansion work [14]. Twice a week in the afternoon, physical exercises for progressive muscle strengthening were performed according to the somatic evaluation. Isometric exercises were performed for the muscles of the trunk, and dynamic exercises with elastic bands were performed for the muscles of the limbs (concentric muscle contractions for the upper limbs and eccentric contractions for the lower limbs, from 6 to 10 repetitions, 3 to 5 sets with recovery of 1 min between sets [11]. Functional exercises included getting up from the floor, chair lifting, walking, and stair practice according to the objective of patient autonomy.

Adapted physical activities were performed 3 times a week, on Mondays, Wednesdays, and Fridays, including 1 h of badminton, initially practiced in a sitting position, then standing, and table tennis, billiards, or archery. Volleyball in the pool and swimming were also proposed, as well as the practice of walking and cycling at the end of the stay according to the weight gain. The exercises were intermittent from 1 to 3 min with a recovery period of at least 3 times the exercise duration (the heart rate should have dropped to less than 120 beats per minute) without exceeding a total practice time of 30 min. A cool-down was then performed with stretching. If the weight goal was not reached or if there was uncontrolled hyperactivity, afternoon physical activities were replaced by a mandatory 1-h rest period followed by a 1-h session of relaxation in hot water balneotherapy (32–34 °C).

The last week was devoted again to the somatic assessment. The length of hospitalization in PMR and the duration of nasogastric refeeding were reported in days, as well as the tolerance to physical activities.

2.4. Psychiatric, Dietetic, and Biological Follow-Up

Throughout the PMR department stay, the patients were followed once a week by a psychiatrist in order to adapt the psychotropic treatment if needed, to provide psychological support, and to help control their weight and possible hyperactivity.

A dietary consultation was performed once a week after medical advice in order to continue the treatment with vitamin and magnesium therapy and gradually introduce oral food, taking into account the reduction of calories provided by the nasogastric tube. The dietician also provided information and advice about nutrition, such as the role of the necessary nutrients for physiological functioning and the need for sufficient nutritional intake in order to achieve the objectives of the hospitalization. The meal times were supervised by a nurse to prevent the possibility of self-induced vomiting.

Various biological parameters were monitored in order to detect a phosphor-calcium disorder (calcium, phosphorus, protein, Vitamin D, and Parathormone) and an inappropriate refeeding syndrome (Hypophosphatemia, liver cytolysis) [9,13,28].

2.5. Somatic Evaluation in the PMR Department

Weight gain was measured to the nearest 0.1 kg twice a week on Monday and Thursday mornings, with an empty stomach and naked (Bathroom scale, SECA 876®, Semur en Auxois, France). The Body Mass Index (BMI) was calculated using the weight-to-height-squared formula. The definition of undernutrition according to the World Health Organization was considered grade V for a BMI < 10 kg/m^2, grade IV for a BMI between 10 and 12.9 kg/m^2, grade III for a BMI between 13 and 14.9 kg/m^2, grade II for a BMI between 15 and 16.9 kg/m^2, and grade I for a BMI between 17 and 18.4 kg/m^2. Only the weight and the BMI at the entry into intensive refeeding care and at the entry and the discharge PMR department were presented in order to assess the evolution of these two parameters.

Knee muscle strength (Extensors and Flexors was measured in a concentric mode using an isokinetic dynamometer (Humac Norm® Medimex, Sainte-Foy-Les-Lyon, France) at an angular speed of 60°/s (3 repetitions) after a warm-up of 5 repetitions performed at 180°/s. The peak force was expressed in Nm/kg. The average of both sides, right and left, was considered. The reproducibility of the measurements is considered good in healthy subjects (ICC: 0.85–0.99) [29]. The muscle strengths of the biceps and triceps brachii were measured elbow flexed at 90° using an isometric dynamometer (MicroFET2®, Biometrics, Orsay, France) to the nearest kg. The results were related to the subjects' weight at the time of the assessment, and the average of both sides was taken into account. The reproducibility of the measurements is considered good in an elderly population (ICC: 0.74–0.85) [30]. The grip strength was measured using a dynamic dynamometer (Jamar®, Madrid, Spain) to the nearest kg. The results were related to the subjects' weight at the time of assessment, and the average of both sides was considered. The reproducibility of the measurements is considered good in healthy or anorexic subjects [31,32]. Endurance of the trunk muscles was measured with a Shirado–Ito test for the abdominal muscles and a Biering–Sorensen test for the spine muscles [33,34]. The Shirado–Ito test was performed in the supine position, maintaining a hip flexion angle of 60° as long as possible (seconds), knees bent at 90°, feet resting on the ground, and upper limbs crossed on the chest. This test was stopped when the patient could no longer maintain this posture or after 180 s. The reproducibility of this test is considered good (ICC: 0.90) [35]. The Biering–Sorensen endurance test was performed in the prone position, trunk in a vacuum, upper limbs crossed over the chest, pelvis and lower limbs held on an examination table. The subjects had to maintain a horizontal posture for as long as possible (seconds). This test was stopped when the patients could no longer maintain this posture or after 180 s. The reproducibility of this test is considered good in healthy subjects (ICC: 0.62–0.93) [36].

The standing balance, eyes open and then eyes closed, was measured using a stabilometric platform (SATEL®, Blagnac, France) focusing on the excursion (sway length in mm) of the center of mass during 25 s, which corresponded to the stabilization of the total body mass exploring the postural responses [37]. These measurements have good reproducibility in healthy subjects (ICC: 0.45–0.86) [38].

The distance (m) achieved during a 6-min walking test was measured during the first and last week of hospitalization in the PMR department under the supervision of a sports instructor [39].

Functional respiratory assessments were performed using a spirometer (Pony FX®, Cosmed, Rome, Italy). The maximum expiratory volume per second (FEV1 in L/s) and the Forced Vital Capacity (FVC in L) were measured according to the recommendations of the American and European Respiratory Society (ATS/ERS) [40]. The FEV1/FVC ratio was calculated to assess restrictive or obstructive pulmonary abnormalities.

Hip bone mineral density (Z-score and T-score) was performed with a densitometer (Lunar Prodigy Advance®, GR Healthcare, Chicago, IL, USA). Results were reported if this assessment had been performed in the year prior to the hospitalization in PMR in order to assess the bone status [41]. To quantify the bodily effects of the treatment in PMR, the fat and lean masses and the bone mineral content in grams were also measured at the level of the whole body, the limbs, and the trunk before and after PMR hospitalization.

The patients were contacted by phone at 12 months in order to know their opinion on the inpatient PMR management and to know if the physical activities were continued. In addition, the number of patients readmitted for a disorder related to anorexia nervosa was collected.

2.6. Statistical Analysis

Statistical analyses were performed using SPSS 23.0® software (Armonk, NY, USA). Quantitative parameters were presented as mean and standard deviation. The normal distribution of the parameters was verified by the Kolgomorov–Smirnoff test. The exercise program was evaluated by a pre/post comparison using a paired *t*-test. The parameters of the subjects who did not complete the first 4 weeks of the contract were included as long as they had been hospitalized for more than 15 days. The comparison between the two subpopulations, hyperactive and non-hyperactive, was performed using a Student's *t*-test or a Mann–Withney test according to the normal distribution of the variables. A repeated measure analysis of variance was carried out in order to compare the evolution of the weight and the BMI of the hyperactive and the non-hyperactive subjects taking into account these variables at the entry into intensive care, at the entry, and at the exit of the PMR department. The assumption of sphericity was assessed and corrected using the epsilon of Greenhouse–Geisser. Effect sizes were assessed by partial eta squared η2, which were defined as trivial, small, moderate, and large for values $\eta^2 \leq 0.1$, ≤ 0.3, ≤ 0.5, and >0.5, respectively. To assess if the improvement of the parameters during hospitalization in PMR was associated with weight gain, a two-tailed Pearson coefficient correlation analysis was performed. The significance level was determined at $p < 0.05$.

3. Results

3.1. Evolution of the Population during the Stay in PRM

We included 37 patients aged 32 ± 11 (34 women and 3 men) hospitalized following a stay in intensive care for refeeding of 21.0 ± 12.0 days. They had been presenting anorexia nervosa since the age of 18.4 ± 5.0 years (duration of anorexia of 13 ± 12 years, from 1 to 36 years). At the entry into intensive care, patients had a weight of 33.9 ± 5.3 kg for a height of 160 ± 8.5 cm [146–190], i.e., a BMI of 12.6 ± 1.5 kg/m^2. Osteopenia or osteoporosis was measured before hospitalization (Table 1), and calcium-vitamin D deficiencies were gradually corrected (Table 2). In total, 13 patients presented with pure restrictive anorexia, 9 had anorexia with purgatory behavior, 11 had anorexia with a history of bulimic episodes, and 4 had anorexia with hyperactivity. Hyperactivity was seen in 17 patients (46%). All the female patients were in amenorrhea and were not taking hormone replacement therapy. Concerning the other parameters, there was no difference according to the sex of the patients.

At the entry into the hospitalization of PMR, the weight was 37.1 ± 5.7 kg for a BMI of 13.8 ± 1.4 kg/m^2. The duration of refeeding by nasogastric tube was 36 ± 16 days during the hospitalization in PMR. The length of stay in the hospital was, on average, 42 ± 18 days. Four patients were discharged between the third and the fourth week for non-compliance with the contract, and one was retransferred to acute care for refeeding syndrome and then returned to PMR hospitalization.

Table 1. Initial bone mineral density (BMD).

Localisation	BMD	Mean (SD)	Min	Max
L1-L4 Spine	T-score	−2.76 ± 1.53	−5.4	0.4
	Z-score	−1.81 ± 1.29	−4.6	0.8
Femoral Neck	T-score	−2.21 ± 1.16	−4.1	0.2
	Z-score	−1.54 ± 1.10	−3.6	0.7
Trochanter	T-score	−2.48 ± 1.18	−4.7	−0.4
	Z-score	−1.80 ± 1.14	−4.1	0.2
Total Body	T-score	−1.51 ± 1.40	−4.2	0.7
	Z-score	−0.57 ± 1.22	−3.3	1.4

Abbreviations: BMD: Bone mineral density; Min: minimum value; Max: maximal value; SD: standard deviation; L: lumbar spine. Z-score: the number of standard deviations above or below the mean for the patient's age, sex, and ethnicity. T-score: the number of standard deviations above or below the mean for a healthy 30-year-old adult of the same sex and ethnicity as the patient. Normal is a T-score of −1.0 or higher, Osteopenia is defined as between −1.0 and −2.5, and Osteoporosis is defined as −2.5 or lower.

Table 2. Biological parameters at the beginning of the PMR hospitalization.

Biological Parameters	Mean	Min	Max
Total Calcium (mmol/L)	2.30 ± 0.09	2.07	2.54
Phosphor (mmol/L)	1.20 ± 0.22	0.80	1.69
Proteins (mmol/L)	63.6 ± 5.7	48	74
D vitamin (N: 30–60 mg/L)	39.2 ± 24.9	6.4	142
Parathormone (N: 30–60 ui/L)	27.9 ± 8.6	15	47.9
Pal (N: 0–120 ui/L)	69.9 ± 52.1	24	250
ALAT (N < 36 ui/L)	45.9 ± 31.7	10	158
ASAT (N < 36 ui/L)	29.8 ± 17.9	12	94

Abbreviations: ALAT: Alanine Transferases; ASAT: Aspartate Amino Transferase; Pal: alkaline phosphatase; N: normal value.

The mean weight gain was 2.7 ± 1.7 kg [95% CI: 2.2–3.2] ($p < 0.0001$). The mean BMI gain was 1.0 ± 0.6 kg/m^2 [95% CI: 0.8–1.2] ($p < 0.001$). Total fat mass increased by 1.7 ± 2.5 kg [95% CI: 0.9–2.6] and body fat percentage increased from 6.9 ± 4.3 to 11.0 ± 8.6% ($p < 0.02$). Fat mass increased significantly in the trunk and upper and lower limbs (40%, 29%, and 47%, respectively) while lean mass did not significantly increase and bone parameters remained unchanged (Table 3).

Table 3. Fat mass, lean mass, and mineral content evolution (Body Dual X-ray Absorptiometry).

	Mass	PMR Entry	PMR Discharge	p	Gain (%)	95% CI
Total Body	Fat mass (kg)	2.49 ± 1.78	4.22 ± 3.52	0.02	1.73 ± 2.57 (69%)	0.9–2.6
	Lean mass (kg)	32.6 ± 3.0	32.9 ± 3.8	0.70	0.2 ± 2.2 (1%)	−0.5–0.9
	BMC (kg)	1.71 ± 0.37	1.61 ± 0.38	0.21	−0.09 ± 0.28 (−5%)	−0.6–0.8
Upper limbs	Fat mass (g)	190.0 ± 162.0	245.0 ± 186.0	0.01	55.0 ± 52.0 (29%)	37.7–72.3
	Lean mass (g)	3139.0 ± 534.0	3295.0 ± 602.0	0.23	160.0 ± 370.0 (5%)	36.6–283.4
	BMC (g)	231.0 ± 53.0	232.0 ± 48.0	0.89	0.78 ± 16.0 (0%)	−4.6–6.1
Lower limbs	Fat mass (g)	1009.0 ± 981.0	1490.0 ± 1078.0	0.002	481.0 ± 332.0 (47%)	370.3–591.7
	Lean mass (g)	10724.0 ± 1579.0	11045.0 ± 1776.0	0.29	320.0 ± 864.0 (2.9%)	31.9–608.0
	BMC (g)	671.0 ± 204.0	658.0 ± 188.0	0.44	−12.7 ± 47.0 (−2%)	−3.0–28.4
Trunk	Fat mass (g)	1150.1 ± 1041.0	1621.0 ± 1313.0	0.04	470.0 ± 579.0 (40%)	279.9–663.0
	Lean mass (g)	16256.0 ± 2261.0	16197.0 ± 1945.0	0.91	−59.0 ± 1512.0 (−1%)	−445.1–563.1
	BMC (g)	396.0 ± 124.0	387.0 ± 129.0	0.61	−9.2 ± 52.0 (−1%)	−8.1–26.5

Abbreviations: BMC: Bone Mineral content; PMR: Physical Medicine and Rehabilitation.

Strength increased significantly in the upper and lower limbs, as well as the endurance in the trunk (Table 4). The walking distance during the 6-min test increased significantly by 90 m ($p < 0.01$), as did the parameters of the balance tests, especially with eyes closed. Respiratory function was significantly improved with a gain in FVC of 200 mL ($p < 0.01$), an improvement of the theoretical values which increased from 82.6 ± 16.4% to 89 ± 16% ($p = 0.004$). The FEV1 also increased ($p = 0.02$), explaining an unchanged FEV1/FVC at 87%, considered non-pathological.

Table 4. Limb and trunk strength, balance, walking, and respiratory evolution during PMR care.

	PMR Entry	PMR Discharge	*p*	Gain (%)
Biceps isometric (kg)	0.31 ± 0.12	0.42 ± 0.16	0.0001	24.8
Triceps isometric (kg)	0.21 ± 0.11	0.27 ± 0.11	0.0001	21.2
Grip (kg)	0.63 ± 0.13	0.67 ± 0.12	0.006	4.6
Quadriceps isometric (kg)	0.41 ± 0.20	0.58 ± 0.22	0.0001	27.8
Quadriceps isokinetic (kg)	1.37 ± 0.34	1.53 ± 0.33	0.001	8.2
Hamstring isometric (kg)	0.29 ± 0.15	0.40 ± 0.16	0.0001	26.7
Hamstring isokinetic (kg)	0.96 ± 0.23	1.03 ± 0.21	0.005	7.4
Abdominal Shirado–Ito test (s)	56.0 ± 61.0	111.0 ± 56.0	0.0001	47.9
Spine Biering–Sorensen test (s)	95.0 ± 67.0	128.0 ± 54.0	0.001	25.9
Balance open eyes (mm)	186.0 ± 86.0	122.0 ± 161.0	0.07	34.0
Balance closed eyes (mm)	424.0 ± 165.0	272.0 ± 164.0	0.001	55.8
6-min walking test (m)	526.0 ± 143.0	617.0 ± 121.0	0.007	17.0
FVC (L)	2.8 ± 0.57	3.02 ± 0.64	0.01	8.0
% predicted value	82.0 ± 17.0	89.0 ± 16.0	0.02	7.0
FEV1 (L/s)	2.46 ± 0.60	2.62 ± 0.61	0.02	6.0
% predicted value	82.0 ± 16.0	90.0 ± 17.0	0.02	8.0
FEV1/FVC (%)	87.4 ± 1.25	87.0 ± 0.09	0.79	0.0

Abbreviations: PMR: Physical Medicine and Rehabilitation; FVC: Forced Vital Capacity; FEV1: Forced Expiratory Volume in one second.

Tolerance to supervised physical activities was good. No stress fracture secondary to supervised physical activity was found in three patients who complained of transient musculoskeletal pain (less than 3 days) related to unusual muscle strain.

3.2. Comparison between Hyperactive and Non-Hyperactive Patients

The population of the 17 hyperactive patients was not different from the non-hyperactive one ($n = 20$) concerning the duration of hospitalization (43.3 ± 18.3 vs. 40.7 ± 18.2 days; $p = 0.66$) and the duration of refeeding by nasal-gastric tube (35.9 ± 17.3 vs. 36.0 ± 15.3 days; $p = 0.98$) (Table 5). The changes in weight and BMI over time were comparable (Weight: F(2.68) = 0.26, $p = 0.67$, $\eta^2 = 0.008$); (BMI: F(2.68) = 0.10, $p = 0.83$, $\eta^2 = 0.003$) (Figure 1a,b). The gains in isometric and isokinetic strength of the limbs and the trunk were comparable, as were gains in balance and gait parameters on the 6-min walking test. The gains of FVC and FEV1 were also no different.

Table 5. Comparison between hyperactive and non-hyperactive patients concerning body weight and BMI.

	Intensive Refeeding Care Entry	PMR Entry	PMR Discharge
Body weight (kg)			
- Hyperactive ($n = 17$)	33.6 ± 5.7	36.4 ± 7.0	38.7 ± 6.1
- Non hyperactive ($n = 20$)	34.3 ± 5.1	37.2 ± 3.6	40.1 ± 3.3
Body Mass Index (kg/m^2)			
- Hyperactive ($n = 17$)	12.8 ± 1.2	13.8 ± 1.7	14.7 ± 1.4
- Non hyperactive ($n = 20$)	12.5 ± 1.8	13.6 ± 1.0	14.6 ± 0.9

Abbreviations: PMR: Physical Medicine and Rehabilitation.

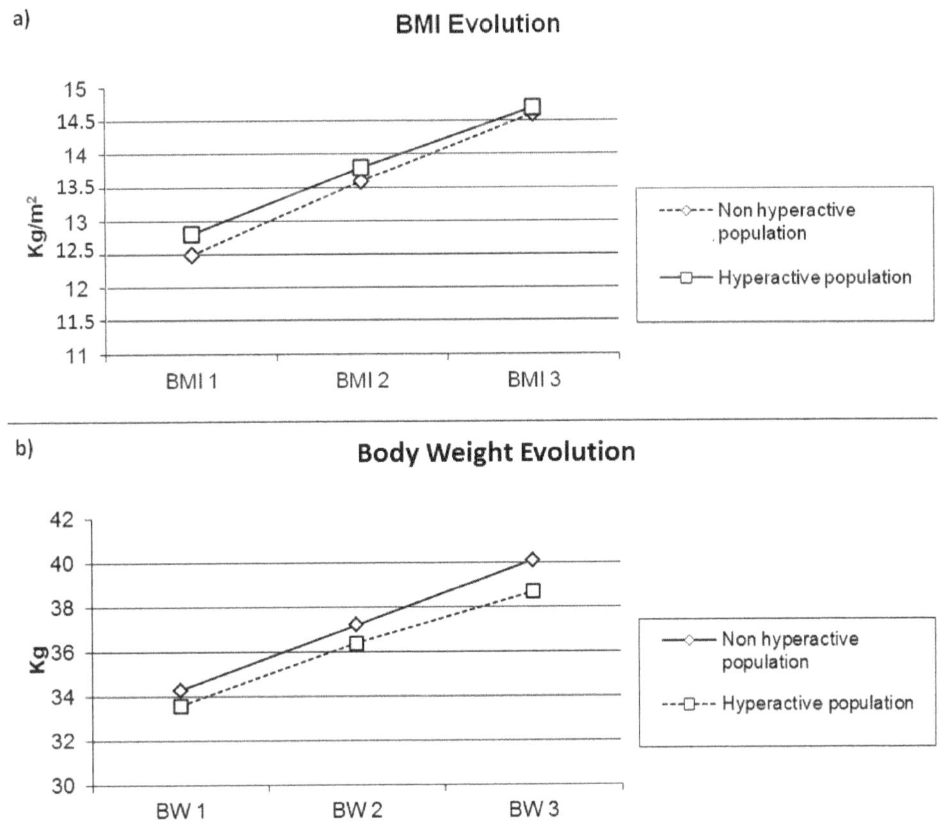

Figure 1. (**a**) Body Mass Index evolution and (**b**) Body Weight evolution according to hyperactivity or not in patients with anorexia nervosa. Abbreviations: BW: Body weight; BMI: Body Mass Index; Evolution 1: Enter in hospital; evolution 2: Enter in PMR; Evolution 3: discharge of MPR.

3.3. Correlations between Clinical Parameters and Weight Gain

Improvement in the 6-min walking test was associated with weight gain (r = 0.432; $p < 0.01$). There was a tendency for an association between weight gain and isokinetic strength gain in the extensors and flexors of the knees (r = 0.392; $p = 0.06$ and r = 0.374; $p = 0.07$, respectively). Improvement in grip strength, endurance of the trunk, isometric strength of the lower and upper limbs, and respiratory function were not associated with weight gain.

3.4. Follow-Up after PMR Hospitalization

The subjective evaluation performed at 12 months of the hospitalization in the PMR department showed that 21 patients were very satisfied ($n = 6$) or satisfied ($n = 15$) because of the medical and paramedical support. Patients reported that this support helped them recover weight, while they perceived progress with a feeling of having more strength. Some of them would have liked the care to last longer, while others felt the care was very strict. Seven subjects were dissatisfied because of the constraints related to the nasogastric tube and the "infantilization" related to the strict framework imposed for weighing.

A total of 17 patients (46%) continued physical activities such as cycling, jogging, fitness, swimming, walking, dancing, and gentle gymnastics. However, among them, 1 patient remained hyperactive (cycling 200 km per week), and another restrictive anorexic patient became hyperactive (running more than 5 times a week). Eleven patients no longer performed physical activities after the PMR treatment. Nine patients did not give their opinion (six non-responders and three dead, including a man and a woman by suicide and a woman by pneumonia).

A total of 8 subjects (21%) were re-hospitalized in the psychiatric service for recurrence, including 6 hyperactive patients. Two patients, a pure restrictive anorexic and an overactive anorexic with purging, were re-hospitalized for consolidation of weight gains.

4. Discussion

Adapted and controlled physical activities during hospitalization in a PMR department were performed safely in severe anorexic subjects (BMI < 14 kg/m^2) with intensive refeeding by nasogastric tube to allow the control of caloric intake. This management required multidisciplinary skills with weekly monitoring of psychiatric care, nutrition, and PMR in order to improve muscle strength, respiratory parameters, balance, and walking while restoring body weight and resuming exclusive oral feeding. Interestingly, we found no differences between the hyperactive and non-hyperactive patients. To our knowledge, this work was the first to propose physical activities during nasogastric refeeding with multiple pre- and post-physical activity assessments while differentiating hyperactive patients from non-hyperactive patients.

Several studies have already shown that it is possible to perform physical activities for anorexic subjects while gaining weight or improving BMI [42–46]. However, no difference has been found compared to control anorexic subjects not performing physical activity [47]. Body fat increase had already been shown in patients with anorexia from Australia aged from 16 to 19 years old (BMI from 14.8 to 15.4 kg/m^2) who gained between 2.5 and 8% of body fat while they performed various anaerobic and aerobic physical activities [48,49]. According to their measurements by DXA, body fat increased in the lower limbs (47%), the trunk (40%), and the upper limbs (29%) in different proportions from those we have shown, certainly due to the predominance of women in our population. Another hypothesis is that the practice of physical activities played a role in the distribution of fatty masses according to the particular demand of certain regions of the body.

One of the objectives of practicing physical activities during refeeding is to gain lean mass by performing muscle strengthening using the anaerobic energetic system [50]. Lean mass gain had previously been reported after calculation and not by direct measurement [49,50]. However, our measures of lean mass by DXA were unmodified at the end of the hospitalization. We certainly did not show an increase in lean mass because a gain in muscle mass undoubtedly requires more time, 20 to 24 weeks of resistance training at a frequency of twice a week in order to allow the synthesis of muscle proteins [51]. Russel et al. used a physical activity program for 10 to 15 weeks [49]. In fact, in healthy Caucasian subjects, the gain in muscle mass is variable depending on the individual (mean gain of 4.8% from −10 to +30%) with the notion of high and low responders (30% of subjects), without the possibility of predicting lean mass gain according to the BMI, the age, and the sex [51]. The relationship between muscle mass and strength is also weak (r = 0.157) [51]. From a physiological point of view, the variations between individuals in lean mass gain are poorly understood, and the participation of different factors are mentioned: genetic, microRNA expression, the phosphorylation status of signaling proteins, androgen receptor concentrations, satellite cell count, mitochondrial function, and inflammatory cytokines [51,52]. In severe anorexic subjects (BMI: 12.6 ± 0.7 kg/m^2), muscle atrophy has been described by MacLoughlin et al. according to a "metabolic myopathy" corresponding to type-2 fiber atrophy with abnormal accumulation of glycogen granules within fibers, which rapidly recovers as the nutrition improves [53,54].

On the other hand, muscle strength and endurance increased significantly in the trunk and limbs. Our results are difficult to compare with those of other studies due to different activities performed in populations of anorexic subjects of different ages and BMIs [47]. Only two medical teams were interested in developing strength during a physical activity program in anorexic patients [11,43,44]. Chantler et al. are the only ones who have studied a population comparable to ours in terms of average age (20 ± 5 years old), while Fernadez del Valle et al. studied 13–14 years old children [11,43,44]. Chantler et al. proposed muscle strengthening exercises against low resistance (2.5 kg dumbbells for the upper body, therapeutic elastic bands for the lower body, and body weight for the back) for 60 min twice a week for 8 weeks [44]. The absolute isokinetic strength of the knee extensors and flexors and the strength of the elbow flexors increased in 7 hospitalized anorexic subjects who ate 2500 calories per day and who had an average BMI of 15.1 ± 1.1 kg/m^2 [44]. From a physiological point of view, several neural factors may be implied, including an increase in motor neuron excitability with inhibition of protective mechanisms to explain the increase in force [44]. This increase in strength was explained by the weight gain (+6 kg) during the refeeding protocol compared with control anorexic subjects (+3.3 kg). Re-nutrition responsible for weight gain was the main factor to explain the increase in strength, while the role of physical activities was difficult to isolate. More recently, Garrido et al. [12] showed that strength was significantly associated to BMI (r = 0.420; $p < 0.01$) before enteral refeeding in 23 severe restrictive anorexics aged 25.6 ± 6.2 years old (BMI: 11.4 ± 1.3 kg/m^2). In the absence of physical activity, muscle strength, which had been manually assessed and summarily rated from 0 to 5, increased in 5 weeks in the trunk and the limbs as well as the body-weight [12]. Unfortunately, no association was sought based on the observed gains. When weight and strength gains were taken into account, we showed that the association was weak between isokinetic strength gain measured at the knee and weight gain. In addition, no significant association was found between isometric strength gain measured at the trunk and the lower limbs or the hand grip. This result suggested a specific role of the practice of adapted physical activities to increase strength. However, we could not confirm this due to the absence of control group.

Concerning bone parameters, it was not surprising to find that the bone mineral content remained unchanged in such a short period of physical activity [55,56]. Moreover, in anorexic subjects, the practice of high-impact physical activities such as repeated jumps was not enough to modify the markers of bone turnover (Bone-specific alkaline phosphatase, N-telopeptide, Osteocalcin) during intensive refeeding [57].

Another goal of physical activities was to improve function. The walking perimeter improved according to our results. We did not find any study that had analyzed this parameter in anorexic subjects, while the expected normal value in healthy subjects was 804 m according to the formula of Enright et al., which includes weight, height, and age [58]. Our population presented impaired walking at entry into PMR, which improved, on average, by 90 m but did not reach the expected standard. Fernandez del Valle et al. [43] studied the interest in 2010 of outpatient resistance training in children aged 14 years old on functional capacity according to the Time Up and Go test of 3 and 10 m and the Time Up and Down Stairs test. Despite an increase in strength, no functional gain was reported, probably due to already normal functional tests before training.

Balance also improved, probably due to a deficit at the entry into hospitalization (186 ± 86 mm with eyes open and 424 ± 165 mm with eyes closed). Indeed, balance with open and closed eyes was altered compared with the results of Fontana et al. [59], who evaluated a population of 15 anorexic subjects comparable to ours (age: 32 ± 11 years and BMI: 15.8 ± 1.8 kg/m^2), hospitalized for a rehabilitation program, including physiotherapy, nutritional and psychological counseling. After our physical activity program, the values were comparable (122 ±161 mm) to those obtained by Fontana et al. eyes open (139 ± 87 mm; healthy subject: 104 ± 30 mm). On the other hand, the values obtained with eyes closed remained high (272 ± 164 mm vs. 160 ± 73 mm; healthy subjects: 124 ± 73 mm) [59]. This altered balance eyes closed may have been related to a state of anxiety present during the test, while strength gains in the lower limbs and trunk may have explained the balance gains. Indeed, anxiety and emotional factors can have a negative influence on the efficiency of human posture control due to interaction between vision and vestibular and somatosensory inputs [59]. In addition, a large variation between individuals was present, evidenced by the standard deviations of the values we reported.

Respiratory capacity also improved. Several studies have shown an alteration of respiratory capacities in anorexic subjects nicknamed "nutritional emphysema-like" [60–62]. However, ventilatory parameters usually remain within the norm, so there is no real "emphysema" [60]. In fact, these parameters undoubtedly depend on the degree of undernutrition. The lower the BMI of the anorexic population is, the lower the respiratory values are. For an average BMI of 18 kg/m^2, the FEV1 and FVC are 106 and 109% of the predicted values, respectively [61], 106 and 100% if the average BMI is 16 kg/m^2 [62], and 91 and 85% if the average BMI is 14.3 kg/m^2 [60]. Before the stay in PMR, we reported values of 82% for a BMI of 13.8 kg/m^2 with an improvement to 89 and 90% when the BMI improved to 14.8 kg/m^2. Therefore, refeeding improved ventilatory parameters. Minano Garrido et al. [12] also showed a significant link between BMI and FEV1 (r = 0.660; $p < 0.01$). However, the practice of physical activities undoubtedly also contributed to ventilatory gain due to work based on the control of breath, with possibly an improvement in anxiety, independently of the weight gain. The improvement in muscle strength contributed to the improvement in respiratory capacities, as already demonstrated by Murciano et al. at the level of the diaphragm during refeeding [63]. The strength improvement of the intercostal muscles and, especially the abdominal muscles, due to an isometric strength gain of 48% during the abdominal Shirado test, undoubtedly contributed to a decrease in the residual volume, evaluated by Pieters et al., to 162% of the predicted values, explaining the use of the term "emphysema-like" [60].

The comparison between hyperactive and non-hyperactive anorexic subjects reported no difference for any of the measured parameters. Therefore, it seems possible to offer adapted and supervised physical activities during inpatient refeeding by nasogastric tube to anorexic subjects with hyperactivity. Few studies have attempted this experience because, most often, the subjects described in the literature are adolescents and present restrictive anorexia [11,42,43,45] or other eating disorders such as bulimia nervosa or Eating Disorder Not Otherwise Specified (EDNOS) [64]. Calogero et al. were, to our knowledge, the first to offer controlled physical activities to treat hyperactivity in patients with eating disorders [21], including multiple supervised exercises including stretching, yoga, Pilates, partner exercises, strength training, aerobic activities, and recreational games, were performed 1 h per session 4 times a week for 6 months. Weight improved by 43% and 38% in restrictive anorexic and bulimic patients, respectively. From a psychological point of view, monitored activities decreased anxiety and increased comfort with gaining weight, reduced anxiety during mealtimes, and increased compliance with the nutritive program [21]. Monitoring and individualizing the practice of physical activities according to weight gain has undoubtedly been successful. Thus, the weight gains were identical between hyperactive and non-hyperactive patients.

However, our results are questionable due to the premature end of the program for five patients, the dissatisfaction of some patients, and the relapses (21%). The three deaths are, of course, not attributable to the program but to the severity of the disease. More positively, 46% of patients continued to practice moderate physical activity, which testifies to the impact of educational advice. Unfortunately, two patients remained hyperactive, highlighting the difficulties in managing anorexia.

Our study has limits, especially concerning the patients' selection, because only the most motivated by this type of PMR care were selected after psychiatric evaluation [21]. In addition, the absence of a control group does not allow us to assess exactly the role of physical activities in weight gain and other parameters improvement [23]. An RCT-type study would have been ideal but would present difficulties related to the definition of hyperactivity in anorexic patients and to the multitude of physical activities that could be offered according to durations, intensities, and frequencies. Indeed, the content of a physical activity program offered to anorexic children should probably be different from the program offered to adolescents or adults [42]. However, our adapted program followed some guidelines described by Cook et al. concerning progression, supervision, individualization, and monitoring according to energy expenditure and calorie intake [65].

The objectives were to gain strength and autonomy while allowing refeeding by nasogastric tube and psychiatric care. The evaluated parameters could have been different, for example, the body image or the evolution of patient anxiety [66].

5. Conclusions

The early return to controlled physical activities in PMR hospitalization did not compromise the efficiency of intensive refeeding in severe anorexia nervosa patients. It allowed an increase in functional performance with a rather good rate of patient satisfaction. However, a very attentive multidisciplinary approach was required in order not to compromise the efficiency of intensive refeeding by nasogastric tube. Further attention should be paid to the program to increase the long-term activity continuation and to avoid the premature ending of the hospitalization or disease relapse.

Author Contributions: Conceptualization, M.D. and P.M.; methodology, M.D. and A.F.-C.; software, M.D.; validation, B.J., S.L. and B.R.; formal analysis, M.D. and A.F.-C.; investigation, M.D., B.J., S.L., M.L.B., A.J., P.G., S.P. and B.R.; resources, B.J., S.L., M.L.B., A.J., P.G., S.P. and B.R.; data curation, M.D., A.F.-C. and P.M.; writing—original draft preparation, M.D. and A.F.-C.; writing—review and editing, P.M., B.J., S.L., M.L.B., A.J., P.G., S.P. and B.R.; supervision, A.F.-C.; project administration, M.D. and A.F.-C. All authors have read and agreed to the published version of the manuscript.

Funding: This research received no external funding.

Institutional Review Board Statement: The local ethics committee (Comité Nantais d'Ethique en Médecine du Sport) approved the protocol under the number of registration CNEMS-2022-001. The study was also declared to the Research Department of the University Hospital. The study was in accordance with the declaration of Helsinki.

Informed Consent Statement: All the patients gave written consent to participate in the study.

Data Availability Statement: The data presented in this study are available on request from the corresponding author. The data are not publicly available due to ethical reasons.

Conflicts of Interest: The authors declare no conflict of interest.

References

1. Smink, F.R.E.; van Hoeken, D.; Hoek, H.W. Epidemiology of Eating Disorders: Incidence, Prevalence and Mortality Rates. *Curr. Psychiatry Rep.* **2012**, *14*, 406–414. [CrossRef] [PubMed]
2. Hudson, J.I.; Hiripi, E.; Pope, H.G.; Kessler, R.C. The Prevalence and Correlates of Eating Disorders in the National Comorbidity Survey Replication. *Biol. Psychiatry* **2007**, *61*, 348–358. [CrossRef]
3. Mustelin, L.; Silén, Y.; Raevuori, A.; Hoek, H.W.; Kaprio, J.; Keski-Rahkonen, A. The DSM-5 Diagnostic Criteria for Anorexia Nervosa May Change Its Population Prevalence and Prognostic Value. *J. Psychiatr. Res.* **2016**, *77*, 85–91. [CrossRef] [PubMed]
4. Arcelus, J.; Mitchell, A.J.; Wales, J.; Nielsen, S. Mortality Rates in Patients with Anorexia Nervosa and Other Eating Disorders. A Meta-Analysis of 36 Studies. *Arch. Gen. Psychiatry* **2011**, *68*, 724–731. [CrossRef] [PubMed]
5. Stheneur, C.; Ali, A.; Tric, L.; Curt, F.; Hubert, T.; Godart, N. Impact of Somatic Severity on Long-Term Mortality in Anorexia Nervosa. *Eat. Weight Disord. EWD* **2017**, *22*, 285–289. [CrossRef]
6. Gjoertz, M.; Wang, J.; Chatelet, S.; Monney Chaubert, C.; Lier, F.; Ambresin, A.-E. Nutrition Approach for Inpatients With Anorexia Nervosa: Impact of a Clinical Refeeding Guideline. *JPEN J. Parenter. Enter. Nutr.* **2020**, *44*, 1124–1139. [CrossRef]
7. Garber, A.K.; Sawyer, S.M.; Golden, N.H.; Guarda, A.S.; Katzman, D.K.; Kohn, M.R.; Le Grange, D.; Madden, S.; Whitelaw, M.; Redgrave, G.W. A Systematic Review of Approaches to Refeeding in Patients with Anorexia Nervosa. *Int. J. Eat. Disord.* **2016**, *49*, 293–310. [CrossRef]
8. Herpertz-Dahlmann, B. Intensive Treatments in Adolescent Anorexia Nervosa. *Nutrients* **2021**, *13*, 1265. [CrossRef]
9. Haas, V.; Kohn, M.; Körner, T.; Cuntz, U.; Garber, A.K.; Le Grange, D.; Voderholzer, U.; Correll, C.U. Practice-Based Evidence and Clinical Guidance to Support Accelerated Re-Nutrition of Patients With Anorexia Nervosa. *J. Am. Acad. Child Adolesc. Psychiatry* **2021**, *60*, 555–561. [CrossRef]
10. Hofer, M.; Pozzi, A.; Joray, M.; Ott, R.; Hähni, F.; Leuenberger, M.; von Känel, R.; Stanga, Z. Safe Refeeding Management of Anorexia Nervosa Inpatients: An Evidence-Based Protocol. *Nutr. Burbank Los Angel. Cty. Calif.* **2014**, *30*, 524–530. [CrossRef]
11. Fernández-del-Valle, M.; Larumbe-Zabala, E.; Villaseñor-Montarroso, A.; Cardona Gonzalez, C.; Diez-Vega, I.; Lopez Mojares, L.M.; Perez Ruiz, M. Resistance Training Enhances Muscular Performance in Patients with Anorexia Nervosa: A Randomized Controlled Trial. *Int. J. Eat. Disord.* **2014**, *47*, 601–609. [CrossRef] [PubMed]

12. Minano Garrido, E.; Di Lodovico, L.; Dicembre, M.; Duquesnoy, M.; Ohanyan, H.; Melchior, J.-C.; Hanachi, M. Evaluation of Muscle-Skeletal Strength and Peak Expiratory Flow in Severely Malnourished Inpatients with Anorexia Nervosa: A Pilot Study. *Nutr. Burbank Los Angel. Cty. Calif.* **2021**, *85*, 111133. [CrossRef]
13. Skowrońska, A.; Sójta, K.; Strzelecki, D. Refeeding Syndrome as Treatment Complication of Anorexia Nervosa. *Psychiatr. Pol.* **2019**, *53*, 1113–1123. [CrossRef] [PubMed]
14. Probst, M.; Majeweski, M.L.; Albertsen, M.N.; Catalan-Matamoros, D.; Danielsen, M.; De Herdt, A.; Duskova Zakova, H.; Fabricius, S.; Joern, C.; Kjölstad, G.; et al. Physiotherapy for Patients with Anorexia Nervosa. *Adv. Eat. Disord.* **2013**, *1*, 224–238. [CrossRef]
15. Blinder, B.J.; Freeman, D.M.; Stunkard, A.J. Behavior Therapy of Anorexia Nervosa: Effectiveness of Activity as a Reinforcer of Weight Gain. *Am. J. Psychiatry* **1970**, *126*, 1093–1098. [CrossRef] [PubMed]
16. Ng, L.W.C.; Ng, D.P.; Wong, W.P. Is Supervised Exercise Training Safe in Patients with Anorexia Nervosa? A Meta-Analysis. *Physiotherapy* **2013**, *99*, 1–11. [CrossRef]
17. Moola, F.J.; Gairdner, S.E.; Amara, C.E. Exercise in the Care of Patients with Anorexia Nervosa: A Systematic Review of the Literature. *Ment. Health Phys. Act.* **2013**, *6*, 59–68. [CrossRef]
18. El Ghoch, M.; Soave, F.; Calugi, S.; Dalle Grave, R. Eating Disorders, Physical Fitness and Sport Performance: A Systematic Review. *Nutrients* **2013**, *5*, 5140–5160. [CrossRef]
19. Hausenblas, H.A.; Cook, B.J.; Chittester, N.I. Can Exercise Treat Eating Disorders? *Exerc. Sport Sci. Rev.* **2008**, *36*, 43–47. [CrossRef]
20. Savidaki, M.; Demirtoka, S.; Rodríguez-Jiménez, R.-M. Re-Inhabiting One's Body: A Pilot Study on the Effects of Dance Movement Therapy on Body Image and Alexithymia in Eating Disorders. *J. Eat. Disord.* **2020**, *8*, 22. [CrossRef]
21. Calogero, R.M.; Pedrotty, K.N. The Practice and Process of Healthy Exercise: An Investigation of the Treatment of Exercise Abuse in Women with Eating Disorders. *Eat. Disord.* **2004**, *12*, 273–291. [CrossRef] [PubMed]
22. Dalle Grave, R.; Calugi, S.; Marchesini, G. Compulsive Exercise to Control Shape or Weight in Eating Disorders: Prevalence, Associated Features, and Treatment Outcome. *Compr. Psychiatry* **2008**, *49*, 346–352. [CrossRef] [PubMed]
23. Kern, L.; Morvan, Y.; Mattar, L.; Molina, E.; Tailhardat, L.; Peguet, A.; De Tournemire, R.; Hirot, F.; Rizk, M.; Godart, N.; et al. Development and Evaluation of an Adapted Physical Activity Program in Anorexia Nervosa Inpatients: A Pilot Study. *Eur. Eat. Disord. Rev. J. Eat. Disord. Assoc.* **2020**, *28*, 687–700. [CrossRef] [PubMed]
24. Brunet, J.; Del Duchetto, F.; Wurz, A. Physical Activity Behaviors and Attitudes among Women with an Eating Disorder: A Qualitative Study. *J. Eat. Disord.* **2021**, *9*, 20. [CrossRef] [PubMed]
25. Meyer, C.; Taranis, L. Exercise in the Eating Disorders: Terms and Definitions. *Eur. Eat. Disord. Rev. J. Eat. Disord. Assoc.* **2011**, *19*, 169–173. [CrossRef]
26. Crocq, M.-A.; Guelfi, J.-D. *DSM-5: Manuel Diagnostique et Statistique des Troubles Mentaux*, 5th ed.; Elsevier Masson: Issy-les-Moulineaux, France, 2015; ISBN 978-2-294-73929-3.
27. Hay, P.; Chinn, D.; Forbes, D.; Madden, S.; Newton, R.; Sugenor, L.; Touyz, S.; Ward, W. Royal Australian and New Zealand College of Psychiatrists Royal Australian and New Zealand College of Psychiatrists Clinical Practice Guidelines for the Treatment of Eating Disorders. *Aust. N. Z. J. Psychiatry* **2014**, *48*, 977–1008. [CrossRef]
28. Mehanna, H.M.; Moledina, J.; Travis, J. Refeeding Syndrome: What It Is, and How to Prevent and Treat It. *BMJ* **2008**, *336*, 1495–1498. [CrossRef]
29. Impellizzeri, F.M.; Bizzini, M.; Rampinini, E.; Cereda, F.; Maffiuletti, N.A. Reliability of Isokinetic Strength Imbalance Ratios Measured Using the Cybex NORM Dynamometer. *Clin. Physiol. Funct. Imaging* **2008**, *28*, 113–119. [CrossRef]
30. Buckinx, F.; Croisier, J.-L.; Reginster, J.-Y.; Dardenne, N.; Beaudart, C.; Slomian, J.; Leonard, S.; Bruyère, O. Reliability of Muscle Strength Measures Obtained with a Hand-Held Dynamometer in an Elderly Population. *Clin. Physiol. Funct. Imaging* **2017**, *37*, 332–340. [CrossRef]
31. Hamilton, G.F.; McDonald, C.; Chenier, T.C. Measurement of Grip Strength: Validity and Reliability of the Sphygmomanometer and Jamar Grip Dynamometer. *J. Orthop. Sports Phys. Ther.* **1992**, *16*, 215–219. [CrossRef]
32. Etemadi, S.; Sun, G.X.; Leung, S.-P.; Siddique, A.; Cooper, S.; Ezenwa, N.C.; Treasure, J.; Robinson, P. The Sit Up Squat Stand Test and Hand Grip Strength: What Is the Role of Tests of Muscle Power in Risk Assessment in Anorexia Nervosa? *Eur. Eat. Disord. Rev. J. Eat. Disord. Assoc.* **2021**, *29*, 670–679. [CrossRef] [PubMed]
33. Ito, T.; Shirado, O.; Suzuki, H.; Takahashi, M.; Kaneda, K.; Strax, T.E. Lumbar Trunk Muscle Endurance Testing: An Inexpensive Alternative to a Machine for Evaluation. *Arch. Phys. Med. Rehabil.* **1996**, *77*, 75–79. [CrossRef]
34. Biering-Sørensen, F. Physical Measurements as Risk Indicators for Low-Back Trouble over a One-Year Period. *Spine* **1984**, *9*, 106–119. [CrossRef] [PubMed]
35. del Pozo-Cruz, B.; Mocholi, M.H.; del Pozo-Cruz, J.; Parraca, J.A.; Adsuar, J.C.; Gusi, N. Reliability and Validity of Lumbar and Abdominal Trunk Muscle Endurance Tests in Office Workers with Nonspecific Subacute Low Back Pain. *J. Back Musculoskelet. Rehabil.* **2014**, *27*, 399–408. [CrossRef]
36. Latimer, J.; Maher, C.G.; Refshauge, K.; Colaco, I. The Reliability and Validity of the Biering-Sorensen Test in Asymptomatic Subjects and Subjects Reporting Current or Previous Nonspecific Low Back Pain. *Spine* **1999**, *24*, 2085–2089, discussion 2090. [CrossRef]
37. Hsu, W.-L.; Scholz, J.P.; Schöner, G.; Jeka, J.J.; Kiemel, T. Control and Estimation of Posture during Quiet Stance Depends on Multijoint Coordination. *J. Neurophysiol.* **2007**, *97*, 3024–3035. [CrossRef]

38. Rodríguez-Rubio, P.R.; Bagur-Calafat, C.; López-de-Celis, C.; Bueno-Gracía, E.; Cabanas-Valdés, R.; Herrera-Pedroviejo, E.; Girabent-Farrés, M. Validity and Reliability of the Satel 40 Hz Stabilometric Force Platform for Measuring Quiet Stance and Dynamic Standing Balance in Healthy Subjects. *Int. J. Environ. Res. Public Health* **2020**, *17*, 7733. [CrossRef]
39. Rikli, R.E.; Jones, C.J. The Reliability and Validity of a 6-Minute Walk Test as a Measure of Physical Endurance in Older Adults. *J. Aging Phys. Act.* **1998**, *6*, 363–375. [CrossRef]
40. Graham, B.L.; Steenbruggen, I.; Miller, M.R.; Barjaktarevic, I.Z.; Cooper, B.G.; Hall, G.L.; Hallstrand, T.S.; Kaminsky, D.A.; McCarthy, K.; McCormack, M.C.; et al. Standardization of Spirometry 2019 Update. An Official American Thoracic Society and European Respiratory Society Technical Statement. *Am. J. Respir. Crit. Care Med.* **2019**, *200*, e70–e88. [CrossRef]
41. Messina, C.; Poloni, A.; Chianca, V.; Albano, D.; Piodi, L.P.; Ulivieri, F.M.; Sconfienza, L.M. Increasing Soft Tissue Thickness Does Not Affect Trabecular Bone Score Reproducibility: A Phantom Study. *Endocrine* **2018**, *61*, 336–342. [CrossRef]
42. Fernández-del-Valle, M.; Larumbe-Zabala, E.; Morande-Lavin, G.; Perez Ruiz, M. Muscle Function and Body Composition Profile in Adolescents with Restrictive Anorexia Nervosa: Does Resistance Training Help? *Disabil. Rehabil.* **2016**, *38*, 346–353. [CrossRef] [PubMed]
43. Fernández del Valle, M.; Pérez, M.; Santana-Sosa, E.; Fiuza-Luces, C.; Bustamante-Ara, N.; Gallardo, C.; Villaseñor, A.; Graell, M.; Morandé, G.; Romo, G.R.; et al. Does Resistance Training Improve the Functional Capacity and Well Being of Very Young Anorexic Patients? A Randomized Controlled Trial. *J. Adolesc. Health Off. Publ. Soc. Adolesc. Med.* **2010**, *46*, 352–358. [CrossRef] [PubMed]
44. Chantler, I.; Szabo, C.P.; Green, K. Muscular Strength Changes in Hospitalized Anorexic Patients after an Eight Week Resistance Training Program. *Int. J. Sports Med.* **2006**, *27*, 660–665. [CrossRef] [PubMed]
45. Tokumura, M.; Yoshiba, S.; Tanaka, T.; Nanri, S.; Watanabe, H. Prescribed Exercise Training Improves Exercise Capacity of Convalescent Children and Adolescents with Anorexia Nervosa. *Eur. J. Pediatr.* **2003**, *162*, 430–431. [CrossRef]
46. Thien, V.; Thomas, A.; Markin, D.; Birmingham, C.L. Pilot Study of a Graded Exercise Program for the Treatment of Anorexia Nervosa. *Int. J. Eat. Disord.* **2000**, *28*, 101–106. [CrossRef]
47. Quiles Marcos, Y.; León Zarceño, E.; López López, J.A. Effectiveness of Exercise-Based Interventions in Patients with Anorexia Nervosa: A Systematic Review. *Eur. Eat. Disord. Rev.* **2021**, *29*, 3–19. [CrossRef]
48. Touyz, S.W.; Lennerts, W.; Arthur, B.; Beumont, P.J.V. Anaerobic Exercise as an Adjunct to Refeeding Patients with Anorexia Nervosa: Does It Compromise Weight Gain? *Eur. Eat. Disord. Rev.* **1993**, *1*, 177–182. [CrossRef]
49. Russell, J.D.; Mira, M.; Allen, B.J.; Stewart, P.J.; Vizzard, J.; Arthur, B.; Beumont, P.J. Effect of Refeeding and Exercise in Restoration of Body Protein in Anorexia Nervosa. *Basic Life Sci.* **1993**, *60*, 207–210. [CrossRef] [PubMed]
50. Szabo, C.P.; Green, K. Hospitalized Anorexics and Resistance Training: Impact on Body Composition and Psychological Well-Being. A Preliminary Study. *Eat. Weight Disord. EWD* **2002**, *7*, 293–297. [CrossRef]
51. Ahtiainen, J.P.; Walker, S.; Peltonen, H.; Holviala, J.; Sillanpää, E.; Karavirta, L.; Sallinen, J.; Mikkola, J.; Valkeinen, H.; Mero, A.; et al. Heterogeneity in Resistance Training-Induced Muscle Strength and Mass Responses in Men and Women of Different Ages. *Age Dordr. Neth.* **2016**, *38*, 10. [CrossRef]
52. Yoo, S.-Z.; No, M.-H.; Heo, J.-W.; Park, D.-H.; Kang, J.-H.; Kim, S.H.; Kwak, H.-B. Role of Exercise in Age-Related Sarcopenia. *J. Exerc. Rehabil.* **2018**, *14*, 551–558. [CrossRef] [PubMed]
53. McLoughlin, D.M.; Spargo, E.; Wassif, W.S.; Newham, D.J.; Peters, T.J.; Lantos, P.L.; Russell, G.F. Structural and Functional Changes in Skeletal Muscle in Anorexia Nervosa. *Acta Neuropathol.* **1998**, *95*, 632–640. [CrossRef]
54. McLoughlin, D.M.; Wassif, W.S.; Morton, J.; Spargo, E.; Peters, T.J.; Russell, G.F. Metabolic Abnormalities Associated with Skeletal Myopathy in Severe Anorexia Nervosa. *Nutr. Burbank Los Angel. Cty. Calif.* **2000**, *16*, 192–196. [CrossRef]
55. Waugh, E.J.; Woodside, D.B.; Beaton, D.E.; Coté, P.; Hawker, G.A. Effects of Exercise on Bone Mass in Young Women with Anorexia Nervosa. *Med. Sci. Sports Exerc.* **2011**, *43*, 755–763. [CrossRef] [PubMed]
56. DiVasta, A.D.; Feldman, H.A.; O'Donnell, J.M.; Long, J.; Leonard, M.B.; Gordon, C.M. Effect of Exercise and Antidepressants on Skeletal Outcomes in Adolescent Girls With Anorexia Nervosa. *J. Adolesc. Health Off. Publ. Soc. Adolesc. Med.* **2017**, *60*, 229–232. [CrossRef] [PubMed]
57. Martin, S.P.K.; Bachrach, L.K.; Golden, N.H. Controlled Pilot Study of High-Impact Low-Frequency Exercise on Bone Loss and Vital-Sign Stabilization in Adolescents With Eating Disorders. *J. Adolesc. Health Off. Publ. Soc. Adolesc. Med.* **2017**, *60*, 33–37. [CrossRef]
58. Enright, P.L.; Sherrill, D.L. Reference Equations for the Six-Minute Walk in Healthy Adults. *Am. J. Respir. Crit. Care Med.* **1998**, *158*, 1384–1387. [CrossRef]
59. Fontana, M.P.; Menegoni, F.; Vismara, L.; Galli, M.; Romei, M.; Bergamini, E.; Petroni, M.L.; Capodaglio, P. Balance in Patients with Anorexia and Bulimia Nervosa. *Eur. J. Phys. Rehabil. Med.* **2009**, *45*, 335–340.
60. Pieters, T.; Boland, B.; Beguin, C.; Veriter, C.; Stanescu, D.; Frans, A.; Lambert, M. Lung Function Study and Diffusion Capacity in Anorexia Nervosa. *J. Intern. Med.* **2000**, *248*, 137–142. [CrossRef]
61. Coxson, H.O.; Chan, I.H.T.; Mayo, J.R.; Hlynsky, J.; Nakano, Y.; Birmingham, C.L. Early Emphysema in Patients with Anorexia Nervosa. *Am. J. Respir. Crit. Care Med.* **2004**, *170*, 748–752. [CrossRef]
62. Gardini Gardenghi, G.; Boni, E.; Todisco, P.; Manara, F.; Borghesi, A.; Tantucci, C. Respiratory Function in Patients with Stable Anorexia Nervosa. *Chest* **2009**, *136*, 1356–1363. [CrossRef] [PubMed]

63. Murciano, D.; Rigaud, D.; Pingleton, S.; Armengaud, M.H.; Melchior, J.C.; Aubier, M. Diaphragmatic Function in Severely Malnourished Patients with Anorexia Nervosa. Effects of Renutrition. *Am. J. Respir. Crit. Care Med.* **1994**, *150*, 1569–1574. [CrossRef] [PubMed]
64. Carei, T.R.; Fyfe-Johnson, A.L.; Breuner, C.C.; Brown, M.A. Randomized Controlled Clinical Trial of Yoga in the Treatment of Eating Disorders. *J. Adolesc. Health Off. Publ. Soc. Adolesc. Med.* **2010**, *46*, 346–351. [CrossRef]
65. Cook, B.J.; Wonderlich, S.A.; Mitchell, J.E.; Thompson, R.; Sherman, R.; McCallum, K. Exercise in Eating Disorders Treatment: Systematic Review and Proposal of Guidelines. *Med. Sci. Sports Exerc.* **2016**, *48*, 1408–1414. [CrossRef] [PubMed]
66. Rizk, M.; Mattar, L.; Kern, L.; Berthoz, S.; Duclos, J.; Viltart, O.; Godart, N. Physical Activity in Eating Disorders: A Systematic Review. *Nutrients* **2020**, *12*, 183. [CrossRef]

nutrients

Review

Neuro-Vulnerability in Energy Metabolism Regulation: A Comprehensive Narrative Review

Vicente Javier Clemente-Suárez [1,2,*], Ana Isabel Beltrán-Velasco [3], Laura Redondo-Flórez [4], Alexandra Martín-Rodríguez [1,*], Rodrigo Yáñez-Sepúlveda [5] and José Francisco Tornero-Aguilera [1]

1 Faculty of Sports Sciences, Universidad Europea de Madrid, Tajo Street, s/n, 28670 Madrid, Spain
2 Grupo de Investigación en Cultura, Educación y Sociedad, Universidad de la Costa, Barranquilla 080002, Colombia
3 Psychology Department, Faculty of Life and Natural Sciences, Nebrija University, 28240 Madrid, Spain
4 Department of Health Sciences, Faculty of Biomedical and Health Sciences, Universidad Europea de Madrid, Tajo Street s/n, 28670 Madrid, Spain
5 Faculty of Education and Social Sciences, Universidad Andres Bello, Viña del Mar 2520000, Chile
* Correspondence: vctxente@yahoo.es (V.J.C.-S.); sandra.martin.rodriguez8@gmail.com (A.M.-R.)

Abstract: This comprehensive narrative review explores the concept of neuro-vulnerability in energy metabolism regulation and its implications for metabolic disorders. The review highlights the complex interactions among the neural, hormonal, and metabolic pathways involved in the regulation of energy metabolism. The key topics discussed include the role of organs, hormones, and neural circuits in maintaining metabolic balance. The review investigates the association between neuro-vulnerability and metabolic disorders, such as obesity, insulin resistance, and eating disorders, considering genetic, epigenetic, and environmental factors that influence neuro-vulnerability and subsequent metabolic dysregulation. Neuroendocrine interactions and the neural regulation of food intake and energy expenditure are examined, with a focus on the impact of neuro-vulnerability on appetite dysregulation and altered energy expenditure. The role of neuroinflammation in metabolic health and neuro-vulnerability is discussed, emphasizing the bidirectional relationship between metabolic dysregulation and neuroinflammatory processes. This review also evaluates the use of neuroimaging techniques in studying neuro-vulnerability and their potential applications in clinical settings. Furthermore, the association between neuro-vulnerability and eating disorders, as well as its contribution to obesity, is examined. Potential therapeutic interventions targeting neuro-vulnerability, including pharmacological treatments and lifestyle modifications, are reviewed. In conclusion, understanding the concept of neuro-vulnerability in energy metabolism regulation is crucial for addressing metabolic disorders. This review provides valuable insights into the underlying neurobiological mechanisms and their implications for metabolic health. Targeting neuro-vulnerability holds promise for developing innovative strategies in the prevention and treatment of metabolic disorders, ultimately improving metabolic health outcomes.

Keywords: neuro-vulnerability; energy metabolism; metabolic disorders; neurobiological mechanisms; neuroendocrine interactions; neuroinflammation; neuroimaging techniques; eating disorders; obesity

1. Introduction

The brain is a highly energy-demanding organ that relies on the precise regulation of energy metabolism for optimal neuronal function and overall brain health. Disruptions in this delicate balance can lead to neuro-vulnerability and contribute to the development of various neurological disorders [1]. This comprehensive narrative review aims to provide an in-depth analysis of the neuro-vulnerability associated with energy metabolism dysregulation. It explores the underlying neurobiological basis, neuroendocrine interactions, neural regulation of food intake and energy expenditure, neuroinflammation, neuroimaging techniques, and their implications in eating disorders and obesity. Additionally, the review discusses therapeutic strategies for modulating neuro-vulnerability.

1.1. Regulation of Brain Metabolism

The human brain relies on the precise regulation of energy metabolism to meet its high metabolic demands. Disruptions in this delicate balance can lead to neuro-vulnerability and contribute to the development of various brain disorders [2]. Impaired glucose metabolism and compromised glucose uptake can result in energy deficits within the brain, compromising neuronal signaling and synaptic plasticity. Furthermore, disturbances in mitochondrial function, including reduced ATP production and increased generation of reactive oxygen species, contribute to energy metabolism dysregulation and neuronal vulnerability [3]. Dysregulated lipid metabolism, characterized by elevated levels of free fatty acids, can induce neuroinflammation, impair insulin signaling, and disrupt neuronal circuitry, exacerbating neuro-vulnerability [4].

Neuroendocrine interactions involving hormones such as leptin, insulin, ghrelin, and glucagon-like peptide-1 (GLP-1), play a crucial role in energy metabolism regulation [5]. Dysregulation of these hormonal signals can disrupt the energy balance and contribute to neuro-vulnerability. Additionally, the neural regulation of food intake and energy expenditure, particularly involving the complex interplay between the hypothalamic and brainstem circuits in appetite control, may contribute to a vulnerability to eating disorders and obesity. Eating disorders, including anorexia nervosa, bulimia nervosa, and binge-eating disorder, involve altered neural circuitry that is related to reward processing, impulse control, and emotion regulation. Disturbances in energy metabolism regulation, neuropeptides involved in appetite regulation, and neurotransmitter abnormalities have been implicated in the neurobiology of eating disorders [6,7]. Understanding the neuro-vulnerability in these disorders is essential for developing targeted interventions that address both the psychological and metabolic aspects. Similarly, neuro-vulnerability has been identified as a contributing factor to the development and progression of obesity. Dysregulated energy metabolism, impaired appetite regulation, altered reward sensitivity, and disruptions in the neural circuits involved in food intake control and energy expenditure have been observed in individuals with obesity [8]. Neuroinflammation and adipose tissue-derived inflammatory factors further contribute to neuro-vulnerability in obesity. Understanding the neurobiological mechanisms underlying neuro-vulnerability in obesity can inform the development of therapeutic strategies aimed at modulating the neural pathways involved in appetite control, energy balance, and metabolic regulation to manage and prevent obesity-related complications [9]. Conversely, compromised energy metabolism can trigger neuroinflammatory responses, creating a detrimental cycle.

This review also examines the potential interventions targeting glucose metabolism, mitochondrial function, neuroinflammation, and neuroendocrine signaling [10]. These interventions hold promise for mitigating neuro-vulnerability and improving neurological outcomes. Additionally, this review emphasizes the importance of neuroimaging techniques, such as positron emission tomography (PET) and functional magnetic resonance imaging (fMRI), in studying energy metabolism dysregulation and its association with neurological disorders. By exploring the neurobiological basis, neuroendocrine interactions, neural regulation of food intake and energy expenditure, neuroinflammation, neuroimaging techniques, and their implications in eating disorders and obesity, this review sheds light on the intricate mechanisms underlying neuro-vulnerability.

In conclusion, understanding the complex mechanisms of energy metabolism dysregulation and its impact on neuro-vulnerability is crucial for unraveling the pathogenesis of brain disorders and developing effective therapeutic interventions. The comprehensive analysis of neurobiological factors, neuroendocrine interactions, neural regulation of food intake and energy expenditure, and the role of neuroinflammation and neuroimaging techniques provides valuable insights into this field of research.

1.2. Methodology of Search

By encompassing both primary and secondary sources, various scientific articles, bibliographic indexes, and databases were utilized, including PubMed, Scopus, Embase, Science Direct, Sports Discuss, ResearchGate, and the Web of Science. The search was conducted using MeSH-compliant keywords to ensure the relevance of the gathered literature. Keywords such as neurological AND energy metabolism, endocrine, regulation, inflammation, imaging, behavior, eating disorder, obesity, and therapy were employed. The search period was limited to articles published between 15 June 2003 and 15 June 2023 to ensure the currency and pertinence of the data included in this review.

To ensure the appropriateness of the studies included in the analysis, the authors of the present review meticulously examined the titles and abstracts of all retrieved manuscripts. Exclusion criteria were applied to filter out studies that utilized outdated data beyond the designated timeframe, studies with unrelated topics that did not align with the specific objectives of this study, and studies not written in the English language. Once the relevant studies were identified, the same team of review authors independently extracted information from the selected articles. This rigorous approach helps maintain the quality and reliability of the data included in this review.

Furthermore, collaborative discussions were conducted among the review authors to synthesize the findings and present the current narrative review. By pooling their expertise and insights, the review authors ensured a comprehensive analysis of the literature and provided a cohesive and informative narrative that addresses the specific objectives of the study.

2. Neurobiological Basis of Energy Metabolism

The neurobiological basis of energy metabolism involves the intricate processes by which the brain regulates and utilizes energy for its proper functioning. Glucose is the primary energy substrate, and its metabolism is crucial for neuronal processes. Astrocytes play a vital role in maintaining energy homeostasis and providing metabolic support to neurons. Other metabolites, such as lactate, are under the focus of research, too [11]. Understanding the mechanisms underlying energy metabolism in the brain is essential for comprehending brain function and developing strategies to address neurological disorders related to energy metabolism dysregulation.

2.1. Metabolic Localization of Glycogen in the Brain

Glycogen plays a crucial role as the primary glucose storage form in human tissues, with diverse functions depending on its location. The liver regulates blood glucose levels by converting glycogen into glucose, which is then released into the circulation during periods of low blood glucose. Skeletal muscles utilize glycogen through glycolysis to meet increased energy demands, particularly during intense physical exercise. While glycogen levels in the brain are lower compared to the liver or muscles, its presence underscores its essential role in supporting neuronal activity. Astrocytes, found in the brain, are actively involved in neuronal metabolic processes, generating lactate and activating glycolysis and glycogen metabolism [11]. However, the extent to which astrocytes consume energy derived from glycogen themselves, rather than providing it to neurons as lactate, is still a subject of debate [12].

In terms of localization in the brain, glycogen exhibits specificity, primarily residing in astrocytes, although it has also been observed in embryonic neurons. However, the variations in glycogen levels among different astrocyte subtypes, distinguished by their morphology and functional characteristics, are not well understood [13]. Yet, glycogen distribution in the brain is not uniform, with higher concentrations observed in regions of dense synaptic activity, suggesting its involvement in synaptic transmission [14]. Gray matter generally contains approximately twice the concentration of glycogen compared to white matter. Significant levels of glycogen are found in regions such as the medulla oblongata, pons, cerebellum, hippocampus, hypothalamus, thalamus, cortex, and striatum [14].

Astrocyte end-feet, which express GLUT1 glucose transporters, extensively cover the capillary surfaces. These end-feet serve as communication sites with capillaries and participate in interactions with neurons and synaptic processes [15]. The collaboration between astrocytes and neurons in metabolic activities forms the foundation of the metabolic brain concept.

Enzymes within astrocytes facilitate glycogen metabolism in the brain, including glycogen phosphorylase (GP) and glycogen synthase (GYS). The brain isoform of GP is predominantly present in astrocytes but has also been identified in other cell types, like choroid plexus cells and ependymal cells. GYS, on the other hand, is found in neurons in the CNS [16]. The brain isoform of GYS shares a high degree of similarity with the muscle isoform and a lesser similarity with the hepatic isoform. GYS is widely distributed in the brain, prominently expressed in regions such as the hippocampus, cerebellum, and olfactory bulbs. It exists in both phosphorylated (inactive) and dephosphorylated (active) forms, allowing for the precise regulation of glycogen metabolism [17]. The interconversion between these forms is controlled by a family of phosphatases.

The brain's energy metabolism is closely linked to compartmentalization, with distinct compartments in neurons and astrocytes characterized by specific conditions. Neurons possess synaptic vesicles exclusive to them [18]. The cytoplasm of brain cells exhibits heterogeneity, with localized high concentrations of metabolites, macromolecules, and ions. Mitochondria, responsible for energy production, also display heterogeneity [19]. Electron microscopy studies have shown the uneven distribution and varying potentials of astrocytic mitochondria within the same cell, indicating differences in their capacity for oxidative metabolism [20]. This suggests that specific mitochondria specialize in ATP production, while others fulfill auxiliary functions, such as the anaplerotic reactions involved in glutamine synthesis and its transport to neurons as precursors for neurotransmitters like glutamate and γ-aminobutyric acid (GABA). Mitochondria within astrocytes demonstrate dynamic behavior, constantly changing in numbers and forming networks [21].

2.2. Regulatory Mechanisms of Glycogen in the Brain

Glycogen metabolism is subject to complex regulation in various tissues, including the brain. Glucose is transported to brain cells through different glucose transporters, with astrocytes and oligodendrocytes utilizing GLUT1 and microglial cells utilizing GLUT5 [22]. Neurons, on the other hand, primarily rely on GLUT3 for glucose uptake. Glycogen synthesis and degradation can occur simultaneously and are tightly regulated processes.

Astrocytes, despite being non-excitable cells, play a crucial role in the absorption of excess potassium ions (K+) released by neurons during synaptic activity [23]. This process involves a mutual relationship between glycogenolysis (glycogen breakdown) and K+ uptake in astrocytes. Studies have shown that glycogen breakdown provides the necessary energy for K+ uptake in astrocyte cultures [24]. Halting glycogenolysis and inhibiting the activity of glycogen phosphorylase (GP) leads to a cessation of K+ ion uptake, indicating that astrocytes are primarily responsible for this activity [25].

The breakdown of glycogen in the brain is regulated by phosphorylation/dephosp horylation and allosteric mechanisms. Phosphorylation activates phosphorylase kinase (PK), which, in turn, phosphorylates GP, converting it from an inactive form (GPb) to an active phosphorylated form (GPa) [26]. PK is controlled by intracellular calcium levels, which can increase during periods of increased K+ uptake. The uptake of K+ also affects the intracellular pH and flow of carbohydrates, triggering the stimulation of adenylate cyclase (AC) and the production of cyclic adenosine monophosphate (cAMP). The subsequent binding of cAMP to protein kinase A (PKA) leads to the phosphorylation of PK. GPb can also be allosterically activated by AMP, which induces a conformational change in GPb, similar to the active GPa form. Glycogen also regulates the activity of AMP-activated protein kinase (AMPK), acting as an allosteric inhibitor of the kinase [27].

Glycogen synthase (GYS) is active in its dephosphorylated form (GYSa) and inactive when phosphorylated (GYSb). Covalent phosphorylation regulates the interconversion between GYSa and GYSb. Both GYS and GP can be simultaneously activated under certain conditions, leading to glycogen synthesis and breakdown [17]. The regulation of carbohydrate transport into the astrocytes is influenced by K+ ions and involves the Na^+/HCO_3^- cotransporter (NBC) [28]. Increased intracellular HCO_3^- stimulates adenylate cyclase, cAMP production, and glycogen breakdown. Bicarbonate-induced glycogenolysis contributes to the activation of PKA and the PK/GP phosphorylation cascade [24].

Glucose in the brain can be oxidized through the pentose-phosphate pathway (PPP), which generates NADPH and 5-carbon sugars [29]. The PPP is crucial for lipid and nucleic acid synthesis, making it particularly important in the developing brain. Additionally, NADPH, derived from the PPP, is involved in metabolizing neurotransmitters and gliotransmitters, as well as in the regeneration of glutathione (GSH). Neuronal glycolysis is dependent on phosphofructokinase B3 (PFKB3), and its absence can lead to neuronal death under conditions of mitochondrial respiration inhibition [24]. Neurons can utilize alternative metabolic pathways, such as the PPP, for glucose oxidation.

Intracellular ascorbic acid has been shown to inhibit glucose uptake in neurons by inhibiting GLUT3, but it stimulates lactate transport through the same transporter [30]. This phenomenon, known as "the ascorbic acid metabolic switch", alters the preference for energy substrates in neurons. Hormones, such as adrenaline, noradrenaline, and insulin, including insulin-like growth factors (IGF I, IGF II), also influence the brain's glycogen levels by regulating glycogenolysis and glycogen synthesis. Additionally, the presence of ascorbic acid and its impact on glucose and lactate transport add another layer of complexity to the energy substrate preferences in the brain [31].

In conclusion, the regulation of glycogen metabolism and K+ uptake in the brain involves intricate mechanisms. Understanding these regulatory processes is crucial for comprehending brain metabolism and its implications in neurological conditions.

2.3. *Lactate as a Metabolite?*

Until recently, it was commonly accepted that neurons primarily generate energy through the oxidative metabolism of glucose, relying on the Krebs cycle and respiratory chain. However, emerging evidence indicates that neurons can efficiently utilize lactate as an energy source and even exhibit a preference for lactate when both glucose and lactate are available [32].

Notably, neurons lack the enzyme phosphofructokinase B3, which is involved in the glycolysis pathway for glucose, due to proteasomal degradation [33]. In contrast, astrocytes express high levels of this enzyme. Additionally, neurons have a slower rate of glycolysis due to their limited production of fructose-2,6-bisphosphate, a potent activator of phosphofructokinase, which is crucial for glycolysis [34]. Conversely, astrocytes have a higher rate of glycolysis, indicating their greater glycolytic capacity compared to neurons [35].

Interestingly, excessive activation of glycolysis in neurons can lead to oxidative stress and neuronal apoptosis, suggesting that neurons cannot sustain a high rate of glycolysis. On the other hand, increasing glucose concentration initiates the hexose monophosphate pathway (HMP) in neurons. Therefore, maintaining a delicate balance between the glycolytic pathway and the HMP cycle is crucial for meeting the energy demands of neurons while preserving their antioxidant status [24]. Utilizing lactate as a substrate may serve as an additional source of ATP production, apart from the glycolytic pathway, allowing neurons to conserve glucose for the HMP cycle and thereby protect themselves.

Astrocytes exhibit a high level of glycolytic activity and preferentially produce and release lactate, which can be further metabolized in the Krebs cycle. Previous assumptions suggested that astrocytes contribute only 5–15% of the brain's energy needs [24]. However, recent evidence challenges this notion, indicating that the role of astrocytes in the brain's energy metabolism processes might have been underestimated [36].

Studies have demonstrated that at rest, astrocytes in the rat brain are responsible for metabolizing approximately 50% of the glucose absorbed by the brain, with this percentage increasing during astrocyte activation [24]. This raises the question of how these findings reconcile with the fact that neurons, not astrocytes, have the highest energy demand. The transfer of energy substrates from astrocytes to neurons provides a plausible explanation for this apparent paradox [18].

Glutamatergic neuron activity leads to an increase in extracellular glutamate concentration, which is taken up by astrocytes through sodium-dependent glutamate transporters, elevating intracellular Na^+ levels [37]. This triggers the activation of Na^+/K^+ ATPase, promoting glucose uptake and glycolysis in astrocytes. Consequently, lactate production increases and is released into the extracellular space [38]. Neurons then acquire lactate through monocarboxylate transporters (MCT) for subsequent metabolism. This concept of lactate transfer, first proposed by George Brooks, extends beyond astrocytes and neurons and encompasses various intracellular, intercellular, and intra-organ lactate transfers [24].

The uptake of glutamate by astrocytes enhances glucose utilization and lactate release. Intriguingly, when neuron and astrocyte cell cultures were exposed to glutamate stimulation, it resulted in increased glucose utilization in the astrocytes but rapidly inhibited glucose transport into the neurons [39]. Notably, this inhibition was more pronounced when lactate was present in the culture medium. The inhibition of glucose transport into neurons, and hence glycolysis by glutamate, necessitates the utilization of lactate as an alternative substrate by neurons.

Under these circumstances, glucose is utilized by neurons through the HMP pathway to generate NADP, which protects neurons against reactive oxygen species [40].

To expand on the topic, recent studies conducted in culture conditions have shown that hippocampal neurons experience a 50% reduction in synaptic transmission during medium glucose deprivation [41]. However, when glucose is supplied to the astrocyte syncytium, neuronal activity is restored. This restorative effect is similarly observed with the delivery of lactate, but it is not observed when a monocarboxylic acid transporter inhibitor, which transports lactate to neurons, is present [42]. This confirms that astrocytes metabolize glucose to lactate, which is subsequently utilized by neurons to maintain their synaptic activity. Numerous studies provide substantial support for the notion of net energy transfer from astrocytes to neurons in the form of lactate, particularly during glutamatergic transmission [11,18].

The transfer of lactate between astrocytes and neurons highlights the significance of glycolysis and lactate production in supporting neuronal activity. While astrocytes primarily engage in glycolysis and lactate generation, neurons primarily rely on oxidative metabolism. The transport of lactate across the blood-brain barrier is facilitated by the monocarboxylate transporter 1 (MCT1) [43]. Lactate uptake by the brain is influenced by the pH gradient between the blood and the brain, with a low pH leading to increased lactate uptake [44]. During exercise, when arterial lactate levels rise, the brain exhibits enhanced lactate uptake, particularly when a favorable H+ gradient is present [45].

Neuronal uptake of lactate primarily occurs through MCT2, a high-affinity isoform, whereas astrocytic uptake involves the expression of MCT1 and MCT4, which are low-affinity carriers with high transport capacities [46]. In the resting brain, neuronal lactate uptake is slower and approximately 60% saturated compared to astrocytic uptake. Intensive exercise, especially involving the legs, leads to increased cerebral lactate uptake [24]. Training can upregulate MCT expression, suggesting that both neurons and astrocytes may enhance their capacity for lactate transport in response to exercise.

During recovery from exercise, the lactate taken up by the brain is metabolized and not released into the blood or accumulated in the cerebrospinal fluid or brain tissue. Lactate may be utilized for synthesis or transported to other brain regions. The glucose-sparing effect of lactate may inhibit glycolysis through the conversion of lactate to pyruvate and subsequent oxidation, although it is still unclear if lactate is preferred over glucose. Lactate oxidation to pyruvate may be advantageous during low energy states, as it does not require ATP for activation [24].

In summary, intense exercise increases arterial lactate levels, decreases the pH, and enhances brain activation, all contributing to a higher cerebral lactate uptake. Lactate metabolism in the brain can account for up to 50% of glucose metabolism during exercise, supporting brain function. The lactate taken up by the brain is likely metabolized rather than released or accumulated. The coupling mechanisms between the neurons and astrocytes are essential for memory formation, with astrocytic glycogen breakdown and lactate release playing a crucial role in long-term memory. Lactate, but not glucose, can rescue amnesia caused by disruptions in astrocytic lactate transporters, highlighting the critical dependence of long-term memory on neuronal lactate uptake.

Thus, the neurobiological basis of energy metabolism involves intricate mechanisms that regulate glycogen metabolism and lactate utilization in the brain. Glycogen, primarily localized in astrocytes, serves as a vital source of energy to support neuronal activity. Astrocytes and neurons collaborate in metabolic processes, with astrocytes generating lactate and providing it to the neurons as an energy substrate. The regulation of glycogen metabolism involves enzymes, such as glycogen phosphorylase and glycogen synthase, as well as complex signaling pathways mediated by calcium levels, cyclic adenosine monophosphate (cAMP), and protein kinases. Furthermore, lactate has emerged as a significant metabolite in the brain, with evidence suggesting that neurons can efficiently utilize lactate as an energy source. Astrocytes exhibit high glycolytic activity and preferentially produce and release lactate, which is then taken up by neurons through monocarboxylate transporters. This lactate transfer from astrocytes to neurons is crucial for maintaining synaptic activity and supporting neuronal function. The regulation of lactate metabolism involves various transporters, pH gradients, and metabolic pathways, such as the hexose monophosphate pathway. Overall, understanding the neurobiological basis of energy metabolism provides valuable insights into brain function and its implications in neurological conditions.

3. Neuro-Vulnerability and Metabolic Dysregulation

The neuronal sensitivity of cell populations is not a field of study that has been widely addressed, although interest has been growing in recent years [47]. The genomic profile of neuronal populations, as well as their structure and functions, is now known, but neuronal adaptive responses to oxidative stress and other neurodegenerative factors are still a developing field of study [48,49].

Due to the blood-brain barrier, the CNS has traditionally been considered a protected system, as this barrier modulates the entry and exit of inflammatory cells and certain chemical mediators [50]. However, recent studies have shown that in healthy patients, reduced numbers of lymphocytes also appear in the cerebrospinal fluid (CSF). Proinflammatory cells or microglia cells that are involved in neuroinflammation and organic inflammatory propagation are present and actively participate in the neuronal sensitivity of acute and chronic pathologies [51,52]. This inflammatory response, which is expressed through the modulation of proinflammatory peripheral cells in the CNS, will favor an increase in the blood-brain barrier [52]. This is possible because the inflammatory mediators, such as prostaglandins and cytokines, induce the expression of these mediators and facilitate the release of harmful molecules to specialized brain cells [53,54].

Microglial cells have a CNS defense functionality and show a morphology that allows controlling the reception and propagation of inflammatory signals [55]. When microglia are activated, their functions are modified and the production of inflammatory cytokines and the presence of antigens as an immune response begins [56]. This is essential when neurological or neurodegenerative pathologies appear where the microglia are activated before a determined stimulus and a diversity of trophic factors and inflammatory mediators are secreted [57,58].

The same is true for astrocytes, as they can express these inflammatory mediators through the increased expression of GFAP or glial fibrillary acidic protein [59]. Astrocytes also secrete Th2-response stimulatory molecules, chemokines, and cytokines, in addition to secreting proteins and enzymes that are involved in neuronal cell damage. Among them are Matrix metalloproteinases (MMPs), the family of enzymes that degrade components of the extracellular matrix and are involved in tissue remodeling. The increased expression and activation of MMPs by astrocytes can contribute to neuronal cell damage [60], as well as phospholipases, since astrocytes can release phospholipases, such as phospholipase A2 (PLA2), which can hydrolyze phospholipids and generate bioactive lipid mediators, including prostaglandins and leukotrienes. These lipid mediators can induce inflammation and contribute to neuronal cell damage [61].

In this line, the accumulation of inflammatory cells and mediators is characterized by the presence of T lymphocytes, NK cells, and leukocytes that secrete cytokines that inflame the brain [62]. Cytokines are peptides that may differ in structure and genetics and act by binding to specific receptors on the cell surface. They are synthesized by different cells and can be classified into lymphokines and monokines, depending on whether they are secreted by macrophages or lymphocytes, and act on different neuronal populations [63]. The most important cytokines involved in the inflammatory processes are interleukins 1, 6, and 10 (IL-1, IL6, and IL-10), tumor necrosis factor-alpha or TNF-α, and growth factor-beta or TGF-β [64,65].

Thus, neuroinflammation, which is often observed in the presence of various pathologies, is associated with changes in the morphology of neuroglial cells and can contribute to tissue destruction [66]. This is closely related to the understanding of the bidirectional relationship expressed through the hypothalamic–pituitary–adrenal (HPA) axis that explains cellular neuroinflammation and the systemic low-grade proinflammatory state that is present when the neuronal vulnerability is identified in certain CNS populations [67,68].

In this line, when the organism presents metabolic alterations, abnormal chemical reactions are produced that hinder the correct functionality of the different organic systems involved in cellular function [69,70]. Among the most frequently diagnosed alterations at present are diabetes, obesity, arterial hypertension, and dyslipidemia [71]. All of them are related to sedentary lifestyles, unhealthy eating habits and high-risk factors for the appearance of cardiovascular pathologies, and although there may be predisposing genetic factors, it is possible to modulate the appearance and maintenance of these risk factors through simple actions in the daily care of the individual [72]. When a series of abnormal characteristics appear in the metabolism and the risk of suffering certain coronary pathologies increases, the physiopathology of the so-called metabolic syndrome or syndrome X is expressed in the organism [73]. These characteristics are increased fasting glycemia, abdominal obesity, increased levels of low-density lipoproteins or LDL in the blood and decreased levels of high-density lipoproteins or HDL, hyperinsulinemia [74].

This is a medical condition that predisposes the person to serious organic diseases, but recent studies have also found a direct relationship between metabolic disorders and mental pathologies [75]. The data collected indicate that, in patients with psychotic disorders, there is a prevalence of metabolic alterations of almost 50% (42.6% men/48.5% women), although it is not yet possible to determine whether the pharmacology used in this type of psychopathology is the cause of the alterations or whether, on the contrary, the metabolic abnormalities were already present before the use of the associated drugs [76].

This is a field of study whose interest has been increasing in recent years and which allows us to identify the synaptic mechanisms of action and the density of receptors to neurotransmitters that are modulated by insulin through different molecular mechanisms, inhibiting the reuptake of noradrenaline and increasing the reuptake of serotonin [77]. In addition, the amount of ionotropic amino-3-hydroxy-5-methyl-4-isoxazolepropionic acid or AMPA, long-term potentiation or LTP and the stimulation of GABA receptors on the postsynaptic membrane are regulated. On the other hand, recent studies indicate that excess insulin in the bloodstream modulates the neuronal metabolism of glucose and GLUT-4 transporters [78]. Animal model studies (neural insulin receptor knockout mice) have shown modifications in neuronal populations of the hypothalamus [79,80].

However, it is important to note that CNS cells maintain a balance of neurotrophic factor signaling aimed at inhibiting the inflammatory immune response of microglia [81]. When a pathogenic stimulus appears and the CNS mononuclear phagocytic cells are activated through cell membrane modification, a series of production and secretion responses of different metabolic enzymes are triggered [82]. This can lead to low-grade systemic inflammation and other pathological manifestations that hamper the homeostasis of microorganisms and the production of reactive oxygen species that promote oxidative stress in the organic cellular environment [83].

Although it is true that not all inflammatory processes are harmful, given the main function of these processes is to limit cell damage, oxidative mechanisms maintained over time favor neuronal damage and the chronification of inflammatory processes [84].

4. Neuroendocrine Interactions in Energy Metabolism

Historically, the study of energy balance has been closely related to the study of obesity. This has made possible an increase in the knowledge of this construct thanks to the initial research in animal models that suggested that the alterations presented in obesity and hyperphagia could be associated with specific brain structures, specifically the hypothalamic nuclei [85]. These structures were affected as the sites involved in appetite control and showed damage in the ventral, dorsomedial and paraventricular areas, as well as in the arcuate nucleus, and thus it was determined that they corresponded to the satiety center [86,87].

Currently, it is known that the cellular, endocrine, immune, and nervous regulatory systems form a unitary system that is maintained and interconnected by neuropeptides—small proteins that have a neurotransmitter function and that are also called polypeptides and that normally act through G protein-coupled receptors [88]. There are more than 100 identified neuropeptides with neurotransmitter functions that are associated with modulation of the sleep–wake cycle, feeding, pain and analgesia, learning, memory, and energy balance [89].

During the last decades, different neuropeptides located in the intestine, brain, and both organ systems have been discovered, all of them involved in the modulation of energy balance [90]. In addition, different cell cultures have been identified that present ample capacity for cell proliferation, as well as cytokines that are produced and secreted in the endothelial reticulum [91]. A clear example of the phenomenon of cell–cell binding by neuropeptides is energy regulation, also known as the diffuse neuroendocrine system (DENS) [92], which presents a wide range of specialized cells that make up such relevant structures as the adrenal medulla, the parathyroid glands, the paraganglia, or the endocrine pancreas, among others [93,94]. It is considered a division of the nervous system and has an essential organic homeostasis function [95].

In this line, neuropeptides have been discovered, which are secreted in the arcuate nucleus and which, thanks to their peripheral or intracranial innervations, send the appetite signal and are called orexigenic [96]. We find here the anabolic neuropeptide Y, composed of 36 amino acids, which is produced in the medulla oblongata, in the dorsomedial nucleus and the arcuate nucleus, and whose secretion to the paraventricular nucleus activates GABA or norepinephrine [97]. In contrast, the appetite regulation and shutdown signal are transmitted by anorexigenics through hypothalamic pathways. Leptin is one of these neuropeptides, secreted in the periphery, specifically by the ob gene of adipocytes, and whose function is the inhibition of neuropeptide Y [98]. It is a neuropeptide containing a peptide containing norepinephrine. It is a peptide containing 167 amino acids and is essential in understanding energy balance [99,100].

Leptin is secreted in the stomach, skeletal muscle, and adipose tissue and, together with cytokines, has a proliferative function on thymocytes [101]. Therefore, it is related to the level of fat in the body, mainly white fat tissue or WAT, and is associated with the energy balance and restriction of energy expenditure. When leptin levels during fasting are decreased, blood insulin levels are also reduced, although the sympathetic inhibition that has been shown in studies with animal models does not appear [102].

In humans, this decrease in leptin produces a reduction in plasma insulin, which leads to metabolic regulation due to a lack of energy and activates gluconeogenesis [103]. Both leptin and insulin produce adipose signals to regulate fat stability by activating receptors in the brain, although they reach the brain by saturation through the cerebrospinal fluid [103,104]. It is now known that leptin is a class of cytokine receptors and belongs to the interleukin-6 family [105]. Signals emitted by leptin receptor activation in skeletal muscle impact fatty acid metabolism and explain insulin sensitivity and glucose metabolism, utilizing the insulin receptor establishment phosphorylation circuits [106].

On the other hand, it is known that nutrients function as regulators of endocrine factors during the development of human beings from the fetal stage, even when it is unnecessary to activate appetite signals. Leptin levels during pregnancy regulate the placental weight and act as a sensor of fatty matter in the central nervous system and, thus, neuroendocrine actions [107,108]. The amount of leptin that reaches the brain will favor modifications in hormone levels that are essential for development, such as growth factors, thyroid hormones, or insulin. All this indicates that leptin functions as an adipostatic signal in the brain in direct relation to body fat and saturates the receptors located in the nuclei of the hypothalamus that regulates food intake [109].

Insulin also functions as an adipostatic signal in the brain and reaches the brain via saturable transport. Glucose stimulates insulin production in the pancreas through body fat levels [110]. Thus, when obesity is present and insulin resistance is established, the pancreas secretes more insulin and excess insulin results in increased fat storage in the adipocytes [111]. Disruption of insulin sensitivity is associated with diabetes, as well. In addition, insulin receptors are present in the same brain structures as leptin, mainly the arcuate nucleus [112]. Both signals are related to modifications in food intake, which are related to hypothalamic neuropeptides [113].

5. Neural Regulation of Food Intake and Satiety

It has been largely proposed by the previous literature how different molecules may modulate the satiety process and consequently regulate food intake. These molecules include motilin, ghrelin, glucagon-like peptide-1 (GLP-1), cholecystokinin, and leptin, among others.

In order to clarify how these different molecules may affect the neural regulation of food intake, it is important to explain the different phases in the cycle of hunger and satiation. Thus, a term in the literature has been proposed as MMC (migrating motor complex), which supposes three different phases. The first one, phase I, in where no contractility exists. In the second one, phase II, contractility starts to become evident, and its frequency and amplitude reach their upper levels. Finally, there is a last step, phase III, in which the maximum levels of contraction occur, and subsequently, the cycle restarts again [114,115]. Thus, the molecule that seems to be most important in MMC regulation is motilin, which is formed in the small intestine and causes gastric contraction [116,117]. In this line, several researchers pointed out how motilin values oscillate depending on the MMC phases, reaching the maximum gastric levels before phase III [118–120].

Another important molecule in the neural regulation of food intake is ghrelin. It is a hormone synthesized in enteroendocrine cells of the gastrointestinal tract, and it is known for its capability of modulating appetite [121,122], as it sends different indications from the gastrointestinal tract to the brain, more specifically to brain nuclei, modulating eating behavior, increasing food intake [122,123]. In this line, the peripheral ghrelin pathways ascend from the vagus nerve to the nucleus of the solitary tract, which is the most important sensory nucleus that collects, among others, cardiovascular and visceral information. From the nucleus of the solitary tract, ghrelin signals climb to the hypothalamic arcuate nucleus through noradrenergic projections synapsis. In the hypothalamus, ghrelin stimulates noradrenergic neurons by way of α1- and β2-adrenergic receptor activation, leading to feeding [124]. Moreover, in the presence of an endogenous ligand for the growth hormone secretagogue receptor, ghrelin is able to enhance food intake as well as it has the ability to promote growth hormone liberation [125]. However, although ghrelin presents certain similarities with motilin, its levels do not oscillate with the different MMC states. In this line, in order to emulate phase III of MMC, it would be necessary during the presence of mealtimes, motilin, or motilin agonist administration [119,126–128]. Moreover, regarding the motilin and ghrelin connection in food intake regulation, recent research conducted in rodents proposed how ghrelin also promotes gastric contractions in vitro in the presence of small motilin doses, as well as motilin encouraging robust gastric contractions under ghrelin during its in vivo presence [117,129]. Ghrelin levels may be modulated by different eating conditions. For example, raised ghrelin levels were found in patients who were suffering from fasting, whereas those levels decreased after oral glucose intake [123]. Hence, ghrelin levels have been found significantly decreased in obese patients [130], and when weight loss occurred, these levels increased, and later they suffered another decrease when the patients suffered weight recuperation [131,132]. These results suggested how the modification in ghrelin levels may modulate different weight variations.

Regarding glucagon-like-peptide-1 (GLP-1), it is a hormone produced by endocrine L-cells originating from the intestinal epithelial in reply to meal intake. GLP-1 enhances insulin secretion as well as reduces glucagon liberation, leading to a reduction in post-prandial glucose and fasting. Concerning its activity in the gut, it has been related to a reduction in its motility, as well as to a reduction in acid secretion. Finally, it modulates food intake and controls appetite [133], as it reduces gastric emptying, inhibiting food intake [134]. It may be explained by its capability of activating brown fat as well as raising energy expenditure through sympathetic nervous system pathways activation [135]. Thus, GLP-1 may cross the blood-brain barrier, accessing the brain through passive diffusion. Then, it may activate the GLP-1 receptors in hypothalamic nuclei, leading to a reduction in weight [136]. In this line, the nucleus of the solitary tract also seems to play an important role in food intake regulation, as it has also been related to GLP-1 activity. Then, it presents neurons that express the proglucagon gene encoding GLP-1 as well as proglucagon-derived peptides. Then, recent studies conducted in murine models proposed how the activation of proglucagon gene-encoding neurons may decrease food consumption, metabolic rate, and glucose production [137]. Similar results were found by other researchers, in which a chemogenetic stimulation of the brainstem nucleus of the solitary tract of the proglucagon gene encoding GLP-1 decreased food intake in high-fat diet-fed mice [138]. GLP-1 involves satiation mechanisms triggering a reduction in food intake. In this line, it has been described how GLP-1 activates the vagus nerve, which in turn excites different sites, such as the nucleus of the solitary tract neurons. Subsequently, these solitary tract neurons activated the discharge of endogenous GLP-1 from their axons, which act in GLP-1 receptors, resulting in meal cessation [139–141].

Cholecystokinin is a hormone produced and liberated by the enteroendocrine cells of the duodenum. It is known for its capability to enhance enzyme and bile discharge, promoting digestion by a reduction in gastric emptying [142]. Furthermore, it also has been pointed out as a useful hormone that may modulate food intake, acting as a satiety signal that modulates the short-term control of food consumption [143–145]. Cholecystokinin involves satiety signaling that is also related to the pathways of the nucleus of the solitary tract, which it reaches via the vagal fibers, and consequently achieves paraventricular nuclei and nuclei of the ventromedial hypothalamus, constituting an autocrine signal mechanism, triggering the satiety effect [146,147].

Leptin is a hormone secreted by the adipose cells. It is known for its capability of reducing fat deposits in the adipocytes as well as reducing appetite [148]. The activity of leptin is mediated by its binding to its receptors, which are extensively expressed both in the brain and peripheral organs. These receptors have been largely described in previous literature due to their important activity in regulating food intake. One of the isoforms, leptin receptor ObRsa or short leptin receptor isoform, is extensively expressed in the brain-blood barrier and allows the pass of leptin to the brain. The other isoform of the receptor, called ObRb, or long leptin receptor isoform, is located in the hypothalamic nuclear groups and controls eating behavior and modulates body weight through signal transduction, primarily the signal transducer and activator of transcription (STAT), which has demonstrated its implication in energy homeostasis regulation [149–151]. Thus, it was described by previous researchers how the administration of leptin in patients who showed decreased leptin levels might inhibit food consumption, enhance satiety pathways, and control body weight [152].

6. Neural Control of Energy Expenditure

Energy expenditure is a highly regulated process that is crucial for maintaining energy balance in the organism. The neural control of energy expenditure plays a fundamental role in orchestrating metabolic processes and ensuring the efficient utilization of energy resources.

Neural control of energy waste involves the activity of different organs, including the gastrointestinal tube, muscle, and adipose storage, such as white adipose tissue (WAT), brown adipose tissue (BAT), and various viscera, such as the liver and pancreas. As a result, the metabolism may be affected in its various stages, including production, depot, mobilization, and usage, enhancing energy source product development [153].

The neural control of energy waste occurs predominantly in the hypothalamus, which is the central axis for coordinating energy balance. More specifically, the regulation of energy expenditure occurs in a specific area, the arcuate nucleus, in which two types of neurons exist and have opposite functions. Firstly, the arcuate nucleus presents orexigenic neurons, which stimulate appetite and increase energy consumption. On the contrary, it also presents the anorexigenic neurons, which suppress appetite and enhance energy expenditure [154]. Thus, depending on the state of fasting or food intake, different hormones may be secreted, promoting the activity of those neurons. In this line, it has been pointed out by previous literature how leptin, which is released by adipose tissue, acts as a satiety signal and inhibits orexigenic neurons while stimulating anorexigenic neurons, whereas ghrelin, produced in the stomach, promotes hunger and stimulates orexigenic neurons [155]. Additionally, other hormones have been highlighted for their capability of modulating neural control of energy expenditure, such as cortisol, TSH, and insulin [156–158].

Regarding leptin, it has been highlighted by its pivotal role in the neural control of energy expenditure [159]. Hence, the previous literature suggested how leptin receptors are expressed in the arcuate nucleus in the hypothalamus, where they interact with different populations of neurons. Thus, by acting on specific receptors within the hypothalamus, leptin influences the appetite and energy balance regulation. In this line, when leptin activates anorexigenic neurons, they produce pro-opiomelanocortin (POMC), a polypeptide precursor of other proteins, which consequently triggers the release of alpha-melanocyte-stimulating hormone (α-MSH). Consequently, α-MSH acts on melanocortin receptors, suppressing appetite and increasing energy expenditure [160]. Nevertheless, when leptin activates orexigenic neurons, they produce neuropeptide Y (NPY) and agouti-related peptide (AgRP) [161,162], two substances involved in the orexigenic processes, as AgRP impedes α-MSH activity and NPY acts on the specific receptors increasing food intake [151,163–165].

Concerning ghrelin, it has been pointed out by its dual activity controlling neural expenditure waste [166,167]. In this line, it has been highlighted as an orexigenic substance, given it stimulates appetite and promotes food intake. Moreover, it has been related to thermogenesis processes regulation, and as a consequence, it has been related to energy metabolism modulation [168]. This modulation has been associated with the fact that ghrelin has been shown to stimulate the release of growth hormone (GH) in the pituitary gland. GH, in turn, has direct effects on energy metabolism by promoting lipolysis and the utilization of fatty acids as an energy source. In addition to its influence on GH release, ghrelin also interacts with other neurotransmitters and signaling systems in the brain that are involved in appetite control and metabolism. For instance, ghrelin has been observed to increase dopamine release in the brain areas associated with reward and motivation, leading to a heightened desire for food consumption and, consequently, an increase in energy expenditure [169]. Regarding ghrelin's activity on thermogenesis, it has been proposed by recent literature how it may activate receptors in the hypothalamus, triggering the release of neuropeptides, including orexin and melanin-concentrating hormone, which have been implicated in the promotion of thermogenesis [170]. Moreover, ghrelin influences thermogenesis through its effects on brown adipose tissue (BAT), a specialized fat tissue that generates heat through the process of uncoupling protein 1 (UCP1)-mediated thermogenesis. Thus, recently it was proposed how ghrelin may enhance UCP1 expression and activity in BAT, thereby increasing energy expenditure and heat production [171,172].

With regard to TSH, it also has been pointed out by its activity, which modulates energy expenditure. TSH, also known as thyrotropin, is a hormone produced by the pituitary gland that plays a central role in the regulation of thyroid function. While its primary function is to stimulate the thyroid gland to produce thyroid hormones, TSH also exerts direct effects on energy expenditure and metabolism [173]. Then, when TSH stimulates the thyroid gland to produce thyroid hormones, it promotes thyroid hormone liberation. Hence, the thyroid hormone modulates metabolism through different organs, including the brain, WAT, BAT, skeletal muscle, liver, and pancreas. Most of the associated processes suppose modulation both in energy storage and expenditure [173]. Furthermore, TSH has been shown to affect energy expenditure through its actions on BAT. BAT is a specialized fat tissue that plays a crucial role in thermogenesis and energy dissipation. TSH receptors are expressed in BAT, and activation of these receptors has been found to stimulate thermogenesis and increase energy expenditure. This process is performed by UCP1 being present in the internal mitochondrial membrane of BAT. Thus, when an adrenergic discharge activates UCP1, it disperses energy as heat by deactivating oxidative phosphorylation [174]. Thus, when TSH activates thermogenesis, there is an increase in energy expenditure due to increased heat production and accelerated nutrient metabolism.

Regarding cortisol, it has been proposed by previous authors how it also may be related to the neural control of energy expenditure. Firstly, cortisol affects appetite and food intake regulation. High levels of cortisol have been associated with increased food intake, particularly a preference for energy-dense foods high in carbohydrates and fats [175–178]. This can lead to an increase in caloric intake and subsequently impact energy expenditure. Moreover, cortisol influences the neural pathways involved in energy homeostasis, particularly those related to the hypothalamus. Cortisol receptors are present in the key hypothalamic areas involved in appetite regulation, including the arcuate nucleus and the paraventricular nucleus, as mentioned above. Hence, cortisol can modulate the activity of these neurons by decreasing leptin's sensitivity in orexigenic and anorexigenic neurons [179]. Subsequently, it could enhance AgRP and NPY activity [180], and as it was explained before, it could increase food intake through α-MSH inhibition due to AGRR activity, as well as by acting on specific receptors as a result of NPY activity.

7. Neuroinflammation and Metabolic Health

Over the past few decades, our understanding of CNS (central nervous system) inflammation has progressed. Whether the disruption to homeostasis originates within or externally, the result is the same: neuroinflammation. Direct and indirect immune-related neuroinflammation plays a role in the pathogenesis of many neurological illnesses, including those caused by trauma, tumors [181], metabolic abnormalities, toxins, infections, autoimmunity, development [182], and degeneration [183]. Brain infiltrates of innate and adaptive immune cells, which produce inflammatory mediators, occur in response to an infectious or noxious substance. Both resident and visiting cells and signals can act as mediators of inflammation. Thus, destructive cytokines, proteases, glutamate, free radicals, and glial cell activation are released when there is an overwhelming inflammatory response in the CNS [184]. Concretely, neuronal loss and an uptick in proinflammatory cytokines like tumor necrosis factor-alpha (TNF-α) and interleukin (IL)-1β, in addition to nitric oxide (NO) are characteristic of the neurodegenerative illnesses associated with abnormal conditions in the microglia [185]. Moreover, the central nervous system's inflammatory response can also be caused by processes resulting from disorders of the central and peripheral nervous systems [183,186]. Likewise, a genetic predisposition [187], environmental factors [8], free radical production [188], excitotoxicity, neuroinflammation, disruption of the calcium regulation system, mitochondrial dysfunction [189,190], and the accumulation of unfolded proteins [191] can all play a role in the progression of neurodegenerative diseases.

Aging and metabolic illnesses, including obesity, hypertension, diabetes, depression, dementia, or brain injury, likely share common cellular and molecular processes that might set off neuroinflammation (Figure 1) [192]. Concretely, epidemiological studies have established a link between diabetes and an increased risk of cognitive decline among the elderly. Several mechanisms have been postulated to explain this association, including central insulin signaling, neurodegeneration, brain amyloidosis, and neuroinflammation, based on animal model research [193]. Concretely, in diabetes patients, hyperglycemia, insulin resistance and altered insulin signaling, neuroinflammation, cerebral microvascular injury, and accumulation of cerebral amyloid and tau proteins are among the postulated pathophysiological mechanisms underlying cognitive decline [193]. In observational studies, those with type 2 diabetes mellitus (T2DM) appear to be at a higher risk of developing Parkinson's disease (PD), as well as experiencing rapid progression and a more severe phenotype of PD, with the effects possibly mediated by several common cellular pathways. By means of insulin dysregulation, amyloid aggregation, neuroinflammation, mitochondrial dysfunction, and altered synaptic plasticity, for instance, the insulin signaling pathway may be responsible for neurodegeneration [15]. Although few conclusive research studies have attempted to identify specific biomarkers, Ehtewish et al. showed that C-reactive protein, tau protein, brain-derived neurotrophic factor, advanced glycation end products, glycosylated hemoglobin, and adipokines should be considered in diabetes-related cognitive decrements [194]. Xu et al. also specified that mild cognitive impairment in type 2 diabetes patients is characterized by aging, peripheral circulating glycogen synthase kinase-3β (GSK-3 β) activation, expression of ApoE ε 4, and an increase in the olfactory score; the combination of these indicators can improve diagnostic accuracy [195].

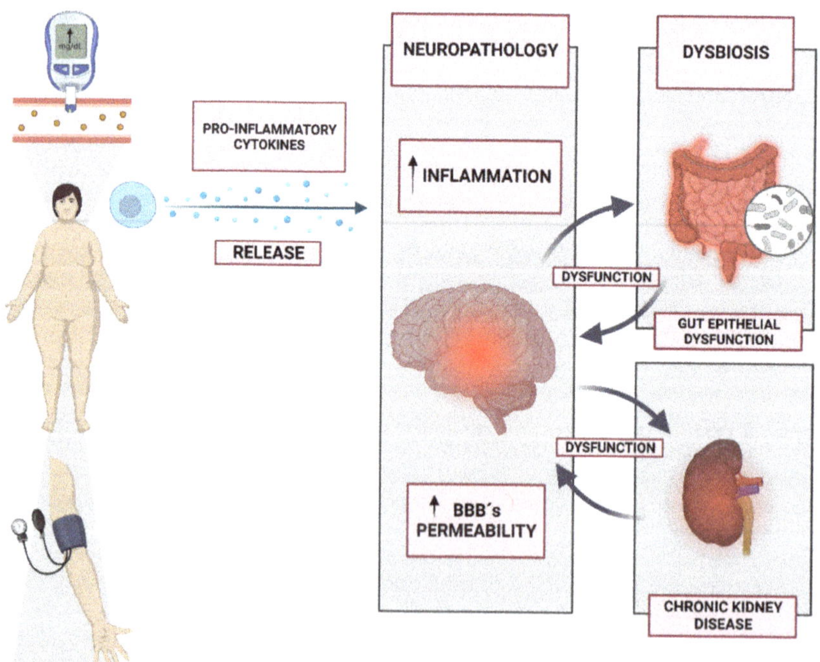

Figure 1. Metabolic complications causing neuroinflammation and the different processes affecting the kidney–brain and gut–brain axis.

In more complex diseases, however, it has been found that nutrition plays a role in the inflammatory processes that can harm the brain. Concretely, systemic inflammation caused by a high-fat diet raises the amounts of proinflammatory cytokines in the blood, which causes inflammation in the center of the body. These moving proinflammatory cytokines move into the brain and hypothalamus by crossing the blood-brain barrier (BBB). This also turns on Nuclear Factor κB (NF-κB) in the microglial cells in the hypothalamus, which causes inflammation and resistance to leptin in the hypothalamus (Figure 1) [196]. The hypothalamus is an important control center for many bodily activities, including energy balance, stress management, reproduction, and even cardiovascular health. Attention, learning, and many facets of memory and cognition are all intricately linked to many of these processes [197,198]. The paraventricular nucleus of the hypothalamus (PVN) is the epicenter of the hypothalamic–pituitary–adrenal axis (HPA), and its dysregulation is linked to memory loss [199]. High morning cortisol levels are strongly tied to the function of the HPA axis, which explains why depressed patients suffer from deficiencies in executive function and memory recall [200]. Specifically, Cope et al. demonstrated that the hippocampus of humans and animal models of Alzheimer's disease (AD) showed signs of diet-induced microgliosis, which suggests a possible mechanistic link between obesity/type 2 diabetes and cognitive impairment/memory decline in this prevalent medical condition [201]. Thus, it has been shown that an excess of saturated fatty acids and simple carbohydrates in the diet is a known environmental risk factor for AD, but a comprehensive understanding of the interdependent processes through which such a diet may contribute to AD pathogenesis is lacking. The Western diet evokes metabolic changes [202], induction of obesity and adipose tissue inflammation, gut microbiota dysbiosis [203], and the acceleration of low-grade systemic inflammation, which causes impairment of the BBB and the development of neuroinflammation, which is accompanied by the accumulation of toxic amyloid [204].

Additionally, one of the most common health problems caused by diet, among other factors, is metabolic syndrome, which encompasses obesity and diabetes [205]. It causes widespread inflammation throughout the body, the full extent of which has yet to be discovered. Increased permeability of the BBB is a common consequence of the neuropathologies produced by metabolic syndrome (Figure 1) [206]. The BBB is critical for healthy brain function because it blocks harmful substances, immune cells, and pathogens from entering the brain. BBB disintegration, poor waste clearance, and increased infiltration of immune cells have all been linked to the local and systemic inflammation brought on by obesity and type 2 diabetes mellitus [207]. Depending on the region of the brain that is impacted, this might lead to hormone imbalance, heightened immunological sensitivity, or cognitive impairment due to glial and neuronal cell disruption [208].

Regarding the gut–brain axis, bidirectional communication between the gut microbiota and the gut epithelium is implicated in the regulation of autonomic nervous system activity and blood pressure control [209]. This dysfunction in the gut–brain axis, characterized by dysbiosis of the gut microbiota, gut epithelial dysfunction, and deranged input to the brain, contributes to the development of hypertension through various mechanisms, including the release of inflammatory mediators, metabolites, and bacteria into the circulation, as well as alterations in afferent information [210]. These processes ultimately lead to neuroinflammation and an imbalance in autonomic nervous system activity, resulting in increased blood pressure. Furthermore, this dysfunction in the gut–brain axis has a negative impact on gastrointestinal function and the composition of the gut microbiota, exacerbating the problem [211]. In relation to hypertension, Richards et al. [211] proposed that immunoglobulin A-coated bacteria originating in the gastrointestinal tract and having access to the brain may play a role. However, it is worth noting that minocycline, known for its anti-inflammatory and antimicrobial properties, is being evaluated as a potential antihypertensive agent targeting the gut–brain axis.

A recent review also specified that chronic kidney disease (CKD) also implies neurodegeneration [212]. Concretely, epidemiologic studies imply that people with CKD at any stage are more likely to acquire neuropsychiatric disorders, cognitive impairment, and dementia. The significant incidence of both symptomatic and subclinical ischemic cerebrovascular lesions explains this risk [213]. It refers to the clinical, metabolic, and hormonal abnormalities that accompany progressive kidney failure [214]. Each patient with uremic syndrome of CKD develops cognitive decline, encephalopathy, seizures, asterixis, myoclonus, restless limb syndrome, central pontine myelinolysis, stroke, extrapyramidal movement disorders, neuropathies, and myopathy being among them (Figure 1). Their pathogenic mechanisms are intricate and varied [212]. In fact, Corona et al. specified that this decline in cognitive function impairs the ability to differentiate between odors in CDK patients. It is unclear whether peritoneal dialysis and hemodialysis enhance olfactory deficits, whereas renal transplants have a significant beneficial effect [214].

Anti-inflammatory medications target various pathways, but because the picture is so complex, it is impossible to foresee what side effects they might induce [215]. Given that some inflammation is required, it is critical to pick the therapeutic targets that will influence the patient's immune response in a safe manner [216]. Resolving metabolic memory may be one of the more important therapeutic options, as it causes ongoing inflammation even after the blood glucose levels are normalized [208,216]. Although some data exist, future research should focus on the impact of specific dietary components, such as fatty acids, cholesterol, and carbohydrates, in the advancement of pathogenesis, which implies neuroinflammation, such as AD. Yet, recent meta-analyses of randomized trials and observational studies have presented intriguing findings regarding the impact of reducing saturated fat intake on CVD and total mortality. These studies have indicated that limiting saturated fat intake may not yield significant beneficial effects in terms of reducing CVD and overall mortality. Conversely, they have revealed potential protective effects against stroke and have shown no increased risk of CVD associated with the consumption of whole-fat dairy or dark chocolate. These important findings challenge the traditional recommendations to restrict saturated fat intake and emphasize the need for a comprehensive reassessment of the relationship between saturated fat and cardiovascular health [204].

Future research should investigate the interaction of environmental and genetic risk factors. The epigenetic modifications that may be caused by environmental risk factors, such as high-fat diets, and the likelihood of their transmission to succeeding generations as disease-promoting vs. disease-protecting predispositions are particularly intriguing.

8. Neuroimaging Techniques in Studying Neuro-Vulnerability

Neuroimaging techniques play a crucial role in studying neuro-vulnerability, which refers to an individual's susceptibility to developing neurological disorders or experiencing changes in brain function [217,218]. These techniques allow researchers to visualize and investigate the structure, function, and connectivity of the brain, providing valuable insights into the underlying mechanisms of neuro-vulnerability [219].

Magnetic resonance imaging (MRI) is a powerful medical imaging technique that uses a strong magnetic field and radio waves to generate detailed images of the internal structures of the body. In this line, MRI plays a crucial role in understanding clinical diagnoses and the treatment of neuro-vulnerability associated with neurodegenerative disease by providing valuable information about the structure and function of the nervous system [220]. Moreover, this technique can help identify structural abnormalities in the brain, such as tumors, vascular malformations, or developmental disorders, which can contribute to neuro-vulnerability [221]. By visualizing these structural changes, MRI helps in the early diagnosis and monitoring of these conditions, allowing for appropriate management and intervention [222].

Thus, Mei et al. [223] used MRI to observe the sex differences in clinical manifestations of males and females with major depressive disorder (MDD). The authors demonstrated that the pathophysiological and developmental mechanisms of MDD differ in male and female patients, which could lead to sex differences in the clinical manifestations of MDD. Furthermore, this has important relevance in the treatment of MDD, given that sex-specific targeted therapies can be developed. Regarding Parkinson's disease (PD), which is characterized by the selective loss of dopaminergic neurons in the substantia nigra, He et al. [224] hypothesized that magnetic resonance imaging could help to differentiate the pathophysiology of this disease from other neurodegenerative diseases. However, the results showed that, although MRI could potentially provide useful disease state biomarkers for clinical trials in the preclinical and early stages of Parkinson's disease, it is insufficient to reliably distinguish atypical Parkinsonian disorders or to monitor the disease's progression in moderate to late-stage patients. Furthermore, Li et al. [225] showed that MRI could be used as a potential biomarker to diagnose preclinical Alzheimer's disease (AD). In this line, Wang et al. [226] stated that MRI is currently the gold standard for the early diagnosis of AD, which is caused by atrophy of the medial temporal lobe.

Apart from MRI, new neuroimaging techniques, such as single photon emission computed tomography (SPECT) and positron emission tomography (PET), have been used for the diagnosis of neurodegenerative diseases. These techniques are a type of imaging technology that involves the use of a specific marker for localization and quantification to show the onset and development of diseases at the molecular level [227]. In terms of PD, the diagnosis was based on the clinical judgment of expert professionals without considering certain biomarkers with high sensitivity and specificity [228]. However, these techniques can be very useful when it comes to an early diagnosis through certain markers, such as the pre-synaptic dopamine transporter (DAT) [227]. Concretely, DAT allows us to evaluate the integrity of the nigrostriatal pathway in vivo, providing an objective measure of neuronal degeneration in PD [229]. However, SPECT has some type of technical limitations due to its hardware design, such as limited spatial resolution and high image noise [230]. For this reason, some researchers have developed algorithms to solve these problems. In this line, Shiiba et al. [231] developed a DAT-SPECT image-derived radiomics signature and reported that their model would be useful for the diagnosis of PD and would have the potential to provide robust diagnostics. In addition, SPECT has been used in the diagnosis of AD due to its potential to provide information on regional cerebral blood flow, which has been postulated as a determinant of this disease. According to this, Höller et al. [232] reported that the quantitative analytical combination of data reported by the electroencephalography and SPECT markers was effective in differentiating AD from other diseases.

Therefore, these techniques can be very useful for the early detection of this type of neurodegenerative disease. However, more in-depth research is needed to provide clinical help and explore the pathophysiological mechanism of these diseases.

9. Neuro-Vulnerability and Eating Disorders

While eating disorders (ED) have psychological and social components, research suggests that they also involve biological and neurological factors. In this line, it has been postulated that eating disorders cause a series of behavioral changes and brain plasticity like those of obesity (Schmidt). In this sense, some research has reported that some temperament disorders and personality traits during childhood can generate a vulnerability to develop eating disorders, such as anorexia nervosa (AN) or bulimia nervosa (BN), during adolescence and adulthood [233].

Several studies have investigated the neurobiological aspects of eating disorders, including brain imaging techniques such as functional magnetic resonance imaging (fMRI). Thus, neuroimaging makes it possible to characterize the neuronal vulnerability factors that increase the risk of weight gain and risky eating behaviors [234]. The results of neuroimaging studies indicate that people with eating disorders present structural and functional alterations in the brain regions involved in reward processing, emotion regulation, body image perception, and cognitive control [234]. Specifically, the most common structural abnormalities found were global reductions in the gray matter and white matter in AN and similar findings in BN [235]. These abnormalities may contribute to the development and maintenance of disordered eating behaviors [236]. However, other investigations have reported a normalization in the volume of gray and white matter in people who have recovered from these pathologies [237].

In addition, it has recently been postulated that certain alterations in the reward mechanisms of the brain could be involved in the pathophysiology of eating disorders [234]. This process is known as anhedonia, which involves a decreased ability of the person to experience the reward. Continuing with the reward system, the visualization of food activates a series of anticipatory responses that condition each person's eating behavior [238]. However, people suffering from these EDs have been shown to have poor visual processing of food [234]. An interesting study carried out by Uher et al. [239], in which the visual response of women with anorexia and bulimia is compared, reported a similar activation of the medial prefrontal cortex and inhibition of the lateral prefrontal cortex.

Another important factor that can increase the neuro-vulnerability of people suffering from eating disorders is their interpretation of body image, usually overestimating it, as well as their body weight. This fact has some repercussions on the activation of brain regions. In this sense, Fladung et al. [240] reported activation of the ventral striatal zone, which is associated with emotional processing, by showing photos of underweight women to patients with AN. This is very interesting since it is possible that the comparison of their body with idealized female bodies elicits reward behavior in patients with eating disorders [234]. Furthermore, excessive physical activity is usually a practice carried out by people who suffer from these disorders since it has been postulated that it helps them reduce anxiety caused by food consumption [241]. In this line, Kullmann et al. [242] observed an increased prefrontal cortex in AN patients after visualizing exercise images in comparison with athletes and non-athletes. As with the visualization of food, the visualization of people undertaking physical exercise can stimulate this reward effect at the brain level in these patients.

The exact relationship between neural vulnerability and eating disorders is complex and not yet fully understood. However, it is believed that genetic, environmental, and even gender factors may contribute to the susceptibility of certain people to developing eating disorders. Thus, it is known that women are at greater risk than men of suffering from eating disorders; this difference increases in adolescence [243]. In this sense, the main factor responsible for this is the difference in sex steroid hormones between both sexes. Specifically, the variability of the risk between sexes and within the sex of those suffering from some type of eating disorder could respond to the modulation of hormones to the neural response of the signals related to eating [244].

Despite all, further research is needed to better understand the specific neuronal vulnerabilities and mechanisms underlying eating disorders. This knowledge could potentially lead to improved diagnostic tools and targeted treatments for the individuals affected by these conditions.

10. Neuro-Vulnerability and Obesity

Obesity is a complex condition that is influenced by a variety of factors, including genetic, environmental, and behavioral factors. Recent research has suggested that neural vulnerability factors may also play a role in the development of obesity. These factors are thought to increase the risk of overeating and weight gain by altering the brain's function and structure [245]. It was found that neurobehavioral correlates of obesity are largely heritable, suggesting that genetic factors may contribute to the neural vulnerability factors that increase the risk of obesity [246]. Other research has shown that obesity and a diet high in sugar and saturated fat may lead to brain changes that hamper impulse control, decision-making, and memory [247]. Brain imaging studies have also shown structural changes in the brains of obese individuals [248]. Once this condition has developed in the subject, it has been demonstrated that whole brain cortical thickness is larger in people who are overweight or obese compared to people who are at a healthy body weight, according to a cross-sectional study involving a diverse sample of ages [249]. There is also a decrease in the structural integrity of the white matter tracts that connect various brain regions. Demyelination of these tissues reduces the anisotropic diffusion of water along the axons, as evidenced by a decrease in fractional anisotropy (FA), which is indicative of a decline in structural integrity as obesity levels rise [250]. In this line, theoretical work has suggested that obesity is related to the enhanced incentive salience of food cues, which may contribute to overeating and weight gain. However, evidence from both behavioral and neuroimaging studies has been mixed, with some studies finding an enhanced neural reactivity to food cues in obese individuals and others finding no differences between obese and non-obese individuals [251].

Due to the results in this field being ambiguous, maybe due to the great phenotypic complexity of addictions and obesity, it should be made clear that the tendency to act quickly without fully considering the implications is referred to as impulsivity [252]. The feature is assumed to be the outcome of a combination of strong arousal responses to possible rewards and poor self-control. According to research, impulsivity makes people more vulnerable to addiction and fat. In this regard, lower self-control, reward sensitivity, and negative affect are three impulsivity-related domains that are particularly relevant for the understanding of the similarities between addiction and obesity (Figure 2) [253]. Individual differences in the neurobiological systems involved in the management of food choices and food intake, on the other hand, are likely to explain why some people are more prone to weight gain than others. Individuals with frequent disinhibited behavior and a heightened sensitivity to possible rewards, for example, may be more sensitive to developing unhealthy weight gain when exposed to an "obesogenic" food-abundant environment [246,254]. Likewise, individual impulsive differences may be a common denominator in obesity and drug addiction. Several research studies have revealed that there are similarities in reward processing between addiction and fat [255].

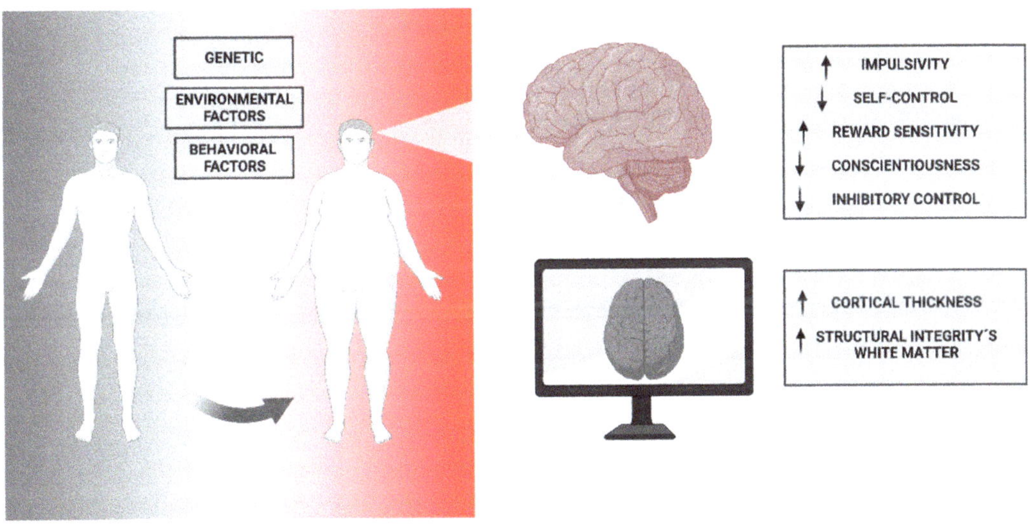

Figure 2. The obesity-related factors that make the obese person vulnerable to various changes at the brain level.

Regarding personality traits, the high disinhibition and low conscientiousness domains of impulsivity are consistently related to a higher risk of addiction, highlighting the need for self-control in avoiding drug misuse [256]. Similarly, obesity has been repeatedly linked to a lower level of conscientiousness [257]. In relation to this, Meule and Blechert discovered that higher attentional and motor impulsivities were predictive of a higher body mass index (BMI) after statistically adjusting for age and gender in a large heterogeneous population. Nevertheless, the effect was minor, and non-planning impulsivity was not found to be significantly related to BMI [258]. However, Hays et al. reported that higher levels of habitual disinhibition, as measured by the Three-Factor Eating Questionnaire, have been linked to long-term body weight growth [259]. Even so, the data remain inconsistent, as a more recent study found no changes between groups in the ability to regulate their impulsive responses [198]. Despite this, disinhibition is an awareness and self-control-related attribute that refers to the tendency to overeat when exposed to appetizing foods or stressful situations. Studies ongoing suggest that obesity is associated with high disinhibition and low conscientiousness. These characteristics may increase a person's propensity to consume in specific situations and make it more challenging for obese individuals to maintain weight loss behaviors [260]. Unlike conscientiousness and disinhibition, the link between neuroticism/negativity in the emotional domain and being overweight is not quite as strong. Adiposity is not guaranteed; however, this personality feature may make a person more prone to binge eating when they are feeling down [261].

Another impulsivity domain is the concept of risk sensitivity. It provides an additional perspective on impetuous decision-making. Risk sensitivity refers to the degree to which an individual is attracted to or repelled by uncertain outcomes [262]. It has been used to define impulsive behavior in addiction and obesity in recent years [263]. Likewise, obesity has been associated with weak inhibitory control. Obese and overweight individuals have inferior inhibitory control performance on food-specific versions of the stop-signal task, according to a comprehensive literature review [264]. For instance, Hall et al. [265] discovered that people with greater degrees of inattention tended to consume more high-calorie snacks. Also, the conventional Stroop test is associated with lower scores in the obese population, as was shown in a recent study [266].

The functional and structural neural correlates of drug abuse and obesity susceptibility have been studied using neuroimaging. Addicts' brains appear to respond to drug signals with heightened activity in the ventral striatum, amygdala, and medial regions of the orbitofrontal cortex, as measured by functional magnetic resonance imaging [267]. Enhanced food reward sensitivity (incentive salience of the cue) and poor inhibitory control may contribute to susceptibility to weight gain and overeating, as suggested by numerous brain imaging studies. The anterior cingulate cortex (ACC), dorsomedial prefrontal cortex (PFC), ventral striatum, para hippocampal gyrus, precentral gyrus, superior/inferior frontal gyrus (IFG), and insula are all more active in obese people than in lean people in response to visual food stimuli. Then, evidence from studies shows that there are common brain processes between obesity and various addictions. Both obesity and addiction illnesses may be associated with impairments in inhibitory control, as well as elevated reward sensitivity and heightened attention to signals (foods or substances) [268]. However, despite the similarities highlighted, there is evidence that obesity and other addictive behaviors are distinct and may only partially overlap [269]. While some studies have found a higher prevalence of addictive disorders in obese populations [270], others have found no correlation between obesity and addiction [271]. Due to this, methodological considerations and the extraordinary intrinsic complexity and heterogeneity of obesity and addiction may help to explain the discrepancies between the studies in understanding the level of neuro-vulnerability experienced by obese and overweight people.

In summary, obesity has been linked to personality modifications, brain structure, and cognitive impairment; however, the processes by which this is achieved remain unclear. Current research suggests that insulin resistance, inflammation, and vascular dysfunction may all play a role. Cognitive impairment due to obesity may be reversible, and there is evidence to suggest that weight loss is linked to improved brain and cognitive results [272]. Psychodynamic (insight-oriented) psychotherapy is helpful in assisting with conflicts regarding excessive weight, body image, relationship to food and disordered eating patterns, and dealing with prejudice and overt discrimination that obese patients may experience [273].

11. Therapeutic Strategies for Modulating Neuro-Vulnerability

Therapeutic strategies for modulating neuro-vulnerability in obesity have been proposed as a potential avenue for preventing and treating obesity. Several psychological treatments have been found to be effective for binge-eating disorder, including cognitive-behavioral therapy (CBT), dialectical behavior therapy (DBT), and behavioral weight loss (BWL) [274]. Research has also identified several neural vulnerability factors that may increase the risk of overeating and weight gain, including emotion reactivity, food cue reactivity, and craving [275]. These factors may be targeted through interventions such as mindfulness-based stress reduction (MBSR), which has been found to reduce food cravings and improve self-regulation in obese individuals [276]. Other potential therapeutic strategies for modulating neuro-vulnerability in obesity include pharmacological interventions and brain stimulation techniques, such as transcranial magnetic stimulation (TMS) and deep brain stimulation (DBS) [277,278]. These interventions have shown promise in reducing food cravings and improving self-regulation in obese individuals, although more research is needed to determine their efficacy and safety. Therapeutic strategies for modulating neuro-vulnerability in obesity are an emerging area of research that holds promise for preventing and treating obesity. Psychological treatments, such as CBT, DBT, and BWL, as well as interventions, such as MBSR, TMS, and DBS, may be effective for targeting the neural vulnerability factors that contribute to overeating and weight gain.

Recent studies have investigated the potential of transcranial direct current stimulation (tDCS) as a therapeutic strategy for modulating neuro-vulnerability in obesity. It was found that tDCS may be effective in reducing food cravings and food intake in individuals affected by obesity and overweight [279]. Other studies have investigated the potential of tDCS to improve lower limb motor performance in healthy adults and people with strokes [280], as well as its effects on self-paced exercise performance and electroencephalographic (EEG) oscillatory brain activity in trained male cyclists [281]. Research has also identified several neural vulnerability factors that may increase the risk of overeating and weight gain, including emotion reactivity, food cue reactivity, and cravings [282]. In this line, neurobehavioral correlates of obesity are largely heritable, suggesting that genetic factors may contribute to the neural vulnerability factors that increase the risk of obesity [246]. Other research has shown that being overweight or obese and having a diet high in sugar and saturated fat may lead to brain changes that hamper impulse control, decision-making, and memory [283].

Other research has shown that food reinforcement and delay discounting are two factors that may contribute to obesity. Food reinforcement refers to the degree to which a person is motivated to eat by the pleasure or reward associated with food, while delay discounting refers to the tendency to choose immediate rewards over delayed rewards, even if the delayed rewards are larger [284]. Studies have found that food reinforcement and delay discounting interact to predict energy intake and that delay discounting moderates the effect of food reinforcement on energy intake among non-obese women [285,286]. These findings suggest that individuals who are highly motivated by the pleasure or reward associated with food and who tend to choose immediate rewards over delayed rewards may be at increased risk for overeating and weight gain. One study found that food reinforcement, delay discounting, and dietary disinhibition were all predictive of weight gain in non-obese adults [287]. The study suggests that these factors may contribute to the development of obesity by promoting overeating and a lack of self-control around food. Overall, research suggests that food reinforcement and delay discounting may be important factors to consider in the prevention and treatment of obesity. Interventions that target these factors, such as mindfulness-based stress reduction (MBSR) and cognitive-behavioral therapy (CBT), may be effective in reducing overeating and promoting healthy eating behaviors.

The significance of multidisciplinary interventions in modulating the psychophysiological response of patients cannot be overstated [288–290]. By bringing together professionals from various disciplines, such as psychiatrists, psychologists, neurologists, and therapists, a comprehensive and holistic approach can be adopted to address the complex interplay between mental and physical health [291–295]. This collaborative effort allows for a more nuanced understanding of the phylogenetic and behavioral bases of the disease, encompassing both genetic predispositions and environmental factors that contribute to its development [296,297]. By gaining insights into these underlying mechanisms, tailored interventions can be implemented to target neuro-vulnerability and promote better outcomes [298,299]. The integration of multiple perspectives and expertise enables a more comprehensive assessment, personalized treatment plans, and improved patient care in the field of mental health [300,301].

12. Future Directions and Research Gaps

While significant progress has been made in understanding the neuro-vulnerability associated with energy metabolism regulation, several important research directions and gaps remain to be addressed:

a. Longitudinal Studies: Conducting longitudinal studies that track individuals over time can provide valuable insights into the temporal dynamics of neuro-vulnerability and its association with metabolic dysregulation. This approach can help identify early markers or predictors of neuro-vulnerability and inform targeted interventions.

b. Genetic and Epigenetic Influences: Investigating the genetic and epigenetic factors underlying neuro-vulnerability can enhance our understanding of individual differences in energy metabolism regulation. Identifying specific genetic variants or epigenetic modifications associated with neuro-vulnerability may open avenues for personalized interventions and precision medicine approaches.

c. Gut–Brain Axis: A further exploration of the bidirectional communication between the gut and the brain, particularly through the gut–brain axis, is crucial for unraveling the mechanisms involved in energy metabolism regulation. Understanding how gut-derived signals modulate the neural circuits involved in metabolic control can pave the way for novel therapeutic strategies.

d. Sex Differences: Examining potential sex differences in neuro-vulnerability and metabolic dysregulation is important, as sex hormones and other sex-specific factors may contribute to variations in energy metabolism regulation. Investigating whether neuro-vulnerability manifests differently between males and females could guide the development of sex-specific interventions.

e. Neuroinflammation and Metabolism: Elucidating the intricate relationship between neuroinflammation and metabolic health is an area of ongoing investigation. Identifying the underlying mechanisms linking neuroinflammation, neuro-vulnerability, and metabolic dysregulation can provide insights into novel therapeutic targets for managing metabolic disorders.

f. Advanced Neuroimaging Techniques: Utilizing advanced neuroimaging techniques, such as functional magnetic resonance imaging (fMRI), positron emission tomography (PET), and magnetic resonance spectroscopy (MRS), can provide more detailed information about neuro-vulnerability and its impact on energy metabolism regulation. These techniques can help elucidate the neural circuits and metabolic pathways involved, allowing for targeted interventions.

g. Neuro-Vulnerability and Aging: Investigating the impact of neuro-vulnerability on energy metabolism regulation in the context of aging is an important area for future research. Understanding how age-related changes in the brain and neuroendocrine systems influence metabolic dysregulation can inform strategies for healthy aging and prevent age-related metabolic disorders.

h. Novel Therapeutic Approaches: Developing innovative therapeutic approaches that specifically target neuro-vulnerability holds promise for improving metabolic health. Exploring neuroprotective agents, neuromodulation techniques, and precision medicine strategies tailored to individuals with neuro-vulnerability can pave the way for more effective interventions.

i. Translational Research: Bridging the gap between basic research and clinical applications is crucial for translating the findings into meaningful interventions. Conducting translational studies that integrate preclinical models, human research, and clinical trials can accelerate the development of targeted therapies for individuals with neuro-vulnerability.

j. Socioeconomic Factors: Considering the influence of socioeconomic factors on neuro-vulnerability and metabolic dysregulation is important for addressing health disparities. Investigating how socioeconomic status, access to healthy food, and environmental factors interact with neuro-vulnerability can inform public health policies and interventions aimed at promoting metabolic health.
k. Comorbidities and Multifactorial Approaches: Given the complex nature of metabolic disorders, exploring the interplay between neuro-vulnerability and comorbid conditions (e.g., cardiovascular disease, diabetes) is necessary. Adopting a multifactorial approach that considers the contributions of both neuro-vulnerability and other systemic factors can enhance our understanding of metabolic dysregulation.
l. Lifestyle Interventions: Investigating the effects of lifestyle interventions, such as dietary modifications, physical activity, and behavioral interventions, on neuro-vulnerability and metabolic health is crucial. Understanding how lifestyle factors interact with neuro-vulnerability can inform evidence-based recommendations for preventing and managing metabolic disorders.
m. Data Sharing and Collaboration: Encouraging data sharing and collaboration among researchers is vital for advancing our knowledge of neuro-vulnerability in energy metabolism regulation. Promoting open science practices and establishing collaborative networks can facilitate the pooling of resources, data, and expertise, leading to more comprehensive and impactful research outcomes.

Addressing these future directions and research gaps will deepen our understanding of neuro-vulnerability in energy metabolism regulation, paving the way for improved diagnostic strategies, targeted interventions, and, ultimately, better metabolic health outcomes.

13. Conclusions

In this comprehensive narrative review, we have delved into the intricate topic of neuro-vulnerability in energy metabolism regulation. By examining the neurobiological basis of energy metabolism, neuroendocrine interactions, neural control of food intake and energy expenditure, and the role of neuroinflammation, we have gained valuable insights into the complex mechanisms underlying metabolic dysregulation.

The findings from this review highlight the crucial role of neural circuits and systems in maintaining metabolic homeostasis. Neuro-vulnerability, characterized by dysfunction and dysregulation within these neural pathways, has emerged as a key factor contributing to the development of metabolic disorders, including obesity, diabetes, and eating disorders. Understanding the underlying mechanisms of neuro-vulnerability is essential for the development of targeted interventions and therapeutic strategies.

This review also emphasizes the importance of interdisciplinary research, bridging knowledge from neurobiology, endocrinology, neuroimaging, and related fields. Future research directions should focus on longitudinal studies to unravel the temporal dynamics of neuro-vulnerability and its association with metabolic dysregulation. Exploring genetic and epigenetic influences, investigating the gut–brain axis, considering sex differences, and examining the impact of neuro-vulnerability on aging are important areas that warrant further investigation. The advancement of neuroimaging techniques, coupled with translational research, holds great promise for deepening our understanding of neuro-vulnerability and its implications for metabolic health. By identifying novel therapeutic approaches and considering the multifactorial nature of metabolic disorders, personalized interventions targeting neuro-vulnerability can be developed to improve outcomes.

It is crucial to acknowledge the research gaps and challenges that lie ahead. Addressing the influence of socioeconomic factors, promoting data sharing and collaboration, and adopting a holistic approach that incorporates lifestyle interventions and comorbidities will further enhance our understanding of neuro-vulnerability and its broader implications.

Author Contributions: Conceptualization, V.J.C.-S.; methodology, J.F.T.-A.; investigation, all authors; writing—original draft preparation, all authors; writing—review and editing, all authors; visualization, all authors; supervision, V.J.C.-S.; project administration, V.J.C.-S. All authors have read and agreed to the published version of the manuscript.

Funding: This research received no external funding.

Institutional Review Board Statement: Not applicable.

Informed Consent Statement: Not applicable.

Data Availability Statement: Not applicable.

Acknowledgments: Figures were created with BioRender.com (accessed on 20 June 2023).

Conflicts of Interest: The authors declare no conflict of interest.

References

1. Traxler, L.; Lagerwall, J.; Eichhorner, S.; Stefanoni, D.; D'Alessandro, A.; Mertens, J. Metabolism Navigates Neural Cell Fate in Development, Aging and Neurodegeneration. *Dis. Model. Mech.* **2021**, *14*, dmm048993. [CrossRef] [PubMed]
2. Mergenthaler, P.; Lindauer, U.; Dienel, G.A.; Meisel, A. Sugar for the Brain: The Role of Glucose in Physiological and Pathological Brain Function. *Trends Neurosci.* **2013**, *36*, 587–597. [CrossRef] [PubMed]
3. Takahashi, S. Metabolic Contribution and Cerebral Blood Flow Regulation by Astrocytes in the Neurovascular Unit. *Cells* **2022**, *11*, 813. [CrossRef] [PubMed]
4. Farooqui, A.A.; Farooqui, T.; Panza, F.; Frisardi, V. Metabolic Syndrome as a Risk Factor for Neurological Disorders. *Cell. Mol. Life Sci.* **2012**, *69*, 741–762. [CrossRef]
5. Boguszewski, C.L.; Paz-Filho, G.; Velloso, L.A. Neuroendocrine Body Weight Regulation: Integration between Fat Tissue, Gastrointestinal Tract, and the Brain. *Endokrynol. Pol.* **2010**, *61*, 194–206.
6. Skowron, K.; Kurnik-Łucka, M.; Dadański, E.; Bętkowska-Korpała, B.; Gil, K. Backstage of Eating Disorder-About the Biological Mechanisms behind the Symptoms of Anorexia Nervosa. *Nutrients* **2020**, *12*, 2604. [CrossRef]
7. Kaye, W. Neurobiology of Anorexia and Bulimia Nervosa. *Physiol. Behav.* **2008**, *94*, 121–135. [CrossRef]
8. Kaye, W.H.; Bailer, U.F. Understanding the Neural Circuitry of Appetitive Regulation in Eating Disorders. *Biol. Psychiatry* **2011**, *70*, 704–705. [CrossRef]
9. Narayanaswami, V.; Dwoskin, L.P. Obesity: Current and Potential Pharmacotherapeutics and Targets. *Pharmacol. Ther.* **2017**, *170*, 116–147. [CrossRef]
10. Cunnane, S.C.; Trushina, E.; Morland, C.; Prigione, A.; Casadesus, G.; Andrews, Z.B.; Beal, M.F.; Bergersen, L.H.; Brinton, R.D.; de la Monte, S.; et al. Brain Energy Rescue: An Emerging Therapeutic Concept for Neurodegenerative Disorders of Ageing. *Nat. Rev. Drug Discov.* **2020**, *19*, 609–633. [CrossRef]
11. Bélanger, M.; Allaman, I.; Magistretti, P.J. Brain Energy Metabolism: Focus on Astrocyte-Neuron Metabolic Cooperation. *Cell Metab.* **2011**, *14*, 724–738. [CrossRef] [PubMed]
12. Brooks, G.A. The Science and Translation of Lactate Shuttle Theory. *Cell Metab.* **2018**, *27*, 757–785. [CrossRef] [PubMed]
13. Obel, L.F.; Müller, M.S.; Walls, A.B.; Sickmann, H.M.; Bak, L.K.; Waagepetersen, H.S.; Schousboe, A. Brain Glycogen-New Perspectives on Its Metabolic Function and Regulation at the Subcellular Level. *Front. Neuroenergetics* **2012**, *4*, 3. [CrossRef] [PubMed]
14. Brown, A.M. Brain Glycogen Re-Awakened. *J. Neurochem.* **2004**, *89*, 537–552. [CrossRef] [PubMed]
15. Garcia, M.A.; Carrasco, M.; Godoy, A.; Reinicke, K.; Montecinos, V.P.; Aguayo, L.G.; Tapia, J.C.; Vera, J.C.; Nualart, F. Elevated Expression of Glucose Transporter-1 in Hypothalamic Ependymal Cells Not Involved in the Formation of the Brain-Cerebrospinal Fluid Barrier. *J. Cell. Biochem.* **2001**, *80*, 491–503. [CrossRef] [PubMed]
16. Brown, A.M.; Ransom, B.R. Astrocyte Glycogen and Brain Energy Metabolism. *Glia* **2007**, *55*, 1263–1271. [CrossRef]
17. Wu, L. Perturbed Brain Energy Metabolism in Alzheimer's Disease and Diabetes. Ph.D. Thesis, University of Kansas, Lawrence, KS, USA, 2017.
18. Pellerin, L.; Bouzier-Sore, A.-K.; Aubert, A.; Serres, S.; Merle, M.; Costalat, R.; Magistretti, P.J. Activity-Dependent Regulation of Energy Metabolism by Astrocytes: An Update. *Glia* **2007**, *55*, 1251–1262. [CrossRef]
19. Gentric, G.; Mieulet, V.; Mechta-Grigoriou, F. Heterogeneity in Cancer Metabolism: New Concepts in an Old Field. *Antioxid. Redox Signal.* **2017**, *26*, 462–485. [CrossRef] [PubMed]
20. Wikstrom, J.D.; Twig, G.; Shirihai, O.S. What Can Mitochondrial Heterogeneity Tell Us about Mitochondrial Dynamics and Autophagy? *Int. J. Biochem. Cell Biol.* **2009**, *41*, 1914–1927. [CrossRef]
21. Murali Mahadevan, H.; Hashemiaghdam, A.; Ashrafi, G.; Harbauer, A.B. Mitochondria in Neuronal Health: From Energy Metabolism to Parkinson's Disease. *Adv. Biol.* **2021**, *5*, e2100663. [CrossRef]
22. Vannucci, S.J.; Maher, F.; Simpson, I.A. Glucose Transporter Proteins in Brain: Delivery of Glucose to Neurons and Glia. *Glia* **1997**, *21*, 2–21. [CrossRef]

23. Lalo, U.; Pankratov, Y.; Parpura, V.; Verkhratsky, A. Ionotropic Receptors in Neuronal-Astroglial Signalling: What Is the Role of "Excitable" Molecules in Non-Excitable Cells. *Biochim. Biophys. Acta* **2011**, *1813*, 992–1002. [CrossRef] [PubMed]
24. Falkowska, A.; Gutowska, I.; Goschorska, M.; Nowacki, P.; Chlubek, D.; Baranowska-Bosiacka, I. Energy Metabolism of the Brain, Including the Cooperation between Astrocytes and Neurons, Especially in the Context of Glycogen Metabolism. *Int. J. Mol. Sci.* **2015**, *16*, 25959–25981. [CrossRef] [PubMed]
25. Tseng, Y.-C.; Huang, C.-J.; Chang, J.C.-H.; Teng, W.-Y.; Baba, O.; Fann, M.-J.; Hwang, P.-P. Glycogen Phosphorylase in Glycogen-Rich Cells Is Involved in the Energy Supply for Ion Regulation in Fish Gill Epithelia. *Am. J. Physiol. Regul. Integr. Comp. Physiol.* **2007**, *293*, R482–R491. [CrossRef] [PubMed]
26. Zois, C.E.; Harris, A.L. Glycogen Metabolism Has a Key Role in the Cancer Microenvironment and Provides New Targets for Cancer Therapy. *J. Mol. Med.* **2016**, *94*, 137–154. [CrossRef]
27. Hardie, D.G.; Carling, D.; Gamblin, S.J. AMP-Activated Protein Kinase: Also Regulated by ADP? *Trends Biochem. Sci.* **2011**, *36*, 470–477. [CrossRef]
28. Oernbo, E.K.; Steffensen, A.B.; Razzaghi Khamesi, P.; Toft-Bertelsen, T.L.; Barbuskaite, D.; Vilhardt, F.; Gerkau, N.J.; Tritsaris, K.; Simonsen, A.H.; Lolansen, S.D.; et al. Membrane Transporters Control Cerebrospinal Fluid Formation Independently of Conventional Osmosis to Modulate Intracranial Pressure. *Fluids Barriers CNS* **2022**, *19*, 65. [CrossRef]
29. Gupta, R.; Gupta, N.; Gupta, R.; Gupta, N. Pentose Phosphate Pathway. In *Fundamentals of Bacterial Physiology and Metabolism*; Springer: Singapore, 2021; pp. 289–305.
30. Castro, M.A.; Angulo, C.; Brauchi, S.; Nualart, F.; Concha, I.I. Ascorbic Acid Participates in a General Mechanism for Concerted Glucose Transport Inhibition and Lactate Transport Stimulation. *Pflugers Arch.* **2008**, *457*, 519–528. [CrossRef]
31. Castro, M.A.; Beltrán, F.A.; Brauchi, S.; Concha, I.I. A Metabolic Switch in Brain: Glucose and Lactate Metabolism Modulation by Ascorbic Acid. *J. Neurochem.* **2009**, *110*, 423–440. [CrossRef]
32. Magistretti, P.J.; Allaman, I. Lactate in the Brain: From Metabolic End-Product to Signalling Molecule. *Nat. Rev. Neurosci.* **2018**, *19*, 235–249. [CrossRef]
33. Duatti, A. Lactate-Induced COL1A1/DDR1 Axis Promotes Prostate Cancer Aggressiveness and Enhances Metastatic Colonization. Ph.D. Thesis, Università di Siena, Siena, Italy, 2023.
34. Wu, C.; Khan, S.A.; Peng, L.-J.; Lange, A.J. Roles for Fructose-2,6-Bisphosphate in the Control of Fuel Metabolism: Beyond Its Allosteric Effects on Glycolytic and Gluconeogenic Enzymes. *Adv. Enzyme Regul.* **2006**, *46*, 72–88. [CrossRef]
35. Allaman, I.; Bélanger, M.; Magistretti, P.J. Methylglyoxal, the Dark Side of Glycolysis. *Front. Neurosci.* **2015**, *9*, 23. [CrossRef] [PubMed]
36. Pestana, F.; Edwards-Faret, G.; Belgard, T.G.; Martirosyan, A.; Holt, M.G. No Longer Underappreciated: The Emerging Concept of Astrocyte Heterogeneity in Neuroscience. *Brain Sci.* **2020**, *10*, 168. [CrossRef] [PubMed]
37. Ye, Z.C.; Rothstein, J.D.; Sontheimer, H. Compromised Glutamate Transport in Human Glioma Cells: Reduction-Mislocalization of Sodium-Dependent Glutamate Transporters and Enhanced Activity of Cystine-Glutamate Exchange. *J. Neurosci.* **1999**, *19*, 10767–10777. [CrossRef]
38. Pellerin, L. How Astrocytes Feed Hungry Neurons. *Mol. Neurobiol.* **2005**, *32*, 59–72. [CrossRef] [PubMed]
39. Díaz-García, C.M.; Mongeon, R.; Lahmann, C.; Koveal, D.; Zucker, H.; Yellen, G. Neuronal Stimulation Triggers Neuronal Glycolysis and Not Lactate Uptake. *Cell Metab.* **2017**, *26*, 361–374.e4. [CrossRef] [PubMed]
40. Bolaños, J.P.; Almeida, A. The Pentose-Phosphate Pathway in Neuronal Survival against Nitrosative Stress. *IUBMB Life* **2010**, *62*, 14–18. [CrossRef]
41. Martín, E.D.; Fernández, M.; Perea, G.; Pascual, O.; Haydon, P.G.; Araque, A.; Ceña, V. Adenosine Released by Astrocytes Contributes to Hypoxia-Induced Modulation of Synaptic Transmission. *Glia* **2007**, *55*, 36–45. [CrossRef]
42. Kambe, Y. Recent Behavioral Findings of Pathophysiological Involvement of Lactate in the Central Nervous System. *Biochim. Biophys. Acta Gen. Subj.* **2022**, *1866*, 130137. [CrossRef]
43. Maurer, M.H.; Canis, M.; Kuschinsky, W.; Duelli, R. Correlation between Local Monocarboxylate Transporter 1 (MCT1) and Glucose Transporter 1 (GLUT1) Densities in the Adult Rat Brain. *Neurosci. Lett.* **2004**, *355*, 105–108. [CrossRef]
44. Hertz, L.; Dienel, G.A. Lactate Transport and Transporters: General Principles and Functional Roles in Brain Cells. *J. Neurosci. Res.* **2005**, *79*, 11–18. [CrossRef] [PubMed]
45. Brooks, G.A.; Arevalo, J.A.; Osmond, A.D.; Leija, R.G.; Curl, C.C.; Tovar, A.P. Lactate in Contemporary Biology: A Phoenix Risen. *J. Physiol.* **2022**, *600*, 1229–1251. [CrossRef]
46. Vijay, N.; Morris, M.E. Role of Monocarboxylate Transporters in Drug Delivery to the Brain. *Curr. Pharm. Des.* **2014**, *20*, 1487–1498. [CrossRef]
47. Sugino, K.; Clark, E.; Schulmann, A.; Shima, Y.; Wang, L.; Hunt, D.L.; Hooks, B.M.; Tränkner, D.; Chandrashekar, J.; Picard, S.; et al. Mapping the Transcriptional Diversity of Genetically and Anatomically Defined Cell Populations in the Mouse Brain. *Elife* **2019**, *8*, e38619. [CrossRef]
48. Frishberg, A.; Peshes-Yaloz, N.; Cohn, O.; Rosentul, D.; Steuerman, Y.; Valadarsky, L.; Yankovitz, G.; Mandelboim, M.; Iraqi, F.A.; Amit, I.; et al. Cell Composition Analysis of Bulk Genomics Using Single-Cell Data. *Nat. Methods* **2019**, *16*, 327–332. [CrossRef]
49. Uhlen, M.; Karlsson, M.J.; Zhong, W.; Tebani, A.; Pou, C.; Mikes, J.; Lakshmikanth, T.; Forsström, B.; Edfors, F.; Odeberg, J.; et al. A Genome-Wide Transcriptomic Analysis of Protein-Coding Genes in Human Blood Cells. *Science* **2019**, *366*, eaax9198. [CrossRef]

50. Rodríguez-Gómez, J.A.; Kavanagh, E.; Engskog-Vlachos, P.; Engskog, M.K.R.; Herrera, A.J.; Espinosa-Oliva, A.M.; Joseph, B.; Hajji, N.; Venero, J.L.; Burguillos, M.A. Microglia: Agents of the CNS Pro-Inflammatory Response. *Cells* **2020**, *9*, 1717. [CrossRef]
51. Marschallinger, J.; Iram, T.; Zardeneta, M.; Lee, S.E.; Lehallier, B.; Haney, M.S.; Pluvinage, J.V.; Mathur, V.; Hahn, O.; Morgens, D.W.; et al. Lipid-Droplet-Accumulating Microglia Represent a Dysfunctional and Proinflammatory State in the Aging Brain. *Nat. Neurosci.* **2020**, *23*, 194–208. [CrossRef]
52. Fan, H.; Tang, H.-B.; Chen, Z.; Wang, H.-Q.; Zhang, L.; Jiang, Y.; Li, T.; Yang, C.-F.; Wang, X.-Y.; Li, X.; et al. Inhibiting HMGB1-RAGE Axis Prevents pro-Inflammatory Macrophages/Microglia Polarization and Affords Neuroprotection after Spinal Cord Injury. *J. Neuroinflamm.* **2020**, *17*, 295. [CrossRef] [PubMed]
53. Bai, Q.; Xue, M.; Yong, V.W. Microglia and Macrophage Phenotypes in Intracerebral Haemorrhage Injury: Therapeutic Opportunities. *Brain* **2020**, *143*, 1297–1314. [CrossRef] [PubMed]
54. Xu, Y.; Li, Y.; Wang, C.; Han, T.; Liu, H.; Sun, L.; Hong, J.; Hashimoto, M.; Wei, J. The Reciprocal Interactions between Microglia and T Cells in Parkinson's Disease: A Double-Edged Sword. *J. Neuroinflammation* **2023**, *20*, 33. [CrossRef]
55. Masuda, T.; Sankowski, R.; Staszewski, O.; Prinz, M. Microglia Heterogeneity in the Single-Cell Era. *Cell Rep.* **2020**, *30*, 1271–1281. [CrossRef]
56. Borst, K.; Dumas, A.A.; Prinz, M. Microglia: Immune and Non-Immune Functions. *Immunity* **2021**, *54*, 2194–2208. [CrossRef] [PubMed]
57. Olah, M.; Menon, V.; Habib, N.; Taga, M.F.; Ma, Y.; Yung, C.J.; Cimpean, M.; Khairallah, A.; Coronas-Samano, G.; Sankowski, R.; et al. Single Cell RNA Sequencing of Human Microglia Uncovers a Subset Associated with Alzheimer's Disease. *Nat. Commun.* **2020**, *11*, 6129. [CrossRef]
58. Chen, X.; Firulyova, M.; Manis, M.; Herz, J.; Smirnov, I.; Aladyeva, E.; Wang, C.; Bao, X.; Finn, M.B.; Hu, H.; et al. Microglia-Mediated T Cell Infiltration Drives Neurodegeneration in Tauopathy. *Nature* **2023**, *615*, 668–677. [CrossRef]
59. Burmeister, A.R.; Johnson, M.B.; Marriott, I. Murine Astrocytes Are Responsive to the Pro-Inflammatory Effects of IL-20. *Neurosci. Lett.* **2019**, *708*, 134334. [CrossRef] [PubMed]
60. Meng, F.; Yao, L. The Role of Inflammation in Epileptogenesis. *Acta Epileptol.* **2020**, *2*, 15. [CrossRef]
61. Araki, T.; Ikegaya, Y.; Koyama, R. The Effects of Microglia- and Astrocyte-Derived Factors on Neurogenesis in Health and Disease. *Eur. J. Neurosci.* **2021**, *54*, 5880–5901. [CrossRef] [PubMed]
62. MacMahon Copas, A.N.; McComish, S.F.; Fletcher, J.M.; Caldwell, M.A. The Pathogenesis of Parkinson's Disease: A Complex Interplay Between Astrocytes, Microglia, and T Lymphocytes? *Front. Neurol.* **2021**, *12*, 666737. [CrossRef]
63. Gharagozloo, M.; Smith, M.D.; Jin, J.; Garton, T.; Taylor, M.; Chao, A.; Meyers, K.; Kornberg, M.D.; Zack, D.J.; Ohayon, J.; et al. Complement Component 3 from Astrocytes Mediates Retinal Ganglion Cell Loss during Neuroinflammation. *Acta Neuropathol.* **2021**, *142*, 899–915. [CrossRef]
64. Raphael, I.; Gomez-Rivera, F.; Raphael, R.A.; Robinson, R.R.; Nalawade, S.; Forsthuber, T.G. TNFR2 Limits Proinflammatory Astrocyte Functions during EAE Induced by Pathogenic DR2b-Restricted T Cells. *JCI Insight* **2019**, *4*, e132527. [CrossRef]
65. Giovannoni, F.; Quintana, F.J. The Role of Astrocytes in CNS Inflammation. *Trends Immunol.* **2020**, *41*, 805–819. [CrossRef] [PubMed]
66. George, S.; Hamblin, M.R.; Abrahamse, H. Differentiation of Mesenchymal Stem Cells to Neuroglia: In the Context of Cell Signalling. *Stem Cell Rev. Rep.* **2019**, *15*, 814–826. [CrossRef]
67. Bakaeva, Z.; Goncharov, M.; Krasilnikova, I.; Zgodova, A.; Frolov, D.; Grebenik, E.; Timashev, P.; Pinelis, V.; Surin, A. Acute and Delayed Effects of Mechanical Injury on Calcium Homeostasis and Mitochondrial Potential of Primary Neuroglial Cell Culture: Potential Causal Contributions to Post-Traumatic Syndrome. *Int. J. Mol. Sci.* **2022**, *23*, 3858. [CrossRef]
68. Wu, Q.; Kong, D.; Peng, W.; Zong, R.; Yu, X.; Feng, S. Deciphering the Biochemical Similarities and Differences Among Human Neuroglial Cells and Glioma Cells Using Fourier Transform Infrared Spectroscopy. *World Neurosurg.* **2022**, *168*, e562–e569. [CrossRef]
69. van Beek, A.A.; Van den Bossche, J.; Mastroberardino, P.G.; de Winther, M.P.J.; Leenen, P.J.M. Metabolic Alterations in Aging Macrophages: Ingredients for Inflammaging? *Trends Immunol.* **2019**, *40*, 113–127. [CrossRef]
70. Lennicke, C.; Cochemé, H.M. Redox Metabolism: ROS as Specific Molecular Regulators of Cell Signaling and Function. *Mol. Cell* **2021**, *81*, 3691–3707. [CrossRef] [PubMed]
71. Greco, E.A.; Lenzi, A.; Migliaccio, S.; Gessani, S. Epigenetic Modifications Induced by Nutrients in Early Life Phases: Gender Differences in Metabolic Alteration in Adulthood. *Front. Genet.* **2019**, *10*, 795. [CrossRef] [PubMed]
72. Kazemian, N.; Mahmoudi, M.; Halperin, F.; Wu, J.C.; Pakpour, S. Gut Microbiota and Cardiovascular Disease: Opportunities and Challenges. *Microbiome* **2020**, *8*, 36. [CrossRef] [PubMed]
73. Chávez-Carbajal, A.; Nirmalkar, K.; Pérez-Lizaur, A.; Hernández-Quiroz, F.; Ramírez-Del-Alto, S.; García-Mena, J.; Hernández-Guerrero, C. Gut Microbiota and Predicted Metabolic Pathways in a Sample of Mexican Women Affected by Obesity and Obesity Plus Metabolic Syndrome. *Int. J. Mol. Sci.* **2019**, *20*, 438. [CrossRef]
74. Vona, R.; Gambardella, L.; Cittadini, C.; Straface, E.; Pietraforte, D. Biomarkers of Oxidative Stress in Metabolic Syndrome and Associated Diseases. *Oxid. Med. Cell. Longev.* **2019**, *2019*, 8267234. [CrossRef] [PubMed]
75. Fahed, G.; Aoun, L.; Bou Zerdan, M.; Allam, S.; Bou Zerdan, M.; Bouferraa, Y.; Assi, H.I. Metabolic Syndrome: Updates on Pathophysiology and Management in 2021. *Int. J. Mol. Sci.* **2022**, *23*, 786. [CrossRef]

76. Son, D.-H.; Lee, H.S.; Lee, Y.-J.; Lee, J.-H.; Han, J.-H. Comparison of Triglyceride-Glucose Index and HOMA-IR for Predicting Prevalence and Incidence of Metabolic Syndrome. *Nutr. Metab. Cardiovasc. Dis.* **2022**, *32*, 596–604. [CrossRef]
77. Maiuolo, J.; Gliozzi, M.; Musolino, V.; Carresi, C.; Scarano, F.; Nucera, S.; Scicchitano, M.; Bosco, F.; Ruga, S.; Zito, M.C.; et al. From Metabolic Syndrome to Neurological Diseases: Role of Autophagy. *Front. Cell Dev. Biol.* **2021**, *9*, 651021. [CrossRef]
78. Barber, T.M.; Kyrou, I.; Randeva, H.S.; Weickert, M.O. Mechanisms of Insulin Resistance at the Crossroad of Obesity with Associated Metabolic Abnormalities and Cognitive Dysfunction. *Int. J. Mol. Sci.* **2021**, *22*, 546. [CrossRef] [PubMed]
79. Patterson, E.; Ryan, P.M.; Wiley, N.; Carafa, I.; Sherwin, E.; Moloney, G.; Franciosi, E.; Mandal, R.; Wishart, D.S.; Tuohy, K.; et al. Gamma-Aminobutyric Acid-Producing Lactobacilli Positively Affect Metabolism and Depressive-like Behaviour in a Mouse Model of Metabolic Syndrome. *Sci. Rep.* **2019**, *9*, 16323. [CrossRef]
80. Polis, B.; Samson, A.O. Role of the Metabolism of Branched-Chain Amino Acids in the Development of Alzheimer's Disease and Other Metabolic Disorders. *Neural Regen. Res.* **2020**, *15*, 1460–1470. [CrossRef] [PubMed]
81. Batlle, E.; Massagué, J. Transforming Growth Factor-β Signaling in Immunity and Cancer. *Immunity* **2019**, *50*, 924–940. [CrossRef]
82. Wang, J.; Li, D.; Cang, H.; Guo, B. Crosstalk between Cancer and Immune Cells: Role of Tumor-Associated Macrophages in the Tumor Microenvironment. *Cancer Med.* **2019**, *8*, 4709–4721. [CrossRef]
83. Schwager, S.; Detmar, M. Inflammation and Lymphatic Function. *Front. Immunol.* **2019**, *10*, 308. [CrossRef]
84. Barker, P.A.; Mantyh, P.; Arendt-Nielsen, L.; Viktrup, L.; Tive, L. Nerve Growth Factor Signaling and Its Contribution to Pain. *J. Pain Res.* **2020**, *13*, 1223–1241. [CrossRef]
85. Delzenne, N.M.; Knudsen, C.; Beaumont, M.; Rodriguez, J.; Neyrinck, A.M.; Bindels, L.B. Contribution of the Gut Microbiota to the Regulation of Host Metabolism and Energy Balance: A Focus on the Gut-Liver Axis. *Proc. Nutr. Soc.* **2019**, *78*, 319–328. [CrossRef]
86. Coll, A.P.; Chen, M.; Taskar, P.; Rimmington, D.; Patel, S.; Tadross, J.A.; Cimino, I.; Yang, M.; Welsh, P.; Virtue, S.; et al. GDF15 Mediates the Effects of Metformin on Body Weight and Energy Balance. *Nature* **2020**, *578*, 444–448. [CrossRef] [PubMed]
87. Hall, K.D.; Farooqi, I.S.; Friedman, J.M.; Klein, S.; Loos, R.J.F.; Mangelsdorf, D.J.; O'Rahilly, S.; Ravussin, E.; Redman, L.M.; Ryan, D.H.; et al. The Energy Balance Model of Obesity: Beyond Calories in, Calories Out. *Am. J. Clin. Nutr.* **2022**, *115*, 1243–1254. [CrossRef]
88. Bitzer-Quintero, O.K.; Ortiz, G.G.; Jaramillo-Bueno, S.; Ramos-González, E.J.; Márquez-Rosales, M.G.; Delgado-Lara, D.L.C.; Torres-Sánchez, E.D.; Tejeda-Martínez, A.R.; Ramirez-Jirano, J. Psycho-Neuro-Endocrine-Immunology: A Role for Melatonin in This New Paradigm. *Molecules* **2022**, *27*, 4888. [CrossRef]
89. Jänig, W. *The Integrative Action of the Autonomic Nervous System: Neurobiology of Homeostasis*; Cambridge University Press: Cambridge, UK, 2022.
90. Dinarello, C.A. Proinflammatory Cytokines. *Chest* **2000**, *118*, 503–508. [CrossRef]
91. Kany, S.; Vollrath, J.T.; Relja, B. Cytokines in Inflammatory Disease. *Int. J. Mol. Sci.* **2019**, *20*, 6008. [CrossRef]
92. Helle, K.B. The Granin Family of Uniquely Acidic Proteins of the Diffuse Neuroendocrine System: Comparative and Functional Aspects. *Biol. Rev. Camb. Philos. Soc.* **2004**, *79*, 769–794. [CrossRef] [PubMed]
93. McLean, R.R. Proinflammatory Cytokines and Osteoporosis. *Curr. Osteoporos. Rep.* **2009**, *7*, 134–139. [CrossRef] [PubMed]
94. Strober, W.; Fuss, I.J. Proinflammatory Cytokines in the Pathogenesis of Inflammatory Bowel Diseases. *Gastroenterology* **2011**, *140*, 1756–1767. [CrossRef]
95. Wieseler-Frank, J.; Maier, S.F.; Watkins, L.R. Central Proinflammatory Cytokines and Pain Enhancement. *Neurosignals* **2005**, *14*, 166–174. [CrossRef]
96. Maley, B.E. Immunohistochemical Localization of Neuropeptides and Neurotransmitters in the Nucleus Solitarius. *Chem. Senses* **1996**, *21*, 367–376. [CrossRef] [PubMed]
97. Xu, H.; Shi, X.; Li, X.; Zou, J.; Zhou, C.; Liu, W.; Shao, H.; Chen, H.; Shi, L. Neurotransmitter and Neuropeptide Regulation of Mast Cell Function: A Systematic Review. *J. Neuroinflamm.* **2020**, *17*, 356. [CrossRef] [PubMed]
98. Benomar, Y.; Taouis, M. Molecular Mechanisms Underlying Obesity-Induced Hypothalamic Inflammation and Insulin Resistance: Pivotal Role of Resistin/TLR4 Pathways. *Front. Endocrinol.* **2019**, *10*, 140. [CrossRef]
99. Ono, H. Molecular Mechanisms of Hypothalamic Insulin Resistance. *Int. J. Mol. Sci.* **2019**, *20*, 1317. [CrossRef]
100. Abuzzahab, M.J.; Roth, C.L.; Shoemaker, A.H. Hypothalamic Obesity: Prologue and Promise. *Horm. Res. Paediatr.* **2019**, *91*, 128–136. [CrossRef]
101. Friedman, J.M. Leptin and the Endocrine Control of Energy Balance. *Nat. Metab.* **2019**, *1*, 754–764. [CrossRef] [PubMed]
102. Poetsch, M.S.; Strano, A.; Guan, K. Role of Leptin in Cardiovascular Diseases. *Front. Endocrinol.* **2020**, *11*, 354. [CrossRef]
103. Varkaneh Kord, H.; Tinsley, G.; Santos, H.O.; Zand, H.; Nazary, A.; Fatahi, S.; Mokhtari, Z.; Salehi-Sahlabadi, A.; Tan, S.C.; Rahmani, J.; et al. The Influence of Fasting and Energy-Restricted Diets on Leptin and Adiponectin Levels in Humans: A Systematic Review and Meta-Analysis. *Clin. Nutr.* **2021**, *40*, 1811–1821. [CrossRef] [PubMed]
104. Dallner, O.S.; Marinis, J.M.; Lu, Y.-H.; Birsoy, K.; Werner, E.; Fayzikhodjaeva, G.; Dill, B.D.; Molina, H.; Moscati, A.; Kutalik, Z.; et al. Dysregulation of a Long Noncoding RNA Reduces Leptin Leading to a Leptin-Responsive Form of Obesity. *Nat. Med.* **2019**, *25*, 507–516. [CrossRef]
105. Butiaeva, L.I.; Slutzki, T.; Swick, H.E.; Bourguignon, C.; Robins, S.C.; Liu, X.; Storch, K.-F.; Kokoeva, M.V. Leptin Receptor-Expressing Pericytes Mediate Access of Hypothalamic Feeding Centers to Circulating Leptin. *Cell Metab.* **2021**, *33*, 1433–1448.e5. [CrossRef]

106. Trinh, T.; Broxmeyer, H.E. Role for Leptin and Leptin Receptors in Stem Cells During Health and Diseases. *Stem Cell Rev. Rep.* **2021**, *17*, 511–522. [CrossRef] [PubMed]
107. Bertucci, J.I.; Blanco, A.M.; Sundarrajan, L.; Rajeswari, J.J.; Velasco, C.; Unniappan, S. Nutrient Regulation of Endocrine Factors Influencing Feeding and Growth in Fish. *Front. Endocrinol.* **2019**, *10*, 83. [CrossRef] [PubMed]
108. Régnier, M.; Van Hul, M.; Knauf, C.; Cani, P.D. Gut Microbiome, Endocrine Control of Gut Barrier Function and Metabolic Diseases. *J. Endocrinol.* **2021**, *248*, R67–R82. [CrossRef] [PubMed]
109. Hill, C.M.; Qualls-Creekmore, E.; Berthoud, H.-R.; Soto, P.; Yu, S.; McDougal, D.H.; Münzberg, H.; Morrison, C.D. FGF21 and the Physiological Regulation of Macronutrient Preference. *Endocrinology* **2020**, *161*, bqaa019. [CrossRef]
110. Becattini, B.; Molinaro, A.; Henricsson, M.; Boren, J.; Solinas, G. Adipocyte PI3K Links Adipostasis with Insulin Secretion through an Adipoincretin Effect. *bioRxiv* **2023**, 2004–2023. [CrossRef]
111. Ghadge, A.A.; Khaire, A.A. Leptin as a Predictive Marker for Metabolic Syndrome. *Cytokine* **2019**, *121*, 154735. [CrossRef]
112. Spezani, R.; da Silva, R.R.; Martins, F.F.; de Souza Marinho, T.; Aguila, M.B.; Mandarim-de-Lacerda, C.A. Intermittent Fasting, Adipokines, Insulin Sensitivity, and Hypothalamic Neuropeptides in a Dietary Overload with High-Fat or High-Fructose Diet in Mice. *J. Nutr. Biochem.* **2020**, *83*, 108419. [CrossRef]
113. García-Carrizo, F.; Picó, C.; Rodríguez, A.M.; Palou, A. High-Esterified Pectin Reverses Metabolic Malprogramming, Improving Sensitivity to Adipostatic/Adipokine Hormones. *J. Agric. Food Chem.* **2019**, *67*, 3633–3642. [CrossRef]
114. Deloose, E.; Janssen, P.; Depoortere, I.; Tack, J. The Migrating Motor Complex: Control Mechanisms and Its Role in Health and Disease. *Nat. Rev. Gastroenterol. Hepatol.* **2012**, *9*, 271–285. [CrossRef]
115. Sakahara, S.; Xie, Z.; Koike, K.; Hoshino, S.; Sakata, I.; Oda, S.; Takahashi, T.; Sakai, T. Physiological Characteristics of Gastric Contractions and Circadian Gastric Motility in the Free-Moving Conscious House Musk Shrew (*Suncus murinus*). *Am. J. Physiol. Regul. Integr. Comp. Physiol.* **2010**, *299*, R1106–R1113. [CrossRef] [PubMed]
116. Mondal, A.; Kawamoto, Y.; Yanaka, T.; Tsutsui, C.; Sakata, I.; Oda, S.-I.; Tanaka, T.; Sakai, T. Myenteric Neural Network Activated by Motilin in the Stomach of *Suncus murinus* (House Musk Shrew). *Neurogastroenterol. Motil.* **2011**, *23*, 1123–1131. [CrossRef] [PubMed]
117. Mondal, A.; Xie, Z.; Miyano, Y.; Tsutsui, C.; Sakata, I.; Kawamoto, Y.; Aizawa, S.; Tanaka, T.; Oda, S.; Sakai, T. Coordination of Motilin and Ghrelin Regulates the Migrating Motor Complex of Gastrointestinal Motility in *Suncus murinus*. *Am. J. Physiol. Gastrointest. Liver Physiol.* **2012**, *302*, G1207–G1215. [CrossRef] [PubMed]
118. Peeters, T.L.; Vantrappen, G.; Janssens, J. Fasting Plasma Motilin Levels Are Related to the Interdigestive Motility Complex. *Gastroenterology* **1980**, *79*, 716–719. [CrossRef] [PubMed]
119. Janssens, J.; Vantrappen, G.; Peeters, T.L. The Activity Front of the Migrating Motor Complex of the Human Stomach but Not of the Small Intestine Is Motilin-Dependent. *Regul. Pept.* **1983**, *6*, 363–369. [CrossRef]
120. Tack, J.; Depoortere, I.; Bisschops, R.; Delporte, C.; Coulie, B.; Meulemans, A.; Janssens, J.; Peeters, T. Influence of Ghrelin on Interdigestive Gastrointestinal Motility in Humans. *Gut* **2006**, *55*, 327–333. [CrossRef]
121. Kojima, M.; Hosoda, H.; Date, Y.; Nakazato, M.; Matsuo, H.; Kangawa, K. Ghrelin Is a Growth-Hormone-Releasing Acylated Peptide from Stomach. *Nature* **1999**, *402*, 656–660. [CrossRef]
122. Wren, A.M.; Small, C.J.; Ward, H.L.; Murphy, K.G.; Dakin, C.L.; Taheri, S.; Kennedy, A.R.; Roberts, G.H.; Morgan, D.G.; Ghatei, M.A.; et al. The Novel Hypothalamic Peptide Ghrelin Stimulates Food Intake and Growth Hormone Secretion. *Endocrinology* **2000**, *141*, 4325–4328. [CrossRef]
123. Tschöp, M.; Smiley, D.L.; Heiman, M.L. Ghrelin Induces Adiposity in Rodents. *Nature* **2000**, *407*, 908–913. [CrossRef]
124. Date, Y.; Shimbara, T.; Koda, S.; Toshinai, K.; Ida, T.; Murakami, N.; Miyazato, M.; Kokame, K.; Ishizuka, Y.; Ishida, Y.; et al. Peripheral Ghrelin Transmits Orexigenic Signals through the Noradrenergic Pathway from the Hindbrain to the Hypothalamus. *Cell Metab.* **2006**, *4*, 323–331. [CrossRef]
125. Kojima, M.; Hosoda, H.; Kangawa, K. Purification and Distribution of Ghrelin: The Natural Endogenous Ligand for the Growth Hormone Secretagogue Receptor. *Horm. Res.* **2001**, *56* (Suppl. S1), 93–97. [CrossRef]
126. Deloose, E.; Vos, R.; Corsetti, M.; Depoortere, I.; Tack, J. Endogenous Motilin, but Not Ghrelin Plasma Levels Fluctuate in Accordance with Gastric Phase III Activity of the Migrating Motor Complex in Man. *Neurogastroenterol. Motil.* **2015**, *27*, 63–71. [CrossRef]
127. Tack, J.; Deloose, E.; Ang, D.; Scarpellini, E.; Vanuytsel, T.; Van Oudenhove, L.; Depoortere, I. Motilin-Induced Gastric Contractions Signal Hunger in Man. *Gut* **2016**, *65*, 214–224. [CrossRef]
128. Deloose, E.; Vos, R.; Janssen, P.; Van den Bergh, O.; Van Oudenhove, L.; Depoortere, I.; Tack, J. The Motilin Receptor Agonist Erythromycin Stimulates Hunger and Food Intake through a Cholinergic Pathway. *Am. J. Clin. Nutr.* **2016**, *103*, 730–737. [CrossRef] [PubMed]
129. Kuroda, K.; Hequing, H.; Mondal, A.; Yoshimura, M.; Ito, K.; Mikami, T.; Takemi, S.; Jogahara, T.; Sakata, I.; Sakai, T. Ghrelin Is an Essential Factor for Motilin-Induced Gastric Contraction in *Suncus murinus*. *Endocrinology* **2015**, *156*, 4437–4447. [CrossRef] [PubMed]
130. Tschöp, M.; Weyer, C.; Tataranni, P.A.; Devanarayan, V.; Ravussin, E.; Heiman, M.L. Circulating Ghrelin Levels Are Decreased in Human Obesity. *Diabetes* **2001**, *50*, 707–709. [CrossRef] [PubMed]
131. Hansen, T.K.; Dall, R.; Hosoda, H.; Kojima, M.; Kangawa, K.; Christiansen, J.S.; Jørgensen, J.O.L. Weight Loss Increases Circulating Levels of Ghrelin in Human Obesity. *Clin. Endocrinol.* **2002**, *56*, 203–206. [CrossRef] [PubMed]

132. Otto, B.; Cuntz, U.; Fruehauf, E.; Wawarta, R.; Folwaczny, C.; Riepl, R.L.; Heiman, M.L.; Lehnert, P.; Fichter, M.; Tschöp, M. Weight Gain Decreases Elevated Plasma Ghrelin Concentrations of Patients with Anorexia Nervosa. *Eur. J. Endocrinol.* **2001**, *145*, 669–673. [CrossRef] [PubMed]
133. Holst, J.J. The Physiology of Glucagon-like Peptide 1. *Physiol. Rev.* **2007**, *87*, 1409–1439. [CrossRef]
134. Drucker, D.J.; Habener, J.F.; Holst, J.J. Discovery, Characterization, and Clinical Development of the Glucagon-like Peptides. *J. Clin. Investig.* **2017**, *127*, 4217–4227. [CrossRef]
135. Nogueiras, R.; Pérez-Tilve, D.; Veyrat-Durebex, C.; Morgan, D.A.; Varela, L.; Haynes, W.G.; Patterson, J.T.; Disse, E.; Pfluger, P.T.; López, M.; et al. Direct Control of Peripheral Lipid Deposition by CNS GLP-1 Receptor Signaling Is Mediated by the Sympathetic Nervous System and Blunted in Diet-Induced Obesity. *J. Neurosci.* **2009**, *29*, 5916–5925. [CrossRef]
136. Baggio, L.L.; Drucker, D.J. Glucagon-like Peptide-1 Receptors in the Brain: Controlling Food Intake and Body Weight. *J. Clin. Investig.* **2014**, *124*, 4223–4226. [CrossRef]
137. Gaykema, R.P.; Newmyer, B.A.; Ottolini, M.; Raje, V.; Warthen, D.M.; Lambeth, P.S.; Niccum, M.; Yao, T.; Huang, Y.; Schulman, I.G.; et al. Activation of Murine Pre-Proglucagon-Producing Neurons Reduces Food Intake and Body Weight. *J. Clin. Investig.* **2017**, *127*, 1031–1045. [CrossRef]
138. Wang, X.-F.; Liu, J.-J.; Xia, J.; Liu, J.; Mirabella, V.; Pang, Z.P. Endogenous Glucagon-like Peptide-1 Suppresses High-Fat Food Intake by Reducing Synaptic Drive onto Mesolimbic Dopamine Neurons. *Cell Rep.* **2015**, *12*, 726–733. [CrossRef] [PubMed]
139. Reiner, D.J.; Leon, R.M.; McGrath, L.E.; Koch-Laskowski, K.; Hahn, J.D.; Kanoski, S.E.; Mietlicki-Baase, E.G.; Hayes, M.R. Glucagon-like Peptide-1 Receptor Signaling in the Lateral Dorsal Tegmental Nucleus Regulates Energy Balance. *Neuropsychopharmacology* **2018**, *43*, 627–637. [CrossRef]
140. Terrill, S.J.; Jackson, C.M.; Greene, H.E.; Lilly, N.; Maske, C.B.; Vallejo, S.; Williams, D.L. Role of Lateral Septum Glucagon-like Peptide 1 Receptors in Food Intake. *Am. J. Physiol. Regul. Integr. Comp. Physiol.* **2016**, *311*, R124–R132. [CrossRef] [PubMed]
141. Ong, Z.Y.; Liu, J.-J.; Pang, Z.P.; Grill, H.J. Paraventricular Thalamic Control of Food Intake and Reward: Role of Glucagon-Like Peptide-1 Receptor Signaling. *Neuropsychopharmacology* **2017**, *42*, 2387–2397. [CrossRef] [PubMed]
142. Rehfeld, J.F.; Friis-Hansen, L.; Goetze, J.P.; Hansen, T.V.O. The Biology of Cholecystokinin and Gastrin Peptides. *Curr. Top. Med. Chem.* **2007**, *7*, 1154–1165. [CrossRef]
143. Chaudhri, O.; Small, C.; Bloom, S. Gastrointestinal Hormones Regulating Appetite. *Philos. Trans. R. Soc. B* **2006**, *361*, 1187–1209. [CrossRef]
144. Crawley, J.N.; Corwin, R.L. Biological Actions of Cholecystokinin. *Peptides* **1994**, *15*, 731–755. [CrossRef]
145. Asin, K.E.; Bednarz, L.; Nikkel, A.L.; Gore, P.A.J.; Nadzan, A.M. A-71623, a Selective CCK-A Receptor Agonist, Suppresses Food Intake in the Mouse, Dog, and Monkey. *Pharmacol. Biochem. Behav.* **1992**, *42*, 699–704. [CrossRef]
146. D'Agostino, G.; Lyons, D.J.; Cristiano, C.; Burke, L.K.; Madara, J.C.; Campbell, J.N.; Garcia, A.P.; Land, B.B.; Lowell, B.B.; Dileone, R.J.; et al. Appetite Controlled by a Cholecystokinin Nucleus of the Solitary Tract to Hypothalamus Neurocircuit. *Elife* **2016**, *5*, e12225. [CrossRef] [PubMed]
147. Peikin, S.R. Role of Cholecystokinin in the Control of Food Intake. *Gastroenterol. Clin. N. Am.* **1989**, *18*, 757–775. [CrossRef]
148. Boden, G.; Chen, X.; Mozzoli, M.; Ryan, I. Effect of Fasting on Serum Leptin in Normal Human Subjects. *J. Clin. Endocrinol. Metab.* **1996**, *81*, 3419–3423. [CrossRef] [PubMed]
149. Bjørbaek, C.; Elmquist, J.K.; Michl, P.; Ahima, R.S.; van Bueren, A.; McCall, A.L.; Flier, J.S. Expression of Leptin Receptor Isoforms in Rat Brain Microvessels. *Endocrinology* **1998**, *139*, 3485–3491. [CrossRef]
150. Elmquist, J.K.; Bjørbaek, C.; Ahima, R.S.; Flier, J.S.; Saper, C.B. Distributions of Leptin Receptor MRNA Isoforms in the Rat Brain. *J. Comp. Neurol.* **1998**, *395*, 535–547. [CrossRef]
151. Bates, S.H.; Stearns, W.H.; Dundon, T.A.; Schubert, M.; Tso, A.W.K.; Wang, Y.; Banks, A.S.; Lavery, H.J.; Haq, A.K.; Maratos-Flier, E.; et al. STAT3 Signalling Is Required for Leptin Regulation of Energy Balance but Not Reproduction. *Nature* **2003**, *421*, 856–859. [CrossRef] [PubMed]
152. Farooqi, I.S.; Bullmore, E.; Keogh, J.; Gillard, J.; O'Rahilly, S.; Fletcher, P.C. Leptin Regulates Striatal Regions and Human Eating Behavior. *Science* **2007**, *317*, 1355. [CrossRef]
153. Münzberg, H.; Qualls-Creekmore, E.; Berthoud, H.-R.; Morrison, C.D.; Yu, S. Neural Control of Energy Expenditure. *Handb. Exp. Pharmacol.* **2016**, *233*, 173–194. [CrossRef]
154. Krashes, M.J.; Shah, B.P.; Madara, J.C.; Olson, D.P.; Strochlic, D.E.; Garfield, A.S.; Vong, L.; Pei, H.; Watabe-Uchida, M.; Uchida, N.; et al. An Excitatory Paraventricular Nucleus to AgRP Neuron Circuit That Drives Hunger. *Nature* **2014**, *507*, 238–242. [CrossRef]
155. Tucker, J.A.L.; Bornath, D.P.D.; McCarthy, S.F.; Hazell, T.J. Leptin and Energy Balance: Exploring Leptin's Role in the Regulation of Energy Intake and Energy Expenditure. *Nutr. Neurosci.* **2022**, 1–9. [CrossRef] [PubMed]
156. Kullmann, S.; Kleinridders, A.; Small, D.M.; Fritsche, A.; Häring, H.-U.; Preissl, H.; Heni, M. Central Nervous Pathways of Insulin Action in the Control of Metabolism and Food Intake. *Lancet Diabetes Endocrinol.* **2020**, *8*, 524–534. [CrossRef]
157. Walczak, K.; Sieminska, L. Obesity and Thyroid Axis. *Int. J. Environ. Res. Public Health* **2021**, *18*, 9434. [CrossRef]
158. Hewagalamulage, S.D.; Lee, T.K.; Clarke, I.J.; Henry, B.A. Stress, Cortisol, and Obesity: A Role for Cortisol Responsiveness in Identifying Individuals Prone to Obesity. *Domest. Anim. Endocrinol.* **2016**, *56*, S112–S120. [CrossRef]
159. Coppari, R.; Bjørbæk, C. Leptin Revisited: Its Mechanism of Action and Potential for Treating Diabetes. *Nat. Rev. Drug Discov.* **2012**, *11*, 692–708. [CrossRef]

160. Myers, M.G.; Cowley, M.A.; Münzberg, H. Mechanisms of Leptin Action and Leptin Resistance. *Annu. Rev. Physiol.* **2008**, *70*, 537–556. [CrossRef] [PubMed]
161. Elmquist, J.K.; Elias, C.F.; Saper, C.B. From Lesions to Leptin: Hypothalamic Control of Food Intake and Body Weight. *Neuron* **1999**, *22*, 221–232. [CrossRef]
162. Liu, L.; Karkanias, G.B.; Morales, J.C.; Hawkins, M.; Barzilai, N.; Wang, J.; Rossetti, L. Intracerebroventricular Leptin Regulates Hepatic but Not Peripheral Glucose Fluxes. *J. Biol. Chem.* **1998**, *273*, 31160–31167. [CrossRef]
163. Heilig, M.; Widerlöv, E. Neuropeptide Y: An Overview of Central Distribution, Functional Aspects, and Possible Involvement in Neuropsychiatric Illnesses. *Acta Psychiatr. Scand.* **1990**, *82*, 95–114. [CrossRef]
164. Kuo, L.E.; Kitlinska, J.B.; Tilan, J.U.; Li, L.; Baker, S.B.; Johnson, M.D.; Lee, E.W.; Burnett, M.S.; Fricke, S.T.; Kvetnansky, R.; et al. Neuropeptide Y Acts Directly in the Periphery on Fat Tissue and Mediates Stress-Induced Obesity and Metabolic Syndrome. *Nat. Med.* **2007**, *13*, 803–811. [CrossRef] [PubMed]
165. Shende, P.; Desai, D. Physiological and Therapeutic Roles of Neuropeptide Y on Biological Functions. *Adv. Exp. Med. Biol.* **2020**, *1237*, 37–47. [CrossRef]
166. Mani, B.K.; Shankar, K.; Zigman, J.M. Ghrelin's Relationship to Blood Glucose. *Endocrinology* **2019**, *160*, 1247–1261. [CrossRef]
167. Müller, T.D.; Nogueiras, R.; Andermann, M.L.; Andrews, Z.B.; Anker, S.D.; Argente, J.; Batterham, R.L.; Benoit, S.C.; Bowers, C.Y.; Broglio, F. Ghrelin. *Mol. Metab.* **2015**, *4*, 437–460. [CrossRef]
168. Cummings, D.E.; Purnell, J.Q.; Frayo, R.S.; Schmidova, K.; Wisse, B.E.; Weigle, D.S. A Preprandial Rise in Plasma Ghrelin Levels Suggests a Role in Meal Initiation in Humans. *Diabetes* **2001**, *50*, 1714–1719. [CrossRef]
169. Perelló, M.; Zigman, J.M. The Role of Ghrelin in Reward-Based Eating. *Biol. Psychiatry* **2012**, *72*, 347–353. [CrossRef] [PubMed]
170. Madden, C.J.; Tupone, D.; Morrison, S.F. Orexin Modulates Brown Adipose Tissue Thermogenesis. *Biomol. Concepts* **2012**, *3*, 381–386. [CrossRef]
171. Lin, L.; Lee, J.H.; Wang, R.; Wang, R.; Sheikh-Hamad, D.; Zang, Q.S.; Sun, Y. AP2-Cre Mediated Ablation of GHS-R Attenuates Adiposity and Improves Insulin Sensitivity during Aging. *Int. J. Mol. Sci.* **2018**, *19*, 3002. [CrossRef] [PubMed]
172. Shabalina, I.G.; Nedergaard, J. Mitochondrial ('mild') Uncoupling and ROS Production: Physiologically Relevant or Not? *Biochem. Soc. Trans.* **2011**, *39*, 1305–1309. [CrossRef]
173. Iwen, K.A.; Schröder, E.; Brabant, G. Thyroid Hormones and the Metabolic Syndrome. *Eur. Thyroid J.* **2013**, *2*, 83–92. [CrossRef] [PubMed]
174. Cannon, B.; Nedergaard, J. Yes, Even Human Brown Fat Is on Fire! *J. Clin. Investig.* **2012**, *122*, 486–489. [CrossRef]
175. Dallman, M.F.; Pecoraro, N.C.; la Fleur, S.E. Chronic Stress and Comfort Foods: Self-Medication and Abdominal Obesity. *Brain. Behav. Immun.* **2005**, *19*, 275–280. [CrossRef] [PubMed]
176. Pecoraro, N.; Reyes, F.; Gomez, F.; Bhargava, A.; Dallman, M.F. Chronic Stress Promotes Palatable Feeding, Which Reduces Signs of Stress: Feedforward and Feedback Effects of Chronic Stress. *Endocrinology* **2004**, *145*, 3754–3762. [CrossRef]
177. Dallman, M.F.; la Fleur, S.E.; Pecoraro, N.C.; Gomez, F.; Houshyar, H.; Akana, S.F. Minireview: Glucocorticoids--Food Intake, Abdominal Obesity, and Wealthy Nations in 2004. *Endocrinology* **2004**, *145*, 2633–2638. [CrossRef]
178. la Fleur, S.E.; Houshyar, H.; Roy, M.; Dallman, M.F. Choice of Lard, but Not Total Lard Calories, Damps Adrenocorticotropin Responses to Restraint. *Endocrinology* **2005**, *146*, 2193–2199. [CrossRef]
179. Jéquier, E. Leptin Signaling, Adiposity, and Energy Balance. *Ann. N. Y. Acad. Sci.* **2002**, *967*, 379–388. [CrossRef] [PubMed]
180. Sinha, R.; Jastreboff, A.M. Stress as a Common Risk Factor for Obesity and Addiction. *Biol. Psychiatry* **2013**, *73*, 827–835. [CrossRef]
181. Mitchell, D.; Shireman, J.; Sierra Potchanant, E.A.; Lara-Velazquez, M.; Dey, M. Neuroinflammation in Autoimmune Disease and Primary Brain Tumors: The Quest for Striking the Right Balance. *Front. Cell. Neurosci.* **2021**, *15*, 716947. [CrossRef] [PubMed]
182. Han, V.X.; Patel, S.; Jones, H.F.; Dale, R.C. Maternal Immune Activation and Neuroinflammation in Human Neurodevelopmental Disorders. *Nat. Rev. Neurol.* **2021**, *17*, 564–579. [CrossRef]
183. Kölliker-Frers, R.; Udovin, L.; Otero-Losada, M.; Kobiec, T.; Herrera, M.I.; Palacios, J.; Razzitte, G.; Capani, F. Neuroinflammation: An Integrating Overview of Reactive-Neuroimmune Cell Interactions in Health and Disease. *Mediators Inflamm.* **2021**, *2021*, 9999146. [CrossRef]
184. Yong, H.Y.F.; Rawji, K.S.; Ghorbani, S.; Xue, M.; Yong, V.W. The Benefits of Neuroinflammation for the Repair of the Injured Central Nervous System. *Cell. Mol. Immunol.* **2019**, *16*, 540–546. [CrossRef]
185. Zhao, J.; Bi, W.; Xiao, S.; Lan, X.; Cheng, X.; Zhang, J.; Lu, D.; Wei, W.; Wang, Y.; Li, H.; et al. Neuroinflammation Induced by Lipopolysaccharide Causes Cognitive Impairment in Mice. *Sci. Rep.* **2019**, *9*, 5790. [CrossRef]
186. Zindler, E.; Zipp, F. Neuronal Injury in Chronic CNS Inflammation. *Best Pract. Res. Clin. Anaesthesiol.* **2010**, *24*, 551–562. [CrossRef]
187. Bertram, L.; Tanzi, R.E. The Genetic Epidemiology of Neurodegenerative Disease. *J. Clin. Investig.* **2005**, *115*, 1449–1457. [CrossRef] [PubMed]
188. Gandhi, S.; Abramov, A.Y. Mechanism of Oxidative Stress in Neurodegeneration. *Oxid. Med. Cell. Longev.* **2012**, *2012*, 428010. [CrossRef] [PubMed]
189. Lezi, E.; Swerdlow, R.H. Mitochondria in Neurodegeneration. *Adv. Exp. Med. Biol.* **2012**, *942*, 269–286. [CrossRef] [PubMed]
190. Müller, M.; Ahumada-Castro, U.; Sanhueza, M.; Gonzalez-Billault, C.; Court, F.A.; Cárdenas, C. Mitochondria and Calcium Regulation as Basis of Neurodegeneration Associated with Aging. *Front. Neurosci.* **2018**, *12*, 470. [CrossRef] [PubMed]
191. Matus, S.; Glimcher, L.H.; Hetz, C. Protein Folding Stress in Neurodegenerative Diseases: A Glimpse into the ER. *Curr. Opin. Cell Biol.* **2011**, *23*, 239–252. [CrossRef]

192. de Araújo Boleti, A.P.; de Oliveira Flores, T.M.; Moreno, S.E.; dos Anjos, L.; Mortari, M.R.; Migliolo, L. Neuroinflammation: An Overview of Neurodegenerative and Metabolic Diseases and of Biotechnological Studies. *Neurochem. Int.* **2020**, *136*, 104714. [CrossRef]
193. Bellia, C.; Lombardo, M.; Meloni, M.; Della-Morte, D.; Bellia, A.; Lauro, D. Diabetes and Cognitive Decline. *Adv. Clin. Chem.* **2022**, *108*, 37–71. [CrossRef]
194. Ehtewish, H.; Arredouani, A.; El-Agnaf, O. Diagnostic, Prognostic, and Mechanistic Biomarkers of Diabetes Mellitus-Associated Cognitive Decline. *Int. J. Mol. Sci.* **2022**, *23*, 6144. [CrossRef] [PubMed]
195. Xu, Z.-P.; Yang, S.-L.; Zhao, S.; Zheng, C.-H.; Li, H.-H.; Zhang, Y.; Huang, R.-X.; Li, M.-Z.; Gao, Y.; Zhang, S.-J.; et al. Biomarkers for Early Diagnostic of Mild Cognitive Impairment in Type-2 Diabetes Patients: A Multicentre, Retrospective, Nested Case-Control Study. *eBioMedicine* **2016**, *5*, 105–113. [CrossRef] [PubMed]
196. Cai, D.; Liu, T. Hypothalamic Inflammation: A Double-Edged Sword to Nutritional Diseases. *Ann. N. Y. Acad. Sci.* **2011**, *1243*, E1–E39. [CrossRef]
197. Miller, A.A.; Spencer, S.J. Obesity and Neuroinflammation: A Pathway to Cognitive Impairment. *Brain. Behav. Immun.* **2014**, *42*, 10–21. [CrossRef] [PubMed]
198. Martín-Rodríguez, A.; Tornero-Aguilera, J.F.; López-Pérez, P.J.; Clemente-Suárez, V.J. Overweight and Executive Functions, Psychological and Behavioral Profile of Spanish Adolescents. *Physiol. Behav.* **2022**, *254*, 113901. [CrossRef] [PubMed]
199. Lara, V.P.; Caramelli, P.; Teixeira, A.L.; Barbosa, M.T.; Carmona, K.C.; Carvalho, M.G.; Fernandes, A.P.; Gomes, K.B. High Cortisol Levels Are Associated with Cognitive Impairment No-Dementia (CIND) and Dementia. *Clin. Chim. Acta.* **2013**, *423*, 18–22. [CrossRef]
200. Rhebergen, D.; Korten, N.C.M.; Penninx, B.W.J.H.; Stek, M.L.; van der Mast, R.C.; Oude Voshaar, R.; Comijs, H.C. Hypothalamic-Pituitary-Adrenal Axis Activity in Older Persons with and without a Depressive Disorder. *Psychoneuroendocrinology* **2015**, *51*, 341–350. [CrossRef] [PubMed]
201. Cope, E.C.; LaMarca, E.A.; Monari, P.K.; Olson, L.B.; Martinez, S.; Zych, A.D.; Katchur, N.J.; Gould, E. Microglia Play an Active Role in Obesity-Associated Cognitive Decline. *J. Neurosci.* **2018**, *38*, 8889–8904. [CrossRef]
202. Adlercreutz, H. Western Diet and Western Diseases: Some Hormonal and Biochemical Mechanisms and Associations. *Scand. J. Clin. Lab. Investig.* **1990**, *201*, 3–23. [CrossRef]
203. Alhabeeb, H.; AlFaiz, A.; Kutbi, E.; AlShahrani, D.; Alsuhail, A.; AlRajhi, S.; Alotaibi, N.; Alotaibi, K.; AlAmri, S.; Alghamdi, S.; et al. Gut Hormones in Health and Obesity: The Upcoming Role of Short Chain Fatty Acids. *Nutrients* **2021**, *13*, 481. [CrossRef]
204. Astrup, A.; Magkos, F.; Bier, D.M.; Brenna, J.T.; de Oliveira Otto, M.C.; Hill, J.O.; King, J.C.; Mente, A.; Ordovas, J.M.; Volek, J.S.; et al. Saturated fats and health: A reassessment of evidence and proposal for food-based recommendations. *J. Am. Coll. Cardiol.* **2020**, *76*, 844–857. [CrossRef] [PubMed]
205. Clifton, P. Metabolic Syndrome-Role of Dietary Fat Type and Quantity. *Nutrients* **2019**, *11*, 1438. [CrossRef] [PubMed]
206. Yamamoto, M.; Guo, D.-H.; Hernandez, C.M.; Stranahan, A.M. Endothelial Adora2a Activation Promotes Blood-Brain Barrier Breakdown and Cognitive Impairment in Mice with Diet-Induced Insulin Resistance. *J. Neurosci.* **2019**, *39*, 4179–4192. [CrossRef]
207. Mauro, C.; De Rosa, V.; Marelli-Berg, F.; Solito, E. Metabolic Syndrome and the Immunological Affair with the Blood-Brain Barrier. *Front. Immunol.* **2014**, *5*, 677. [CrossRef] [PubMed]
208. Van Dyken, P.; Lacoste, B. Impact of Metabolic Syndrome on Neuroinflammation and the Blood-Brain Barrier. *Front. Neurosci.* **2018**, *12*, 930. [CrossRef]
209. Kwon, Y.N.; Kim, Y.-J. Gut-Brain-Microbiota Axis and Hypertension: A Literature Review. *Curr. Pharm. Des.* **2021**, *27*, 3939–3946. [CrossRef]
210. Sharma, R.K.; Yang, T.; Oliveira, A.C.; Lobaton, G.O.; Aquino, V.; Kim, S.; Richards, E.M.; Pepine, C.J.; Sumners, C.; Raizada, M.K. Microglial Cells Impact Gut Microbiota and Gut Pathology in Angiotensin II-Induced Hypertension. *Circ. Res.* **2019**, *124*, 727–736. [CrossRef]
211. Richards, E.M.; Li, J.; Stevens, B.R.; Pepine, C.J.; Raizada, M.K. Gut Microbiome and Neuroinflammation in Hypertension. *Circ. Res.* **2022**, *130*, 401–417. [CrossRef] [PubMed]
212. Hamed, S.A. Neurologic Conditions and Disorders of Uremic Syndrome of Chronic Kidney Disease: Presentations, Causes, and Treatment Strategies. *Expert Rev. Clin. Pharmacol.* **2019**, *12*, 61–90. [CrossRef]
213. Miranda, A.S.; Cordeiro, T.M.; Dos Santos Lacerda Soares, T.M.; Ferreira, R.N.; Simões e Silva, A.C. Kidney-Brain Axis Inflammatory Cross-Talk: From Bench to Bedside. *Clin. Sci.* **2017**, *131*, 1093–1105. [CrossRef] [PubMed]
214. Corona, R.; Ordaz, B.; Robles-Osorio, L.; Sabath, E.; Morales, T. Neuroimmunoendocrine Link Between Chronic Kidney Disease and Olfactory Deficits. *Front. Integr. Neurosci.* **2022**, *16*, 763986. [CrossRef]
215. Moalem, G.; Leibowitz-Amit, R.; Yoles, E.; Mor, F.; Cohen, I.R.; Schwartz, M. Autoimmune T Cells Protect Neurons from Secondary Degeneration after Central Nervous System Axotomy. *Nat. Med.* **1999**, *5*, 49–55. [CrossRef]
216. Ceriello, A. The Emerging Challenge in Diabetes: The "Metabolic Memory". *Vascul. Pharmacol.* **2012**, *57*, 133–138. [CrossRef] [PubMed]
217. Wong, Y.C.; Luk, K.; Purtell, K.; Burke Nanni, S.; Stoessl, A.J.; Trudeau, L.-E.; Yue, Z.; Krainc, D.; Oertel, W.; Obeso, J.A.; et al. Neuronal Vulnerability in Parkinson Disease: Should the Focus Be on Axons and Synaptic Terminals? *Mov. Disord.* **2019**, *34*, 1406–1422. [CrossRef] [PubMed]

218. Jordan, L.C.; DeBaun, M.R.; Donahue, M.J. Advances in Neuroimaging to Improve Care in Sickle Cell Disease. *Lancet. Neurol.* **2021**, *20*, 398–408. [CrossRef] [PubMed]
219. Shimizu, S.; Hirose, D.; Hatanaka, H.; Takenoshita, N.; Kaneko, Y.; Ogawa, Y.; Sakurai, H.; Hanyu, H. Role of Neuroimaging as a Biomarker for Neurodegenerative Diseases. *Front. Neurol.* **2018**, *9*, 265. [CrossRef]
220. McKhann, G.M.; Knopman, D.S.; Chertkow, H.; Hyman, B.T.; Jack, C.R.J.; Kawas, C.H.; Klunk, W.E.; Koroshetz, W.J.; Manly, J.J.; Mayeux, R.; et al. The Diagnosis of Dementia Due to Alzheimer's Disease: Recommendations from the National Institute on Aging-Alzheimer's Association Workgroups on Diagnostic Guidelines for Alzheimer's Disease. *Alzheimers. Dement.* **2011**, *7*, 263–269. [CrossRef] [PubMed]
221. Zhao, X.; Zhao, X.-M. Deep Learning of Brain Magnetic Resonance Images: A Brief Review. *Methods* **2021**, *192*, 131–140. [CrossRef] [PubMed]
222. Wilson, D.; Ambler, G.; Lee, K.-J.; Lim, J.-S.; Shiozawa, M.; Koga, M.; Li, L.; Lovelock, C.; Chabriat, H.; Hennerici, M. Cerebral Microbleeds and Stroke Risk after Ischaemic Stroke or Transient Ischaemic Attack: A Pooled Analysis of Individual Patient Data from Cohort Studies. *Lancet Neurol.* **2019**, *18*, 653–665. [CrossRef]
223. Mei, L.; Wang, Y.; Liu, C.; Mou, J.; Yuan, Y.; Qiu, L.; Gong, Q. Study of Sex Differences in Unmedicated Patients with Major Depressive Disorder by Using Resting State Brain Functional Magnetic Resonance Imaging. *Front. Neurosci.* **2022**, *16*, 814410. [CrossRef]
224. He, N.; Chen, Y.; LeWitt, P.A.; Yan, F.; Haacke, E.M. Application of Neuromelanin MR Imaging in Parkinson Disease. *J. Magn. Reson. Imaging* **2023**, *57*, 337–352. [CrossRef]
225. Li, T.-R.; Wu, Y.; Jiang, J.-J.; Lin, H.; Han, C.-L.; Jiang, J.-H.; Han, Y. Radiomics Analysis of Magnetic Resonance Imaging Facilitates the Identification of Preclinical Alzheimer's Disease: An Exploratory Study. *Front. Cell Dev. Biol.* **2020**, *8*, 605734. [CrossRef] [PubMed]
226. Wang, W.-Y.; Yu, J.-T.; Liu, Y.; Yin, R.-H.; Wang, H.-F.; Wang, J.; Tan, L.; Radua, J.; Tan, L. Voxel-Based Meta-Analysis of Grey Matter Changes in Alzheimer's Disease. *Transl. Neurodegener.* **2015**, *4*, 6. [CrossRef] [PubMed]
227. Yao, N.-T.; Zheng, Q.; Xu, Z.-Q.; Yin, J.-H.; Lu, L.-G.; Zuo, Q.; Yang, S.; Zhang, C.-L.; Jiao, L. Positron Emission Computed Tomography/Single Photon Emission Computed Tomography in Parkinson Disease. *Chin. Med. J.* **2020**, *133*, 1448–1455. [CrossRef]
228. Bhat, S.; Acharya, U.R.; Hagiwara, Y.; Dadmehr, N.; Adeli, H. Parkinson's Disease: Cause Factors, Measurable Indicators, and Early Diagnosis. *Comput. Biol. Med.* **2018**, *102*, 234–241. [CrossRef] [PubMed]
229. Kägi, G.; Bhatia, K.P.; Tolosa, E. The Role of DAT-SPECT in Movement Disorders. *J. Neurol. Neurosurg. Psychiatry* **2010**, *81*, 5–12. [CrossRef]
230. Shao, W.; Rowe, S.P.; Du, Y. Artificial Intelligence in Single Photon Emission Computed Tomography (SPECT) Imaging: A Narrative Review. *Ann. Transl. Med.* **2021**, *9*, 820. [CrossRef] [PubMed]
231. Shiiba, T.; Takano, K.; Takaki, A.; Suwazono, S. Dopamine Transporter Single-Photon Emission Computed Tomography-Derived Radiomics Signature for Detecting Parkinson's Disease. *EJNMMI Res.* **2022**, *12*, 39. [CrossRef]
232. Höller, Y.; Bathke, A.C.; Uhl, A.; Strobl, N.; Lang, A.; Bergmann, J.; Nardone, R.; Rossini, F.; Zauner, H.; Kirschner, M.; et al. Combining SPECT and Quantitative EEG Analysis for the Automated Differential Diagnosis of Disorders with Amnestic Symptoms. *Front. Aging Neurosci.* **2017**, *9*, 290. [CrossRef]
233. Lilenfeld, L.R.R.; Wonderlich, S.; Riso, L.P.; Crosby, R.; Mitchell, J. Eating Disorders and Personality: A Methodological and Empirical Review. *Clin. Psychol. Rev.* **2006**, *26*, 299–320. [CrossRef]
234. Monteleone, A.M.; Castellini, G.; Volpe, U.; Ricca, V.; Lelli, L.; Monteleone, P.; Maj, M. Neuroendocrinology and Brain Imaging of Reward in Eating Disorders: A Possible Key to the Treatment of Anorexia Nervosa and Bulimia Nervosa. *Prog. Neuropsychopharmacol. Biol. Psychiatry* **2018**, *80 Pt B*, 132–142. [CrossRef]
235. Frank, G.K.; Bailer, U.F.; Henry, S.; Wagner, A.; Kaye, W.H. Neuroimaging Studies in Eating Disorders. *CNS Spectr.* **2004**, *9*, 539–548. [CrossRef] [PubMed]
236. Frank, G.K.W. Advances from Neuroimaging Studies in Eating Disorders. *CNS Spectr.* **2015**, *20*, 391–400. [CrossRef] [PubMed]
237. Wagner, A.; Greer, P.; Bailer, U.F.; Frank, G.K.; Henry, S.E.; Putnam, K.; Meltzer, C.C.; Ziolko, S.K.; Hoge, J.; McConaha, C.; et al. Normal Brain Tissue Volumes after Long-Term Recovery in Anorexia and Bulimia Nervosa. *Biol. Psychiatry* **2006**, *59*, 291–293. [CrossRef] [PubMed]
238. Stice, E.; Spoor, S.; Ng, J.; Zald, D.H. Relation of Obesity to Consummatory and Anticipatory Food Reward. *Physiol. Behav.* **2009**, *97*, 551–560. [CrossRef] [PubMed]
239. Uher, R.; Murphy, T.; Brammer, M.J.; Dalgleish, T.; Phillips, M.L.; Ng, V.W.; Andrew, C.M.; Williams, S.C.R.; Campbell, I.C.; Treasure, J. Medial Prefrontal Cortex Activity Associated with Symptom Provocation in Eating Disorders. *Am. J. Psychiatry* **2004**, *161*, 1238–1246. [CrossRef] [PubMed]
240. Fladung, A.-K.; Grön, G.; Grammer, K.; Herrnberger, B.; Schilly, E.; Grasteit, S.; Wolf, R.C.; Walter, H.; von Wietersheim, J. A Neural Signature of Anorexia Nervosa in the Ventral Striatal Reward System. *Am. J. Psychiatry* **2010**, *167*, 206–212. [CrossRef]
241. Keating, C.; Tilbrook, A.J.; Rossell, S.L.; Enticott, P.G.; Fitzgerald, P.B. Reward Processing in Anorexia Nervosa. *Neuropsychologia* **2012**, *50*, 567–575. [CrossRef]

242. Kullmann, S.; Pape, A.-A.; Heni, M.; Ketterer, C.; Schick, F.; Häring, H.-U.; Fritsche, A.; Preissl, H.; Veit, R. Functional Network Connectivity Underlying Food Processing: Disturbed Salience and Visual Processing in Overweight and Obese Adults. *Cereb. Cortex* **2013**, *23*, 1247–1256. [CrossRef]
243. Culbert, K.M.; Sisk, C.L.; Klump, K.L. A Narrative Review of Sex Differences in Eating Disorders: Is There a Biological Basis? *Clin. Ther.* **2021**, *43*, 95–111. [CrossRef]
244. Asarian, L.; Geary, N. Sex Differences in the Physiology of Eating. *Am. J. Physiol. Regul. Integr. Comp. Physiol.* **2013**, *305*, R1215-67. [CrossRef]
245. Pursey, K.M.; Stanwell, P.; Callister, R.J.; Brain, K.; Collins, C.E.; Burrows, T.L. Neural Responses to Visual Food Cues According to Weight Status: A Systematic Review of Functional Magnetic Resonance Imaging Studies. *Front. Nutr.* **2014**, *1*, 7. [CrossRef] [PubMed]
246. Vainik, U.; Baker, T.E.; Dadar, M.; Zeighami, Y.; Michaud, A.; Zhang, Y.; García Alanis, J.C.; Misic, B.; Collins, D.L.; Dagher, A. Neurobehavioral Correlates of Obesity Are Largely Heritable. *Proc. Natl. Acad. Sci. USA* **2018**, *115*, 9312–9317. [CrossRef] [PubMed]
247. Fotuhi, M.; Lubinski, B. The Effects of Obesity on Brain Structure and Size. *Pract. Neurol.* **2013**. Available online: https://neurogrow.com/wp-content/uploads/2020/07/2013_-_fotuhi_-_practical_neurology.pdf (accessed on 20 June 2023).
248. Stice, E.; Yokum, S. Neural Vulnerability Factors That Increase Risk for Future Weight Gain. *Psychol. Bull.* **2016**, *142*, 447–471. [CrossRef] [PubMed]
249. Ronan, L.; Alexander-Bloch, A.F.; Wagstyl, K.; Farooqi, S.; Brayne, C.; Tyler, L.K.; Fletcher, P.C. Obesity Associated with Increased Brain Age from Midlife. *Neurobiol. Aging* **2016**, *47*, 63–70. [CrossRef] [PubMed]
250. Kullmann, S.; Schweizer, F.; Veit, R.; Fritsche, A.; Preissl, H. Compromised White Matter Integrity in Obesity. *Obes. Rev. Off. J. Int. Assoc. Study Obes.* **2015**, *16*, 273–281. [CrossRef]
251. Morys, F.; García-García, I.; Dagher, A. Is Obesity Related to Enhanced Neural Reactivity to Visual Food Cues? A Review and Meta-Analysis. *Soc. Cogn. Affect. Neurosci.* **2020**, *18*, 1438. [CrossRef]
252. Sharma, L.; Markon, K.E.; Clark, L.A. Toward a Theory of Distinct Types of "Impulsive" Behaviors: A Meta-Analysis of Self-Report and Behavioral Measures. *Psychol. Bull.* **2014**, *140*, 374–408. [CrossRef]
253. Michaud, A.; Vainik, U.; Garcia-Garcia, I.; Dagher, A. Overlapping Neural Endophenotypes in Addiction and Obesity. *Front. Endocrinol.* **2017**, *8*, 127. [CrossRef]
254. Bryant, E.J.; King, N.A.; Blundell, J.E. Disinhibition: Its Effects on Appetite and Weight Regulation. *Obes. Rev.* **2008**, *9*, 409–419. [CrossRef]
255. Davis, C.; Curtis, C.; Levitan, R.D.; Carter, J.C.; Kaplan, A.S.; Kennedy, J.L. Evidence That "food Addiction" Is a Valid Phenotype of Obesity. *Appetite* **2011**, *57*, 711–717. [CrossRef] [PubMed]
256. Torres, A.; Catena, A.; Megías, A.; Maldonado, A.; Cándido, A.; Verdejo-García, A.; Perales, J.C. Emotional and Non-Emotional Pathways to Impulsive Behavior and Addiction. *Front. Hum. Neurosci.* **2013**, *7*, 43. [CrossRef] [PubMed]
257. Gerlach, G.; Herpertz, S.; Loeber, S. Personality Traits and Obesity: A Systematic Review. *Obes. Rev.* **2015**, *16*, 32–63. [CrossRef] [PubMed]
258. Meule, A.; Blechert, J. Trait Impulsivity and Body Mass Index: A Cross-Sectional Investigation in 3073 Individuals Reveals Positive, but Very Small Relationships. *Health Psychol. Open* **2016**, *3*, 2055102916659164. [CrossRef]
259. Hays, N.P.; Roberts, S.B. Aspects of Eating Behaviors "Disinhibition" and "Restraint" Are Related to Weight Gain and BMI in Women. *Obesity* **2008**, *16*, 52–58. [CrossRef]
260. Bryant, E.J.; Rehman, J.; Pepper, L.B.; Walters, E.R. Obesity and Eating Disturbance: The Role of TFEQ Restraint and Disinhibition. *Curr. Obes. Rep.* **2019**, *8*, 363–372. [CrossRef]
261. Emery, R.L.; King, K.M.; Fischer, S.F.; Davis, K.R. The Moderating Role of Negative Urgency on the Prospective Association between Dietary Restraint and Binge Eating. *Appetite* **2013**, *71*, 113–119. [CrossRef]
262. Platt, M.L.; Watson, K.K.; Hayden, B.Y.; Shepherd, S.V.; Klein, J.T. *Neuroeconomics: Implications for Understanding the Neurobiology of Addiction*; Kuhn, C.M., Koob, G.F., Eds.; CRC Press: Boca Raton, FL, USA, 2010.
263. Brogan, A.; Hevey, D.; O'Callaghan, G.; Yoder, R.; O'Shea, D. Impaired Decision Making among Morbidly Obese Adults. *J. Psychosom. Res.* **2011**, *70*, 189–196. [CrossRef]
264. Bartholdy, S.; Dalton, B.; O'Daly, O.G.; Campbell, I.C.; Schmidt, U. A Systematic Review of the Relationship between Eating, Weight and Inhibitory Control Using the Stop Signal Task. *Neurosci. Biobehav. Rev.* **2016**, *64*, 35–62. [CrossRef]
265. Hall, P.A.; Lowe, C.; Vincent, C. Executive Control Resources and Snack Food Consumption in the Presence of Restraining versus Facilitating Cues. *J. Behav. Med.* **2014**, *37*, 587–594. [CrossRef]
266. Wu, X.; Nussbaum, M.A.; Madigan, M.L. Executive Function and Measures of Fall Risk Among People with Obesity. *Percept. Mot. Skills* **2016**, *122*, 825–839. [CrossRef]
267. Chase, H.W.; Eickhoff, S.B.; Laird, A.R.; Hogarth, L. The Neural Basis of Drug Stimulus Processing and Craving: An Activation Likelihood Estimation Meta-Analysis. *Biol. Psychiatry* **2011**, *70*, 785–793. [CrossRef] [PubMed]
268. García-García, I.; Horstmann, A.; Jurado, M.A.; Garolera, M.; Chaudhry, S.J.; Margulies, D.S.; Villringer, A.; Neumann, J. Reward Processing in Obesity, Substance Addiction and Non-Substance Addiction. *Obes. Rev.* **2014**, *15*, 853–869. [CrossRef]
269. Barry, D.; Clarke, M.; Petry, N.M. Obesity and Its Relationship to Addictions: Is Overeating a Form of Addictive Behavior? *Am. J. Addict.* **2009**, *18*, 439–451. [CrossRef]

270. Barry, D.; Petry, N.M. Associations between Body Mass Index and Substance Use Disorders Differ by Gender: Results from the National Epidemiologic Survey on Alcohol and Related Conditions. *Addict. Behav.* **2009**, *34*, 51–60. [CrossRef] [PubMed]
271. Sansone, R.A.; Sansone, L.A. Obesity and Substance Misuse: Is There a Relationship? *Innov. Clin. Neurosci.* **2013**, *10*, 30–35.
272. Tanaka, H.; Gourley, D.D.; Dekhtyar, M.; Haley, A.P. Cognition, Brain Structure, and Brain Function in Individuals with Obesity and Related Disorders. *Curr. Obes. Rep.* **2020**, *9*, 544–549. [CrossRef]
273. Karasu, S.R. Psychotherapy-Lite: Obesity and the Role of the Mental Health Practitioner. *Am. J. Psychother.* **2013**, *67*, 3–22. [CrossRef] [PubMed]
274. Brownell, K.D.; Walsh, B.T. *Eating Disorders and Obesity: A Comprehensive Handbook*; Guilford Publications: New York, NY, USA, 2017.
275. Daubenmier, J.; Moran, P.J.; Kristeller, J.; Acree, M.; Bacchetti, P.; Kemeny, M.E.; Dallman, M.; Lustig, R.H.; Grunfeld, C.; Nixon, D.F.; et al. Effects of a Mindfulness-Based Weight Loss Intervention in Adults with Obesity: A Randomized Clinical Trial. *Obesity* **2016**, *24*, 794–804. [CrossRef]
276. Kober, H.; Boswell, R.G. Potential Psychological & Neural Mechanisms in Binge Eating Disorder: Implications for Treatment. *Clin. Psychol. Rev.* **2018**, *60*, 32–44. [CrossRef]
277. Volkow, N.D.; Wise, R.A. How Can Drug Addiction Help Us Understand Obesity? *Nat. Neurosci.* **2005**, *8*, 555–560. [CrossRef] [PubMed]
278. Formolo, D.A.; Gaspar, J.M.; Melo, H.M.; Eichwald, T.; Zepeda, R.J.; Latini, A.; Okun, M.S.; Walz, R. Deep Brain Stimulation for Obesity: A Review and Future Directions. *Front. Neurosci.* **2019**, *13*, 323. [CrossRef]
279. Orrù, G.; Cesari, V.; Malloggi, E.; Conversano, C.; Menicucci, D.; Rotondo, A.; Scarpazza, C.; Marchi, L.; Gemignani, A. The Effects of Transcranial Direct Current Stimulation on Food Craving and Food Intake in Individuals Affected by Obesity and Overweight: A Mini Review of the Magnitude of the Effects. *AIMS Neurosci.* **2022**, *9*, 358–372. [CrossRef] [PubMed]
280. Figlewski, K.; Blicher, J.U.; Mortensen, J.; Severinsen, K.E.; Nielsen, J.F.; Andersen, H. Transcranial Direct Current Stimulation Potentiates Improvements in Functional Ability in Patients with Chronic Stroke Receiving Constraint-Induced Movement Therapy. *Stroke* **2017**, *48*, 229–232. [CrossRef] [PubMed]
281. Gallo, G.; Geda, E.; Codella, R.; Faelli, E.; Panascì, M.; Ranieri, L.E.; Pollastri, L.; Brighenti, S.; Molino, L.; Riba, U.; et al. Effects of Bilateral Dorsolateral Prefrontal Cortex High-Definition Transcranial Direct-Current Stimulation on Physiological and Performance Responses at Severe-Intensity Exercise Domain in Elite Road Cyclists. *Int. J. Sports Physiol. Perform.* **2022**, *17*, 1085–1093. [CrossRef]
282. Gadde, K.M.; Martin, C.K.; Berthoud, H.-R.; Heymsfield, S.B. Obesity: Pathophysiology and Management. *J. Am. Coll. Cardiol.* **2018**, *71*, 69–84. [CrossRef] [PubMed]
283. de Ceglia, M.; Decara, J.; Gaetani, S.; Rodríguez de Fonseca, F. Obesity as a Condition Determined by Food Addiction: Should Brain Endocannabinoid System Alterations Be the Cause and Its Modulation the Solution? *Pharmaceuticals* **2021**, *14*, 1002. [CrossRef]
284. Epstein, L.H.; Salvy, S.J.; Carr, K.A.; Dearing, K.K.; Bickel, W.K. Food Reinforcement, Delay Discounting and Obesity. *Physiol. Behav.* **2010**, *100*, 438–445. [CrossRef]
285. Carr, K.A.; Daniel, T.O.; Lin, H.; Epstein, L.H. Reinforcement Pathology and Obesity. *Curr. Drug Abuse Rev.* **2011**, *4*, 190–196. [CrossRef]
286. Rollins, B.Y.; Dearing, K.K.; Epstein, L.H. Delay Discounting Moderates the Effect of Food Reinforcement on Energy Intake among Non-Obese Women. *Appetite* **2010**, *55*, 420–425. [CrossRef]
287. Carr, K.A.; Lin, H.; Fletcher, K.D.; Epstein, L.H. Food Reinforcement, Dietary Disinhibition and Weight Gain in Nonobese Adults. *Obesity* **2014**, *22*, 254–259. [CrossRef] [PubMed]
288. Clemente-Suárez, V.J. Multidisciplinary intervention in the treatment of mixed anxiety and depression disorder. *Physiol. Behav.* **2020**, *219*, 112858. [CrossRef] [PubMed]
289. Carreira-Míguez, M.; Navarro-Jiménez, E.; Clemente-Suárez, V.J. Behavioral Patterns of Depression Patients and Control Population. *Int. J. Environ. Res. Public Health* **2022**, *19*, 9506. [CrossRef]
290. Clemente-Suárez, V.J.; Bustamante-Sanchez, Á.; Tornero-Aguilera, J.F.; Ruisoto, P.; Mielgo-Ayuso, J. Inflammation in COVID-19 and the effects of non-pharmacological interventions during the pandemic: A review. *Int. J. Mol. Sci.* **2022**, *23*, 15584. [CrossRef] [PubMed]
291. Clemente-Suárez, V.J.; Ramírez-Goerke, M.I.; Redondo-Flórez, L.; Beltrán-Velasco, A.I.; Martín-Rodríguez, A.; Ramos-Campo, D.J.; Navarro-Jiménez, E.; Yáñez-Sepúlveda, R.; Tornero-Aguilera, J.F. The Impact of Anorexia Nervosa and the Basis for Non-Pharmacological Interventions. *Nutrients* **2023**, *15*, 2594. [CrossRef]
292. Clemente-Suárez, V.J.; Beltrán-Velasco, A.I.; Redondo-Flórez, L.; Martín-Rodríguez, A.; Tornero-Aguilera, J.F. Global Impacts of Western Diet and Its Effects on Metabolism and Health: A Narrative Review. *Nutrients* **2023**, *15*, 2749. [CrossRef]
293. Clemente-Suárez, V.J.; Martín-Rodríguez, A.; Redondo-Flórez, L.; López-Mora, C.; Yáñez-Sepúlveda, R.; Tornero-Aguilera, J.F. New Insights and Potential Therapeutic Interventions in Metabolic Diseases. *Int. J. Mol. Sci.* **2023**, *24*, 10672. [CrossRef]
294. Clemente-Suárez, V.J.; Martín-Rodríguez, A.; Redondo-Flórez, L.; Ruisoto, P.; Navarro-Jiménez, E.; Ramos-Campo, D.J.; Tornero-Aguilera, J.F. Metabolic health, mitochondrial fitness, physical activity, and cancer. *Cancers* **2023**, *15*, 814. [CrossRef]
295. Carreira-Míguez, M.; Belinchón-deMiguel, P.P.; Clemente-Suárez, V.J. Behavioural, odontological and physical activity patterns of hypertense and control population. *Physiol. Behav.* **2022**, *252*, 113841. [CrossRef]

296. Bustamante-Sanchez, A.; Villegas-Mora, B.E.; Martínez-Guardado, I.; Tornero-Aguilera, J.F.; Ardigò, L.P.; Nobari, H.; Clemente-Suárez, V.J. Physical activity and nutritional pattern related to maturation and development. *Sustainability* **2022**, *14*, 16958. [CrossRef]
297. Ciccozzi, M.; Lai, A.; Zehender, G.; Borsetti, A.; Cella, E.; Ciotti, M.; Sagnelli, E.; Sagnelli, C.; Angeletti, S. The phylogenetic approach for viral infectious disease evolution and epidemiology: An updating review. *J. Med. Virol.* **2019**, *91*, 1707–1724. [CrossRef] [PubMed]
298. Carreira Míguez, M.; Clemente Suárez, V.J. Physical activity levels affect mental health and behavior in men. *J. Men's Health* **2023**, *1*, 12. [CrossRef]
299. Carreira-Míguez, M.; Ramos-Campo, D.J.; Clemente-Suárez, V.J. Differences in Nutritional and Psychological Habits in Hypertension Patients. *BioMed Res. Int.* **2022**, *2022*, 1920996. [CrossRef]
300. Clemente-Suárez, V.J.; Navarro-Jiménez, E.; Jimenez, M.; Hormeño-Holgado, A.; Martinez-Gonzalez, M.B.; Benitez-Agudelo, J.C.; Perez-Palencia, N.; Laborde-Cárdenas, C.C.; Tornero-Aguilera, J.F. Impact of COVID-19 pandemic in public mental health: An extensive narrative review. *Sustainability* **2021**, *13*, 3221. [CrossRef]
301. Martín-Rodríguez, A.; Tornero-Aguilera, J.F.; López-Pérez, P.J.; Clemente-Suárez, V.J. The effect of loneliness in psychological and behavioral profile among high school students in Spain. *Sustainability* **2021**, *14*, 168. [CrossRef]

nutrients

MDPI

Review

New Perspective on Anorexia Nervosa: Tryptophan-Kynurenine Pathway Hypothesis

Charl Alberts [1], Maja Owe-Larsson [2,3] and Ewa M. Urbanska [4,*]

1 Department of Experimental and Clinical Pharmacology, Medical University of Lublin, Jaczewskiego 8B, 20-059 Lublin, Poland
2 Department of Histology and Embryology, Center of Biostructure Research, Medical University of Warsaw, Chałubińskiego 5, 02-004 Warsaw, Poland
3 Laboratory of Center for Preclinical Research, Department of Experimental and Clinical Physiology, Medical University of Warsaw, Banacha 1B, 02-097 Warsaw, Poland
4 Laboratory of Cellular and Molecular Pharmacology, Department of Experimental and Clinical Pharmacology, Medical University of Lublin, Jaczewskiego 8B, 20-059 Lublin, Poland
* Correspondence: ewa.urbanska@umlub.pl

Abstract: Anorexia nervosa (AN), affecting up to 4% of all females and 0.3% of all males globally, remains the neuropsychiatric disorder with the highest mortality rate. However, the response to the current therapeutic options is rarely satisfactory. Considering the devastating prognosis of survival among patients with AN, further research aimed at developing novel, more effective therapies for AN is essential. Brain and serum tryptophan is mostly converted along the kynurenine pathway into multiple neuroactive derivatives, whereas only 1–2% is used for the synthesis of serotonin. This narrative review provides an update on the experimental and clinical research data concerning the metabolism of tryptophan along the kynurenine pathway in anorexia nervosa based on the available literature. We propose that in AN, lower levels of L-kynurenine and kynurenic acid result in diminished stimulation of the aryl hydrocarbon receptor, which could contribute to abnormally low body weight. The impact of L-kynurenine supplementation on anorexia in animal models and the effects of changes in tryptophan and downstream kynurenines on the clinical progression of AN require further investigation. Moreover, prospective clinical studies on larger cohorts of restrictive and binge-eating/purging AN patients and assessing the potential benefit of L-kynurenine as an add-on therapeutic agent, should follow.

Keywords: anorexia nervosa; L-kynurenine; kynurenic acid; quinolinic acid; aryl hydrocarbon receptor; kynurenine aminotransferase; exercise

1. Introduction

Anorexia nervosa (AN), commonly manifesting with self-starvation, extreme anxiety, hyperactivity, and amenorrhea, remains the psychiatric disorder with the highest mortality rate. It affects up to 4% of all females and 0.3% of all males globally, and recent studies indicate an increasing incidence in younger people aged <15 years [1,2]. A recent review analyzing the data from 2013 to 2022 demonstrates that 5.5–17.9% of young women and 0.6–2.4% of young men have experienced a DSM-5 eating disorder by early adulthood. Lifetime DSM-5 anorexia nervosa was reported by 0.8–6.3% of women and 0.1–0.3% of men, with gender and sexual minorities at particularly high risk. Emerging studies from Eastern Europe, Asia, and Latin America show a similarly high prevalence. During the COVID-19 pandemic, the incidence of eating disorders increased [2]. A large meta-analysis of 42 anorexia-related mortality studies (with follow-up periods from 1.7 to 33 years and a total of 3006 subjects) revealed a crude death rate in AN of 5.9%, with an aggregate mortality rate of 5.6% per decade. Suicide rates were 200-fold more likely among patients with AN than in the general population [3]. The majority of AN outpatients are readmitted five or more years after presentation [4]. Some 20-year follow-up studies revealed that full recovery was achieved in 27.5–50.6% of patients and that 15.6–17.5% had died from causes related to the disease [5,6].

AN is a disorder with a very complex etiology, including congenital and environmental factors. Patients typically present with major depressive disorder or generalized anxiety disorder, among others, as psychiatric comorbidities [7]. Behavioral dysfunction includes pathological reward and eating habits, impaired appetite, altered impulse control, neuroticism, anxiety, and lowered mood. Low body mass is achieved with pathological dieting, purging, binge eating, or excessive physical exercise. Accordingly, AN is categorized into two major subtypes: restrictive and binge-eating/purging [8,9]. In the brain, profound changes in the connectivity and neurotransmission within the dopaminergic and serotoninergic systems are frequently observed [7]. Morphological assessments indicate brain atrophy involving gray and white matter volume reductions [10,11]. However, the findings are inconsistent, as the location and extent of changes are highly variable. Following the body weight restoration, brain volume reductions may be reversible, and it is unclear whether long-term morphological complications persist in severe AN [12,13].

The disturbed function of the serotoninergic system in the etiology of AN is substantiated by a number of experimental and clinical data. However, the results are conflicting, and it is uncertain whether the changes are of a causative or symptomatic nature [14]. Serotonin is synthesized in the brain and periphery from tryptophan (TRP), yet only a minor part of the TRP pool enters this metabolic pathway. TRP depletion stimulated by stress and inflammation lowers peripheral and central serotonin levels [15], and a majority of research in AN focuses on this aspect of TRP metabolism. It was suggested that there is a correlation between pathological behavioral traits, such as anxiety, obsessions, or harm avoidance, and serotonin. Thus, starvation may be used by patients with AN to decrease dysphoria. On the other hand, the deficient serotoninergic transmission may result in a depressive mood and further aggravate the course of the disease [16].

Noteworthy, a majority of serum TRP is converted along the kynurenine pathway (KP) into multiple neuroactive derivatives termed collectively as kynurenines. Accumulated evidence clearly indicates the importance of bilateral interactions between TRP metabolism along the KP and inflammatory pathways [17]. Furthermore, the majority of brain kynurenines are generated within glial cells, and there is increasing evidence of the role of glial cells in the pathophysiology of eating disorders, including anorexia nervosa [18]. Yet, the potential contribution of disturbed TRP metabolism along the KP to the development of AN is poorly understood. Thus, we aimed to review the available data on TRP and its metabolism along the KP in AN. We searched articles published in English that appeared in Medline/Pubmed using key terms relating to anorexia nervosa, the metabolites of TRP along the KP, and the pathway enzymes. The accumulated evidence is scarce, yet it supports the notion that AN is an illness in which the deficiency of dietary TRP lessens not only the synthesis of serotonin but also hampers kynurenine synthesis. This, in turn, may further contribute to troubled emotions and disturbed eating behaviors. We highlight the possible association between glia, inflammation, and kynurenines in AN. The KP emerges as an important link integrating environmental and inflammation-related changes with the clinical course of AN.

2. The Kynurenine Pathway

In humans, TRP supplied with food is incorporated into structural and enzymatic proteins, serves as a source of serotonin and melatonin, or is converted along the kynurenine pathway (KP) into a number of bioactive molecules [19–21] (Figure 1).

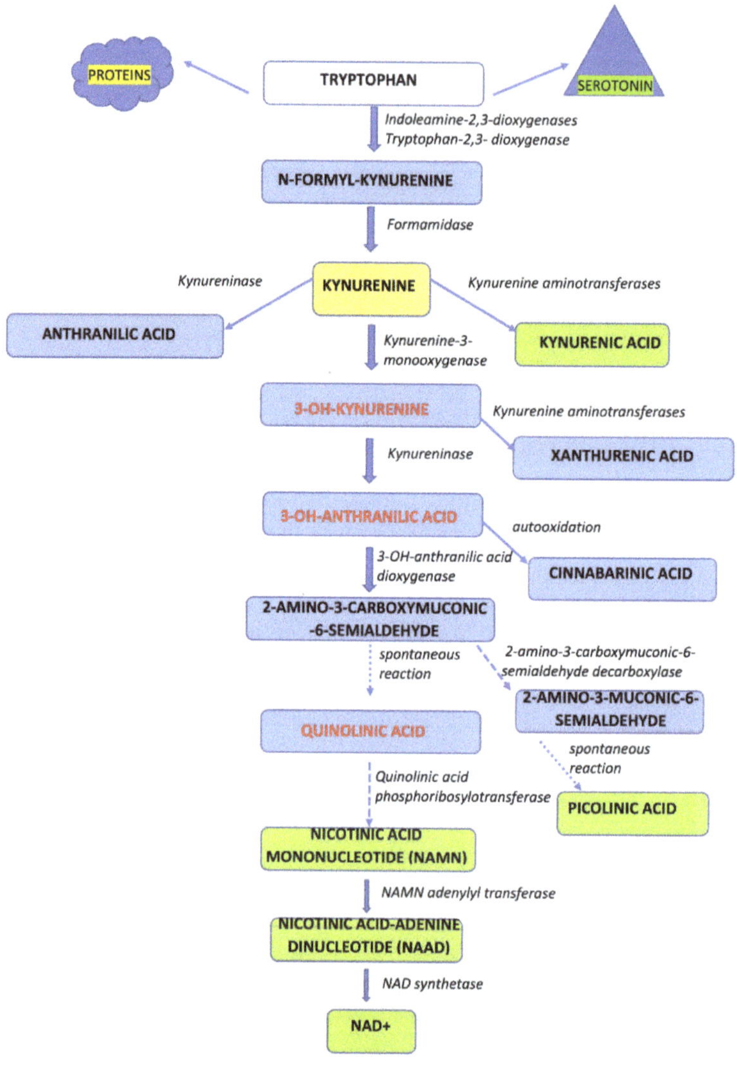

Figure 1. The scheme of tryptophan metabolism along the kynurenine pathway (KP). The majority of available serum tryptophan enters the KP. IDOs or TDO convert tryptophan into L-kynurenine, which is further catabolized by kynurenine aminotransferases to kynurenic acid, kynurenine-3-monooxygenase to 3-OH-L-kynurenine, or kynureninase to anthranilic acid. Kynurenine aminotransferases may convert 3-OH-L-kynurenine to xanthurenic acid or kynureninase to form 3-OH-anthranilic acid. Further, 3-OH-anthranilic acid is converted into quinolinic or picolinic acid by a series of enzymatic conversions.

Approximately 95% of serum TRP enters the KP, whereas only a minor proportion of this amino acid yields serotonin and other products. The first step of the pathway is catabolized by tryptophan 2,3-dioxygenase (TDO) or indoleamine 2,3-dioxygenases (IDO1 and IDO2), forming N-formylkynurenine, which is subsequently converted into L-kynurenine [19–21]. TDO, expressed mostly in hepatocytes, is strongly upregulated by tryptophan itself and glucocorticoids [22]. IDO-1 expression was detected in microglia, neurons, and astrocytes, as well as in macrophages, epithelial cells, and fibroblasts. During inflammation, either overt or low-grade, released cytokines such as interleukin-1 (IL-1), IL-6, interferon-γ (IFN-γ), or tumor necrosis factor-α (TNF-α) and they act as molecular signals activating IDO via pathways involving a signal transducer and an activator of transcription (STAT)-1, IFN-regulatory factor-1, p38 mitogen-activated protein kinase (MAPK), and NF-κB [23–25]. However, due to rather low activities of IDOs and TDO in the brain, a substantial amount of the central pool of L-kynurenine originates from peripheral sources (60–70%), whereas the remaining 30–40% is produced in situ [26]. An increase in L-kynurenine local biosynthesis has been observed in neuroinflammation and is presumed to occur partly due to the immune stimulation of IDO [17,25]. Inflammation has been linked to altered eating habits under pathological conditions, with cytokines such as, e.g., IFN-γ modulate food intake regulation and wasting [27,28].

L-kynurenine is further catabolized into various metabolites displaying numerous and often opposing biological properties. Kynurenines were shown to exert pro- and anti-inflammatory effects, to either cause cytotoxicity or prevent it, or to act as free radical scavengers or a source of free radicals. Considering its central position in the KP, L-kynurenine serves as a switch point, directing the metabolic fate of TRP in three directions.

The first route of L-kynurenine metabolism, considered neuroprotective, is catalyzed by four distinct aminotransferases (KATs I-IV), generating kynurenic acid (KYNA). KAT I [glutamine transaminase K (GTK)/cysteine conjugate beta-lyase (CCBL) 1], KAT II [aminoadipate aminotransferase (AADAT)], KAT III (CCBL2), and KAT IV [glutamic-oxaloacetic transaminase (GOT) 2/mitochondrial aspartate aminotransferase (mASPAT)] were detected in rodent and human brains [29]. Due to its polar structure, KYNA does not easily cross the blood–brain barrier. In contrast, TRP and L-kynurenine are actively transported from the periphery into the brain via the large neutral amino acid (LNAA) transport system [26]. Furthermore, diverse substrate profiles, dissimilar optimal pH ranges, and various region-specific activities are characteristic for KATs. Overall, the local regulation of KYNA synthesis seems finely tuned and precisely controlled [21].

The second route yields 3-OH-kynurenine through the activity of kynurenine 3-monooxygenase (KMO). Indirectly, the activity of KMO, which displays a much lower K_m value for L-kynurenine, also impacts the synthesis of KYNA. 3-OH-kynurenine is further metabolized to quinolinic acid (QUIN) through initial conversion by kynureninase into 3-hydroxyanthranilic acid (3-HAA) and subsequent breakdown into unstable ACMS by 3-hydroxyanthranilic acid oxygenase [20,21]. QUIN is a source of nicotinamide adenine dinucleotide$^+$ (NAD^+), which is essential in cellular metabolism. The third possible route of L-kynurenine metabolism results from kynureninase-mediated conversion, which yields anthranilic acid, which may further generate 3-hyroxyanthranilic acid. Enzymatic conversion by KATs can occur for 3-OH-kynurenine into xanthurenic acid [30].

Experimental data from in vitro and in vivo studies clearly demonstrated the neuroprotective properties of KYNA and the neurotoxic effects of such derivatives as 3-OH-kynurenine or QUIN. Furthermore, a number of generated kynurenines also manifest potent immunomodulatory properties [17]. L-kynurenine, KYNA, and xanthurenic acid act as ligands of the aryl hydrocarbon receptor (AhR), known to play an essential role in limiting immune response and the induction of immune tolerance, partly through the conversion of naive T cells to the anti-inflammatory Treg phenotype [17,31,32].

KYNA is considered a unique TRP metabolite due to its pleiotropic effects [21,33]. This compound was initially identified as an endogenous nonselective antagonist of all 3 ionotropic excitatory amino acid receptors: N-methyl-D-aspartate (NMDA), α-amino-3-hydroxy-5-methyl-4-isoxazole propionic acid ((R,S)-AMPA), and kainate type. KYNA displays the highest affinity for the strychnine-insensitive glycine site of the NMDA receptor [21]. Furthermore, KYNA, apart from being an agonist of AhR, is also an agonist of the orphan receptor GP35 and an antagonist of α-7 nicotinic cholinergic receptors, although data concerning the latter effect are unclear [21,33,34]. Moreover, KYNA plays a role as a direct reactive oxygen species (ROS) scavenger [21,33].

Another product of the KP, QUIN, is a potent agonist of excitatory amino acid receptors of the NMDA type. It is produced in the brain mostly by microglia and macrophages [35]. QUIN is well known to cause neuronal cell death through excitotoxic processes. Furthermore, it may increase free radical production by inducing NOS activity in astrocytes and neurons, inhibit succinate dehydrogenase, thus impairing the mitochondrial respiratory chain, or induce cytoskeletal disruption [35]. Thus, increased availability of L-kynurenine may result in two opposite scenarios: neuroprotective and neurotoxic. Cellular protection would be linked mostly to the higher availability of KYNA. KYNA would be produced at the expense of the other two routes, and an increase in the KYNA/3-OH-kynurenine and KYNA/QUIN ratios would follow.

The hypothesis linking neuroinflammation with increased metabolism of TRP along the KP and its shift towards neurotoxic kynurenines is well substantiated [17,36,37]. An increasing number of data suggest that an elevated expression of pro-inflammatory cytokines, such as TNFα, IFNγ, IL-1, and IL-6, may favor catabolic reactions and cachexia. IL-1, IFNγ, and TNFα were shown to affect the hypothalamic neurons implicated in the regulation of eating behavior and appetite [38]. It is unclear whether the disturbed cytokine profile detected in patients with AN results from impaired nutrition, psychopathological, and neuroendocrine factors or inherited genetic disturbances [38]. In most of the prospective studies, initially altered cytokine serum levels returned to normal values after re-nutrition [38], thus suggesting their temporary nature. However, the sequel of changes linking altered immune responses with pathological eating behaviors is still unclear. We suggest that in AN, the environment promoting neuronal damage and oxidative stress, resulting in sustained neuroinflammation, may cause mood disturbances and dysfunction of hypothalamic anorexigenic pathways, in part through the alterations in kynurenine synthesis and function.

3. Tryptophan and Kynurenines in Anorexia Nervosa

In the following sections, we present the available data on TRP and its metabolites along the KP in AN (Table 1).

Table 1. Tryptophan, kynurenines, and the kynurenine pathway enzymes in experimental and clinical studies on anorexia nervosa.

Metabolites/Enzymes	Conditions	Type of Samples	Results	Reference Number
Tryptophan	Four-day starvation in rats	Brain	↓	[39,40]
	Four-week starvation in rats	Plasma	↓	[41]
		Brain (hypothalamus)	↓	[41]
	Caenorhabditis elegans, in culture, 2 h fasting	Extracts from *C. elegans*	←→	[42]
	AN (n = 35)	Plasma	←→	[43]
	AN (n = 16)	Blood	←→	[44]
	Anorectic, dialyzed (n = 13)	Plasma	←→	[45]
	AN (n = 26)	Plasma	↓	[46]
	Acute AN (n = 32), Recovered AN (n = 32)	Plasma	↓	[47]
	AN (n = 42)	Plasma	↓	[48]
	AN (n = 19)	Whole blood	↓	[49]
	AN (n = 16)	Serum	↓	[50]
	Acute AN (n = 14), Recovered AN (n = 14)	Plasma	↓ acute AN vs. recovered ←→ vs. CTR	[51]

Table 1. *Cont.*

Metabolites/Enzymes	Conditions	Type of Samples	Results	Reference Number
	Medication-free AN (*n* = 10)	CSF	←→	[52]
	Restrictive AN (*n* = 20)	Serum	←→	[53]
	Purging AN (*n* = 21)	Serum	↑	[54]
Tryptophan/LNAA ratio	AN (*n* = 16)	Blood	↑ in more severe catabolic status	[44]
	Anorectic, dialyzed (*n* = 13)	Plasma	←→	[45]
	AN (*n* = 19)	Whole blood	↓	[49]
	Acute AN (*n* = 14), Recovered AN (*n* = 14)	Plasma	↑	[51]
	AN (*n* = 42)	Plasma	↓	[48]
L-kynurenine	*Caenorhabditis elegans*, in culture, 2 h fasting	Extracts from *C. elegans*	↓	[42]
	Medication-free AN (*n* = 10)	CSF	←→	[52]
	Restrictive AN (*n* = 20)	Serum	←→	[53]
	Restrictive AN (*n* = 45), purging AN (*n* = 21)	Serum	←→	[54]
3-OH-kynurenine	*Caenorhabditis elegans*, in culture, 2 h fasting	Extracts from *C. elegans*	↓	[42]
	Restrictive AN (*n* = 20)	Serum	←→	[53]
Kynurenic acid	Medication-free AN (*n* = 10)	CSF	↓	[52]
	Restrictive AN (*n* = 20)	Serum	←→	[53]
Quinolinic acid	Medication-free AN (*n* = 10)	CSF	←→	[52]
KAT1 gene expression	Restrictive AN (*n* = 20)	Serum	←→	[53]
KAT2 gene expression	Restrictive AN (*n* = 20)	Serum	←→	[53]
KAT3 gene expression	C57BL/6 mice, activity-based anorexia	Muscles	↑	[55]
	Restrictive AN (*n* = 20)	Serum	↑	[53]
KAT4 gene expression	C57BL/6 mice, activity-based anorexia	Muscles	↑	[55]

↓—decrease; ↑—increase; and ←→—no change. AN—anorexia nervosa; CSF—cerebrospinal fluid; CTR—control; KAT—kynurenine aminotransferase; and LNAA—large neutral amino acids.

3.1. *Tryptophan*

The role of TRP in the control of food intake and its correlation with brain serotonin was the subject of several studies in experimental animals [56]. In animals receiving protein-poor but rich in carbohydrate foods or injected with insulin, plasma and brain TRP levels increased with a subsequent transient rise in serotonin levels [57]. However, when even larger elevations of plasma TRP are generated by the ingestion of protein-containing diets, no changes in the brain levels of TRP and serotonin occur [58]. The plasma amino acid pattern modulates the uptake of TRP into the brain through competition with other LNAA for their transporter. Paradoxically, an increase in brain TRP is evoked by dietary carbohydrates, whereas protein-rich foods containing TRP fail to do so. Most probably, insulin markedly lowers the plasma level of LNAA, which allows more TRP to enter the brain. Dietary proteins raise plasma TRP levels, but due to the rather low content of TRP, this rise is small in comparison with that of more abundant amino acids, such as leucine, isoleucine, and valine, which compete for the LNAA transporter [59].

Following an acute IL-1 injection in rats, food intake significantly declined, which was paralleled by a decrease in plasma-free TRP and an increase in plasma LNAA. In contrast, IL-1 significantly increased the concentration of TRP in rodents' CSF [60]. Similarly, after peripheral or intra-hypothalamic administration of cytokines, feeding behavior is hindered via a mechanism linked with an enhanced expression and release of leptin [61,62].

The above changes are characteristic only of short-lasting changes in eating patterns and seem to serve as a protective mechanism, allowing the individual to maintain relatively undisturbed serotoninergic neurotransmission. During extended starvation, an actual decline in the brain's TRP and serotonin levels is frequently observed. A study comparing rats subjected to either a 4-day restricted diet or a 4-day restricted diet and subsequent feeding for 2 days revealed that starvation lowers brain TRP levels [39,40]. The same group reported that prolonged starvation results in disparate effects concerning TRP levels in male and female rats. Restricted feeding decreased plasma TRP concentration in starved and starved/re-fed females and starved males. Hypothalamic TRP levels were lower in starved and starved/re-fed female rats and starved/re-fed males. Serotonin decreased in both starved and starved/re-fed male and female rats. Food restriction decreased serotonin levels in other brain areas of male but not female rats [41].

Clinical evidence mostly demonstrates the deficiency of TRP and LNAA in the blood of AN patients. Therefore, it is generally assumed that during either evident AN or restored nutrition, the TRP level merely represents nutritional status in anorectics. However, the results of the clinical studies are puzzling because both normal and reduced levels of TRP were detected. Considering that TRP and LNAA compete for the transporter that shifts amino acids across the blood–brain barrier, the peripheral TRP/LNAA ratio can indicate the quantities of TRP that enter the brain [63]. Thus, it is often measured as a peripheral parameter reflecting the status of brain TRP availability. However, the results are also perplexing, as normal, lower, or higher TRP/LNAA ratios were found in AN.

In a group of 35 patients with AN, plasma TRP levels did not differ from controls [43]. Similarly, the study in 16 anorectic patients revealed that blood TRP and LNAA levels were within normal ranges. There was no correlation between the TRP/LNAA ratios and the Hopkins Symptom Checklist (HSCL) and Eating Disorders Inventory (EDI). However, the TRP/LNAA ratio seemed to be higher in patients exercising excessively, with a more severe catabolic status. The ratio was inversely correlated with the body mass index, body fat, muscle mass, daily energy intake, and daily TRP intake. Thus, it was suggested that the TRP/LNAA ratio is not controlled only by the diet but is associated with the status of catabolism [44]. Likewise, a cross-sectional study including 59 dialyzed patients, of which 13 manifested poor appetite and malnutrition, revealed that the plasma levels of free TRP, LNAA, and TRP/LNAA ratios were similar between anorectic and well-nourished patients [45]. Similarly, a study of 20 female patients with restrictive AN revealed no changes in serum TRP compared to 24 control individuals [53].

In contrast, others showed a decrease in TRP levels in the blood of anorectic patients. A study of 26 female AN patients and 15 control subjects revealed that plasma TRP is significantly lower in low-weight patients [46]. Data from 19 anorectic patients, 10 of whom presented with associated bulimic features, demonstrated lower TRP or TRP/LNAA ratios as opposed to 12 healthy controls [46]. Similarly, a study comprising 32 patients who recovered from severe AN, 32 acutely underweight patients with AN, and 32 healthy individuals showed significantly lower plasma levels of TRP among anorectics [47]. Serum levels of TRP in 16 patients with AN were significantly lower than in control groups [50]. A study of 34 patients with acute AN, 19 weight-recovered patients, and 35 healthy control women revealed lower plasma TRP and detected a positive correlation between TRP and S100B, a small calcium-binding protein [64].

During the recovery period, plasma TRP usually increases in AN. A study of 14 women with symptomatic AN, 14 women who recovered from AN, and 15 healthy control individuals revealed that both groups of anorectic women had significantly higher mean baseline TRP/LNAA ratios compared with the control [51]. In a cohort of 26 female patients with

AN and 15 control subjects, plasma TRP, LNAA, and the TRP/LNAA ratio increased significantly during refeeding [46]. Similarly, in 42 anorectic patients, the levels of serotonin, TRP, LNAA, and the TRP/LNAA ratio were considerably lower than in the control, both at admission and after refeeding. During the refeeding, the levels of measured metabolites increased significantly in comparison with admission but did not reach control values [48].

No difference in the CSF TRP level was found between 33 anorexic and 14 healthy women [65]. Similarly, a study analyzing the levels of kynurenines in the CSF samples obtained from 10 medication-free female patients with AN, 22 normal-weight bulimia nervosa patients, and 8 healthy females revealed that the level of TRP was not altered in the AN group [52]. The TRP level was negatively associated with the body mass index (BMI) in AN [52].

3.2. L-Kynurenine and Kynurenic Acid

Experimental data support the notion that kynurenines may modify feeding behavior. A number of studies were performed on animal models of anorexia. One of the models employs the administration of polyinosino:polycytidylic acid (Poly I:C) viral mimic that is a synthetic double-stranded RNA. It is a strong inducer of an immune response that produces profound anorexia in mice [66,67]. Poly I:C-treated mice maintain muscle strength and motor coordination, along with the ability to climb and rear; however, they manifest weight loss, which seems to result from a decreased drive to eat [66,68]. It was demonstrated that Poly I:C evokes a potent rise in L-kynurenine levels and an increase in the L-kynurenine/TRP ratio [66]. Thus, activation of the KP seems to be linked with anorectic behavior. Metabolomic analysis of 391 metabolites during hunger and satiety in *Drosophila melanogaster* revealed that, in response to eating, metabolic profiles change in a distinct way. L-kynurenine depletion was detected in the heads of flies on a high-sugar diet, supporting the view that the L-kynurenine level is correlated with the brain energy state and feeding behavior [69]. These observations suggest that higher L-kynurenine levels may contribute to decreased food intake, whereas lower L-kynurenine is associated with feeding. However, it cannot be excluded that the observed changes are not the cause but the result of a disturbed eating pattern.

In fact, others reported that in *Caenorhabditis elegans* displaying food-related behavioral plasticity, fasting depletes L-kynurenine and KYNA levels but not TRP levels [42]. In *C. elegans*, NKAT-1 and NKAT-3 are homologous to mammalian KATs. In *nkat-1* mutants, depletion of KYNA during fasting was shown to be a regulatory factor needed for the hyperactivation of feeding in *C. elegans* when they re-encounter food. KYNA depletion leads to reduced stimulation of NMDA receptors on neurons that communicate with serotonergic sensory neurons. Upon refeeding, KYNA levels are eventually replenished, ending the elevated feeding period. These data suggest the role of KYNA as a measure conveying the peripheral metabolic state that controls serotonin signaling in *C. elegans* [42]. A similar mechanism may also exist in humans and participate in the regulation of food intake during anorectic conditions.

So far, only three clinical studies have evaluated the downstream metabolites of TRP along the KP in AN. A study of 10 medication-free female patients with AN revealed reduced CSF levels of KYNA but not of kynurenine among underweight anorectic patients as opposed to normal-weight females. KYNA deficiency normalized as the body weight increased [52]. A quarter of a century later, the peripheral levels of kynurenines were investigated in 20 female patients with restrictive AN (mostly drug-free, all during the first episode of the disease) and compared with 24 controls [53]. We detected neither changes in serum L-kynurenine, KYNA, nor in the ratios TRP/L-kynurenine or L-kynurenine/KYNA. Thus, our investigation did not confirm the presence of KP changes in peripheral blood among AN patients, in contrast, to study in CSF [52]. However, their studies were performed in CSF samples, reflecting the condition of the TRP metabolism along the KP in the brain tissue. Very recently, DNA methylation profiles at promoter-associated CpG sites of the *SCL6A4* gene, encoding for the serotonin transporter (SERT), and the serum

KYN/TRP ratio were studied in a cohort of eating disorders patients, including 45 patients with restrictive AN, 21 with purging AN, 21 with bulimia (BN), 31 with binge eating disorders, 23 with unspecified feeding or eating disorders, 14 with other specified eating disorders, and 34 healthy controls. Anorectic and bulimic patients did not manifest changes in L-kynurenine levels compared to controls. There was a small but significant increase in the TRP level among purging AN, as well as a small decrease in the L-kynurenine/TRP ratio [54]. Excessive physical activity in both groups of patients with AN resulted in a lower L-kynurenine level and higher TRP compared to non-exercising patients [54].

3.3. *3-Hydroxykynurenine and Quinolinic Acid*

Neither 3-OH-kynurenine levels nor L-kynurenine/3-OH-kynurenine and KYNA/3-OH-kynurenine ratios were altered in the serum of 20 females with restrictive AN [53]. In 10 medication-free female patients with AN, CSF QUIN levels were within the control range, yet the ratio QUIN/KYNA was significantly higher during the underweight phase of AN [52]. Furthermore, a correlation between urinary cortisol excretion and the QUIN/KYNA ratio in CSF was observed. Considering that hypercortisolism can induce TDO activity and increase systemic production of kynurenines [70], this mechanism could be responsible for enhanced conversion of TRP towards QUIN. On the other hand, the effects of glucocorticoids on QUIN levels are not straightforward, as both a decrease or no change in QUIN levels were observed after glucocorticoid administration [71,72]. In contrast, it is well documented that immune stimulation and stress may increase the conversion of TRP along the branch of the KP leading to QUIN, with distinct effects in various structures of the brain [73,74]. Possibly, QUIN levels are strongly increased due to genetic errors prior to the overt development of AN. Then, during the fully active phase of AN, the attenuating effects of hypercortisolism could lower the QUIN level. However, considering the concomitant decrease of KYNA, the ratio QUIN/KYNA would still be higher, as observed [52].

3.4. *Enzymes of the Kynurenine Pathway*

The results of Demitrack and co-workers indicated impaired KYNA generation in the CSF of AN patients with a concurrent lack of changes in the concentration of its direct bioprecursor, L-kynurenine [52]. Thus, it was suggested that KYNA deficiency occurred due to altered activity of biosynthetic enzymes, KATs [52]. The probable decline in KATs activity could result from deficient nutrition, including an inappropriate supply of enzymatic cofactors, such as vitamin B6 (pyridoxal 5′-phosphate) and pyruvate [52]. However, the authors did not measure the actual activity of KAT enzymes.

The expression of mRNA for *KAT1–3* was studied in 20 female patients with restrictive AN and in 24 controls [53]. The expression of the gene encoding *KAT3*, but not of the genes encoding *KAT1* and *KAT2*, was higher in 20 patients with restrictive AN. KYNA is produced mainly within astrocytes, primarily by KAT2 [75]. Interestingly, in animal models of AN, the density of astrocytic cells, as well as the expression of glial fibrillary acidic protein (GFAP), glutamate transporters (GLT-1 and GLAST), and glutamine synthetase, are reduced [18,76]. It was recently suggested that glial function is compromised by anorexia [77]. Therefore, it seems probable that dysfunctional glial cells produce lower quantities of KYNA. Lower KYNA levels in CSF would reflect region-specific and restricted to changes in TRP metabolism in the brain among AN patients. The peripheral metabolism of TRP may be affected differently and influenced by various factors able to restore/maintain KYNA levels within normal values.

Noteworthy, in C57BL/6 mice during activity-based anorexia, an additional physical exercise during the refeeding period resulted in an increased expression of muscle *KAT3* and *KAT4* mRNA levels, in contrast to re-fed mice without access to a running wheel [55]. Moreover, KYNA synthesis from L-kynurenine in muscle tissue was stimulated during the recovery from a malnourished state, but only in physically active animals [55]. Physical exercise was shown to stimulate the expression of muscle *KAT1*, *3*, and *4* in humans [78].

Similarly, a significantly higher expression of the *KAT3* gene was found in a cohort of patients with restrictive AN who exercised excessively prior to their admission [53]. Thus, it is very likely that the observed increase in *KAT3* expression is a consequence of patients' intense physical activity, which in turn may reverse the initial deficit of KYNA synthesis.

4. Dietary Interventions

The administration of TRP was evaluated as a means to affect the processes regulating food intake. A study in animals, either stress-free or subjected to short-duration immobilization stress, showed that TRP (300 mg/kg, orally) increased peripheral levels of serotonin and leptin while decreasing ghrelin levels in rats not exposed to stress [79]. There were no changes in 24-h cumulative food intake and elevated plus maze performance. In contrast, animals subjected to 2-h of stress manifested a decreased 24-h food intake, increased anxiety, lower serum serotonin, and increased leptin. TRP pre-treatment prevented the occurrence of behavioral and biochemical alterations [79]. Others have shown that subcutaneous application of TRP (100 mg/kg, for 2 days) increased both free and total TRP but did not change food intake, body weight, carcass adiposity, or leptin levels. Plasma-free TRP, but not total TRP, was significantly negatively correlated with food intake [80].

Intraperitoneal TRP administration after food deprivation evokes a hypothalamic serotonin increase, similar to exposure to the smell of food, eating a meal, or application of d-fenfluramine, as shown by a microdialysis study in rats. These data imply that TRP, among other factors, can be used to preferentially modify hypothalamic serotonin [81].

The beneficial effects of TRP were also shown in a rat model of immobilization stress-induced anorexia. TRP administration attenuated the impairment of food intake and ameliorated depressive symptoms [40]. Interestingly, TRP-fed animals did not manifest increased brain TRP, possibly due to a prominent peripheral metabolism. Alternatively, it can be assumed that as stress increases TRP hydroxylase activity, even a minor rise in brain TRP leads to its immediate conversion into serotonin and 5-hydroxyindoleacetic acid. Chronic intraperitoneal TRP administration attenuated the hyperactivity associated with a 38-day starvation in rats [82]. TRP treatment in starving rats normalized the declining levels of dopamine, serotonin, and their metabolites in the striatum [82].

The impact of TRP on eating habits in healthy and anorectic patients has been the subject of some studies. A high dose of TRP given to healthy individuals decreased the total caloric, carbohydrate, and protein intakes, whereas a smaller dose of TRP increased caloric and protein intakes but decreased carbohydrate intake [83]. Similarly, TRP administration to healthy volunteers in a high-protein serving was shown to decrease the intake of carbohydrates during the following free-choice meal [84]. A clinical randomized controlled trial in 29 healthy subjects allocated to a high- (n = 14) or low-protein diet (n = 15) for 2 weeks has shown a decreased plasma KYNA, but not TRP or L-kynurenine, on a low-protein diet. Plasma QUIN levels were below the detection limit. In urine, the levels of KYNA and QUIN, but not of L-kynurenine, were reduced on a low-protein diet. Surprisingly, metabolite changes were markedly different between human subjects and mice. The authors also conducted research on 20 wild-type FVB mice who were randomly assigned a high-protein or control diet for 21 days. In contrast to humans, a high-protein diet resulted in lower TRP and L-kynurenine levels than in controls. However, the authors did not assess the effect of a low-protein diet in experimental animals. Thus, it is rather difficult to draw a clear conclusion [85].

Another study investigated 22 healthy subjects (11 males and 11 females, aged 25.9 $\pm$ 4.2 years), and a total of 92 biomarkers were measured before a standardized meal as well as 30 and 120 min afterward. The only studied marker relevant to the KP was kynureninase. No changes were detected in its protein level, but a correlation with BMI was found [86]. The co-administration of a nutritional supplement containing 2,3 g of TRP with fluoxetine (5–26 weeks) was studied in a double-blind, placebo-controlled manner in a group of 26 subjects with AN. No effect of supplementation on weight gain, anxiety, or obsessive-compulsive symptoms in AN was observed [87].

As shown in a cohort of 42 individuals with AN, an increase in the TRP/LNAA ratio during refeeding correlated with a decrease in depressive symptoms [48]. On the other hand, increased anxiety was frequently linked with higher TRP levels. Intravenous TRP blunted growth hormone secretion and augmented the anxiety levels in AN [88]. Consequently, several studies have aimed at assessing the potential anxiolytic effects of TRP depletion. However, the results concerning the status of behavioral and biochemical parameters after TRP depletion in various neuropsychiatric conditions, such as depression, bulimia nervosa, autism, aggression, and substance dependence, are inconsistent [89].

In terms of AN, the data on TRP depletion are rather limited. The study performed on 14 women with symptomatic AN and 14 women who recovered from AN demonstrated that TRP depletion leads to a significantly greater reduction in the TRP/LNAA among anorectics. Patients from both AN groups also experienced a significant reduction in anxiety on the TRP depletion day compared with the placebo [51]. Acute TRP depletion in AN increased resting-state functional connectivity in patients recovered from AN (n= 22) in a similar manner to control individuals (n = 22) [90]. The same group reported that, despite the reduction of TRP/LNAA ratio, there was no difference in anxiety and mood between recovered AN (n = 22) and healthy controls (n = 25) exposed to TRP depletion [91]. Finally, based on functional magnetic resonance imaging, acute TRP depletion was shown to normalize the reward-related neural responses in recovered AN (n = 22) compared to controls (n = 25) [92].

Thus, the possibility of using TRP as a supplementary therapy in AN remains open and requires further detailed studies.

5. Concluding Remarks and Future Directions

Experimental and clinical research data indicate that TRP metabolism along the KP is disturbed in anorexia. However, the available research is limited, and the results are not clear-cut. Furthermore, the data originate mostly from studies in the peripheral compartment, and the analyses in the brain or CSF of patients with AN are scarce.

The available data concerning the effects of TRP loading or depletion seem to support the hypotheses that, among individuals predisposed toward or recovered from AN and manifesting excessive serotoninergic transmission, the restricted TRP supply, through a reduction in serotonin availability, may alleviate dysphoric moods.

Furthermore, careful interpretation of the evidence suggests that the central deficit of L-kynurenine supply as well as an impaired astrocytic production of KYNA are associated with AN. L-kynurenine and KYNA are both agonists of AHR. In experimental animals fed a Western diet, the AHR may disrupt fat metabolism and contribute to obesity [93,94]. Mice deficient in IDO1, an enzyme that metabolizes TRP, were resistant to obesity. At physiological levels, L-kynurenine was shown to activate AHR-directed luciferase expression. As enhanced IDO1 activity may increase L-kynurenine levels, this might activate the AHR and cause weight gain. In contrast, a deficiency of L-kynurenine and insufficient stimulation of the AHR may lead to weight loss [93,94]. Indeed, AHR-knockout mice tend to exhibit extreme physiologic abnormalities, including a reduction in body weight [32]. We propose that among AN patients manifesting lower levels of L-kynurenine and KYNA, the stimulation of AHR is impaired, which could contribute to the abnormally low body weight.

In conclusion, there is a great need for basic science research assessing enzymes and metabolites of the KP, including their temporal pattern, in the ontogeny of AN. The impact of changed TRP and L-kynurenine levels on anorexia and the effects of alterations in other downstream kynurenines on the clinical progression of AN require further investigation. Furthermore, prospective clinical studies on larger cohorts of restrictive and binge-eating/purging AN patients, assessing the potential benefit of modulation of TRP and L-kynurenine levels as add-on therapy, should follow. Finally, detailed studies on the links between excessive physical activity and higher expression of KAT3 are needed. Considering the devastating prognosis for survival among patients with AN, further research aimed at developing novel, more effective therapies for AN is essential.

Author Contributions: Conceptualization, C.A., and E.M.U.; writing—original draft preparation, C.A., M.O.-L.; writing—review and editing, E.M.U.; funding acquisition, E.M.U. All authors have read and agreed to the published version of the manuscript.

Funding: This research was financed by statutory grants from the Medical University in Lublin (DS. 450/22, 450/23) to E.M.U.

Data Availability Statement: No new data were created.

Conflicts of Interest: The authors declare that they do not have any conflicts of interest.

References

1. van Eeden, A.E.; van Hoeken, D.; Hoek, H.W. Incidence, prevalence and mortality of anorexia nervosa and bulimia nervosa. *Curr. Opin. Psychiatry* **2021**, *34*, 515–524. [CrossRef] [PubMed]
2. Silén, Y.; Keski-Rahkonen, A. Worldwide prevalence of DSM-5 eating disorders among young people. *Curr. Opin. Psychiatry* **2022**, *35*, 362–371. [CrossRef] [PubMed]
3. Sullivan, P.F. Mortality in anorexia nervosa. *Am. J. Psychiatry* **1995**, *152*, 1073–1074. [CrossRef]
4. Keel, P.K.; Brown, T.A. Update on course and outcome in eating disorders. *Int. J. Eat. Disord.* **2010**, *43*, 195–204. [CrossRef] [PubMed]
5. Ratnasuriya, R.H.; Eisler, I.; Szmukler, G.I.; Russell, G.F. Anorexia nervosa: Outcome and prognostic factors after 20 years. *Br. J. Psychiatry* **1991**, *158*, 495–502. [CrossRef]
6. Zipfel, S.; Löwe, B.; Reas, D.L.; Deter, H.C.; Herzog, W. Long-term prognosis in anorexia nervosa: Lessons from a 21-year follow-up study. *Lancet* **2000**, *355*, 721–722. [CrossRef]
7. Moore, C.A.; Bokor, B.R. Anorexia Nervosa. In *StatPearls*; StatPearls Publishing. Copyright © 2022; StatPearls Publishing LLC.: Treasure Island, FL, USA, 2022.
8. Walsh, B.T. The enigmatic persistence of anorexia nervosa. *Am. J. Psychiatry* **2013**, *170*, 477–484. [CrossRef]
9. Di Lodovico, L.; Hanachi, M.; Duriez, P.; Gorwood, P. The Fitter I Am, the Larger I Feel-The Vicious Circle of Physical Exercise in Anorexia Nervosa. *Nutrients* **2022**, *14*, 4507. [CrossRef]
10. Titova, O.E.; Hjorth, O.C.; Schiöth, H.B.; Brooks, S.J. Anorexia nervosa is linked to reduced brain structure in reward and somatosensory regions: A meta-analysis of VBM studies. *BMC Psychiatry* **2013**, *13*, 110. [CrossRef]
11. Seitz, J.; Bühren, K.; von Polier, G.G.; Heussen, N.; Herpertz-Dahlmann, B.; Konrad, K. Morphological changes in the brain of acutely ill and weight-recovered patients with anorexia nervosa. A meta-analysis and qualitative review. *Z Kinder Jugendpsychiatr. Psychother.* **2014**, *42*, 7–17; quiz 17–18. [CrossRef]
12. King, J.A.; Geisler, D.; Ritschel, F.; Boehm, I.; Seidel, M.; Roschinski, B.; Soltwedel, L.; Zwipp, J.; Pfuhl, G.; Marxen, M.; et al. Global cortical thinning in acute anorexia nervosa normalizes following long-term weight restoration. *Biol. Psychiatry* **2015**, *77*, 624–632. [CrossRef]
13. Nickel, K.; Joos, A.; Tebartz van Elst, L.; Matthis, J.; Holovics, L.; Endres, D.; Zeeck, A.; Hartmann, A.; Tüscher, O.; Maier, S. Recovery of cortical volume and thickness after remission from acute anorexia nervosa. *Int. J. Eat. Disord.* **2018**, *51*, 1056–1069. [CrossRef]
14. Riva, G. Neurobiology of Anorexia Nervosa: Serotonin Dysfunctions Link Self-Starvation with Body Image Disturbances through an Impaired Body Memory. *Front. Hum. Neurosci.* **2016**, *10*, 600. [CrossRef]
15. Russo, S.; Kema, I.P.; Bosker, F.; Haavik, J.; Korf, J. Tryptophan as an evolutionarily conserved signal to brain serotonin: Molecular evidence and psychiatric implications. *World J. Biol. Psychiatry* **2009**, *10*, 258–268. [CrossRef] [PubMed]
16. Kaye, W.H.; Fudge, J.L.; Paulus, M. New insights into symptoms and neurocircuit function of anorexia nervosa. *Nat. Rev. Neurosci.* **2009**, *10*, 573–584. [CrossRef] [PubMed]
17. Tanaka, M.; Tóth, F.; Polyák, H.; Szabó, Á.; Mándi, Y.; Vécsei, L. Immune Influencers in Action: Metabolites and Enzymes of the Tryptophan-Kynurenine Metabolic Pathway. *Biomedicines* **2021**, *9*, 734. [CrossRef]
18. Frintrop, L.; Trinh, S.; Seitz, J.; Kipp, M. The Role of Glial Cells in Regulating Feeding Behavior: Potential Relevance to Anorexia Nervosa. *J. Clin. Med.* **2021**, *11*, 186. [CrossRef] [PubMed]
19. Schwarcz, R.; Bruno, J.P.; Muchowski, P.J.; Wu, H.Q. Kynurenines in the mammalian brain: When physiology meets pathology. *Nat. Rev. Neurosci.* **2012**, *13*, 465–477. [CrossRef] [PubMed]
20. Huang, Y.S.; Ogbechi, J.; Clanchy, F.I.; Williams, R.O.; Stone, T.W. IDO and Kynurenine Metabolites in Peripheral and CNS Disorders. *Front. Immunol.* **2020**, *11*, 388. [CrossRef]
21. Ostapiuk, A.; Urbanska, E.M. Kynurenic acid in neurodegenerative disorders-unique neuroprotection or double-edged sword? *CNS Neurosci.* **2022**, *28*, 19–35. [CrossRef]
22. Chen, Y.; Guillemin, G.J. Kynurenine pathway metabolites in humans: Disease and healthy States. *Int. J. Tryptophan Res.* **2009**, *2*, IJTR-S2097. [CrossRef]

23. Fujigaki, H.; Saito, K.; Fujigaki, S.; Takemura, M.; Sudo, K.; Ishiguro, H.; Seishima, M. The signal transducer and activator of transcription 1alpha and interferon regulatory factor 1 are not essential for the induction of indoleamine 2,3-dioxygenase by lipopolysaccharide: Involvement of p38 mitogen-activated protein kinase and nuclear factor-kappaB pathways, and synergistic effect of several proinflammatory cytokines. *J. Biochem.* **2006**, *139*, 655–662. [CrossRef]
24. Asp, L.; Johansson, A.S.; Mann, A.; Owe-Larsson, B.; Urbanska, E.M.; Kocki, T.; Kegel, M.; Engberg, G.; Lundkvist, G.B.; Karlsson, H. Effects of pro-inflammatory cytokines on expression of kynurenine pathway enzymes in human dermal fibroblasts. *J. Inflamm. (Lond)* **2011**, *8*, 25. [CrossRef] [PubMed]
25. Haroon, E.; Raison, C.L.; Miller, A.H. Psychoneuroimmunology meets neuropsychopharmacology: Translational implications of the impact of inflammation on behavior. *Neuropsychopharmacology* **2012**, *37*, 137–162. [CrossRef] [PubMed]
26. Fukui, S.; Schwarcz, R.; Rapoport, S.I.; Takada, Y.; Smith, Q.R. Blood-brain barrier transport of kynurenines: Implications for brain synthesis and metabolism. *J. Neurochem.* **1991**, *56*, 2007–2017. [CrossRef]
27. Acharyya, S.; Ladner, K.J.; Nelsen, L.L.; Damrauer, J.; Reiser, P.J.; Swoap, S.; Guttridge, D.C. Cancer cachexia is regulated by selective targeting of skeletal muscle gene products. *J. Clin. Invest.* **2004**, *114*, 370–378. [CrossRef]
28. Dafny, N.; Yang, P.B. Interferon and the central nervous system. *Eur. J. Pharm.* **2005**, *523*, 1–15. [CrossRef] [PubMed]
29. Han, Q.; Cai, T.; Tagle, D.A.; Li, J. Structure, expression, and function of kynurenine aminotransferases in human and rodent brains. *Cell. Mol. Life Sci.* **2010**, *67*, 353–368. [CrossRef]
30. Sathyasaikumar, K.V.; Tararina, M.; Wu, H.Q.; Neale, S.A.; Weisz, F.; Salt, T.E.; Schwarcz, R. Xanthurenic Acid Formation from 3-Hydroxykynurenine in the Mammalian Brain: Neurochemical Characterization and Physiological Effects. *Neuroscience* **2017**, *367*, 85–97. [CrossRef] [PubMed]
31. Veldhoen, M.; Hirota, K.; Christensen, J.; O'Garra, A.; Stockinger, B. Natural agonists for aryl hydrocarbon receptor in culture medium are essential for optimal differentiation of Th17 T cells. *J. Exp. Med.* **2009**, *206*, 43–49. [CrossRef]
32. DiNatale, B.C.; Murray, I.A.; Schroeder, J.C.; Flaveny, C.A.; Lahoti, T.S.; Laurenzana, E.M.; Omiecinski, C.J.; Perdew, G.H. Kynurenic acid is a potent endogenous aryl hydrocarbon receptor ligand that synergistically induces interleukin-6 in the presence of inflammatory signaling. *Toxicol. Sci.* **2010**, *115*, 89–97. [CrossRef]
33. Rossi, F.; Miggiano, R.; Ferraris, D.M.; Rizzi, M. The Synthesis of Kynurenic Acid in Mammals: An Updated Kynurenine Aminotransferase Structural KATalogue. *Front. Mol. Biosci.* **2019**, *6*, 7. [CrossRef]
34. Stone, T.W. Does kynurenic acid act on nicotinic receptors? An assessment of the evidence. *J. Neurochem.* **2020**, *152*, 627–649. [CrossRef] [PubMed]
35. Lugo-Huitrón, R.; Ugalde Muñiz, P.; Pineda, B.; Pedraza-Chaverrí, J.; Ríos, C.; Pérez-de la Cruz, V. Quinolinic acid: An endogenous neurotoxin with multiple targets. *Oxid. Med. Cell Longev.* **2013**, *2013*, 104024. [CrossRef]
36. Fellendorf, F.T.; Bonkat, N.; Dalkner, N.; Schönthaler, E.M.D.; Manchia, M.; Fuchs, D.; Reininghaus, E.Z. Indoleamine 2,3-dioxygenase (IDO)-activity in Severe Psychiatric Disorders: A Systemic Review. *Curr. Top Med. Chem.* **2022**, *22*, 2107–2118. [CrossRef] [PubMed]
37. Mithaiwala, M.N.; Santana-Coelho, D.; Porter, G.A.; O'Connor, J.C. Neuroinflammation and the Kynurenine Pathway in CNS Disease: Molecular Mechanisms and Therapeutic Implications. *Cells* **2021**, *10*, 1548. [CrossRef] [PubMed]
38. Corcos, M.; Guilbaud, O.; Paterniti, S.; Moussa, M.; Chambry, J.; Chaouat, G.; Consoli, S.M.; Jeammet, P. Involvement of cytokines in eating disorders: A critical review of the human literature. *Psychoneuroendocrinology* **2003**, *28*, 229–249. [CrossRef]
39. Haleem, D.J. Decreases of plasma tryptophan concentrations following restricted feeding do not decrease serotonin and its metabolite in rat brain. *Nahrung* **1994**, *38*, 606–611. [CrossRef]
40. Haleem, D.J.; Jabeen, B.; Parveen, T. Inhibition of restraint-induced anorexia by injected tryptophan. *Life Sci.* **1998**, *63*, PL205–PL212. [CrossRef]
41. Haider, S.; Haleem, D.J. Decreases of brain serotonin following a food restriction schedule of 4 weeks in male and female rats. *Med. Sci. Monit.* **2000**, *6*, 1061–1067.
42. Lemieux, G.A.; Cunningham, K.A.; Lin, L.; Mayer, F.; Werb, Z.; Ashrafi, K. Kynurenic acid is a nutritional cue that enables behavioral plasticity. *Cell* **2015**, *160*, 119–131. [CrossRef]
43. Hassanyeh, F.; Marshall, E.F. Measures of serotonin metabolism in anorexia nervosa. *Acta Psychiatr. Scand.* **1991**, *84*, 561–563. [CrossRef]
44. Favaro, A.; Caregaro, L.; Burlina, A.B.; Santonastaso, P. Tryptophan levels, excessive exercise, and nutritional status in anorexia nervosa. *Psychosom. Med.* **2000**, *62*, 535–538. [CrossRef]
45. Bossola, M.; Scribano, D.; Colacicco, L.; Tavazzi, B.; Giungi, S.; Zuppi, C.; Luciani, G.; Tazza, L. Anorexia and plasma levels of free tryptophan, branched chain amino acids, and ghrelin in hemodialysis patients. *J. Ren. Nutr.* **2009**, *19*, 248–255. [CrossRef]
46. Attia, E.; Wolk, S.; Cooper, T.; Glasofer, D.; Walsh, B.T. Plasma tryptophan during weight restoration in patients with anorexia nervosa. *Biol. Psychiatry* **2005**, *57*, 674–678. [CrossRef] [PubMed]
47. Ehrlich, S.; Franke, L.; Schneider, N.; Salbach-Andrae, H.; Schott, R.; Craciun, E.M.; Pfeiffer, E.; Uebelhack, R.; Lehmkuhl, U. Aromatic amino acids in weight-recovered females with anorexia nervosa. *Int. J. Eat. Disord.* **2009**, *42*, 166–172. [CrossRef] [PubMed]
48. Gauthier, C.; Hassler, C.; Mattar, L.; Launay, J.M.; Callebert, J.; Steiger, H.; Melchior, J.C.; Falissard, B.; Berthoz, S.; Mourier-Soleillant, V.; et al. Symptoms of depression and anxiety in anorexia nervosa: Links with plasma tryptophan and serotonin metabolism. *Psychoneuroendocrinology* **2014**, *39*, 170–178. [CrossRef] [PubMed]

49. Askenazy, F.; Candito, M.; Caci, H.; Myquel, M.; Chambon, P.; Darcourt, G.; Puech, A.J. Whole blood serotonin content, tryptophan concentrations, and impulsivity in anorexia nervosa. *Biol. Psychiatry* **1998**, *43*, 188–195. [CrossRef]
50. Comai, S.; Bertazzo, A.; Carretti, N.; Podfigurna-Stopa, A.; Luisi, S.; Costa, C.V. Serum levels of tryptophan, 5-hydroxytryptophan and serotonin in patients affected with different forms of amenorrhea. *Int. J. Tryptophan Res.* **2010**, *3*, 69–75. [CrossRef] [PubMed]
51. Kaye, W.H.; Barbarich, N.C.; Putnam, K.; Gendall, K.A.; Fernstrom, J.; Fernstrom, M.; McConaha, C.W.; Kishore, A. Anxiolytic effects of acute tryptophan depletion in anorexia nervosa. *Int. J. Eat. Disord.* **2003**, *33*, 257–267. [CrossRef]
52. Demitrack, M.A.; Heyes, M.P.; Altemus, M.; Pigott, T.A.; Gold, P.W. Cerebrospinal fluid levels of kynurenine pathway metabolites in patients with eating disorders: Relation to clinical and biochemical variable. *Biol. Psychiatry* **1995**, *37*, 512–520. [CrossRef]
53. Dudzińska, E.; Szymona, K.; Kloc, R.; Kocki, T.; Gil-Kulik, P.; Bogucki, J.; Kocki, J.; Paduch, R.; Urbańska, E.M. Fractalkine, sICAM-1 and Kynurenine Pathway in Restrictive Anorexia Nervosa-Exploratory Study. *Nutrients* **2021**, *13*, 339. [CrossRef]
54. Franzago, M.; Orecchini, E.; Porreca, A.; Mondanelli, G.; Orabona, C.; Dalla Ragione, L.; Di Nicola, M.; Stuppia, L.; Vitacolonna, E.; Beccari, T.; et al. SLC6A4 DNA Methylation Levels and Serum Kynurenine/Tryptophan Ratio in Eating Disorders: A Possible Link with Psychopathological Traits? *Nutrients* **2023**, *15*, 406. [CrossRef] [PubMed]
55. Achamrah, N.; Nobis, S.; Breton, J.; Jésus, P.; Belmonte, L.; Maurer, B.; Legrand, R.; Bôle-Feysot, C.; do Rego, J.L.; Goichon, A.; et al. Maintaining physical activity during refeeding improves body composition, intestinal hyperpermeability and behavior in anorectic mice. *Sci. Rep.* **2016**, *6*, 21887. [CrossRef] [PubMed]
56. Höglund, E.; Øverli, Ø.; Winberg, S. Tryptophan Metabolic Pathways and Brain Serotonergic Activity: A Comparative Review. *Front. Endocrinol. (Lausanne)* **2019**, *10*, 158. [CrossRef]
57. Fernstrom, J.D.; Wurtman, R.J. Brain serotonin content: Increase following ingestion of carbohydrate diet. *Science* **1971**, *174*, 1023–1025. [CrossRef]
58. Fernstrom, J.D.; Wurtman, R.J. Brain serotonin content: Physiological regulation by plasma neutral amino acids. *Science* **1972**, *178*, 414–416. [CrossRef] [PubMed]
59. Wurtman, R.J.; Wurtman, J.J. Brain serotonin, carbohydrate-craving, obesity and depression. *Obes. Res.* **1995**, *3* (Suppl. 4), 477s–480s. [CrossRef]
60. Molfino, A.; Muscaritoli, M.; Cascino, A.; Fanfarillo, F.; Fava, A.; Bertini, G.; Citro, G.; Rossi Fanelli, F.; Laviano, A. Free tryptophan/large neutral amino acids ratios in blood plasma do not predict cerebral spinal fluid tryptophan concentrations in interleukin-1-induced anorexia. *Pharm. Biochem. Behav.* **2008**, *89*, 31–35. [CrossRef]
61. Pajak, B.; Orzechowska, S.; Pijet, B.; Pijet, M.; Pogorzelska, A.; Gajkowska, B.; Orzechowski, A. Crossroads of cytokine signaling–the chase to stop muscle cachexia. *J. Physiol. Pharm.* **2008**, *59* (Suppl. 9), 251–264.
62. Asarian, L.; Langhans, W. A new look on brain mechanisms of acute illness anorexia. *Physiol. Behav.* **2010**, *100*, 464–471. [CrossRef]
63. van Donkelaar, E.L.; Blokland, A.; Ferrington, L.; Kelly, P.A.; Steinbusch, H.W.; Prickaerts, J. Mechanism of acute tryptophan depletion: Is it only serotonin? *Mol. Psychiatry* **2011**, *16*, 695–713. [CrossRef]
64. Ehrlich, S.; Salbach-Andrae, H.; Weiss, D.; Burghardt, R.; Goldhahn, K.; Craciun, E.M.; Franke, L.; Uebelhack, R.; Klapp, B.F.; Lehmkuhl, U. S100B in underweight and weight-recovered patients with anorexia nervosa. *Psychoneuroendocrinology* **2008**, *33*, 782–788. [CrossRef]
65. Gerner, R.H.; Cohen, D.J.; Fairbanks, L.; Anderson, G.M.; Young, J.G.; Scheinin, M.; Linnoila, M.; Shaywitz, B.A.; Hare, T.A. CSF neurochemistry of women with anorexia nervosa and normal women. *Am. J. Psychiatry* **1984**, *141*, 1441–1444. [CrossRef] [PubMed]
66. Murray, C.; Griffin, É.W.; O'Loughlin, E.; Lyons, A.; Sherwin, E.; Ahmed, S.; Stevenson, N.J.; Harkin, A.; Cunningham, C. Interdependent and independent roles of type I interferons and IL-6 in innate immune, neuroinflammatory and sickness behaviour responses to systemic poly I:C. *Brain Behav. Immun.* **2015**, *48*, 274–286. [CrossRef] [PubMed]
67. Cunningham, C.; Campion, S.; Teeling, J.; Felton, L.; Perry, V.H. The sickness behaviour and CNS inflammatory mediator profile induced by systemic challenge of mice with synthetic double-stranded RNA (poly I:C). *Brain Behav. Immun.* **2007**, *21*, 490–502. [CrossRef]
68. Field, R.; Campion, S.; Warren, C.; Murray, C.; Cunningham, C. Systemic challenge with the TLR3 agonist poly I:C induces amplified IFNalpha/beta and IL-1beta responses in the diseased brain and exacerbates chronic neurodegeneration. *Brain Behav. Immun.* **2010**, *24*, 996–1007. [CrossRef]
69. Wilinski, D.; Winzeler, J.; Duren, W.; Persons, J.L.; Holme, K.J.; Mosquera, J.; Khabiri, M.; Kinchen, J.M.; Freddolino, P.L.; Karnovsky, A.; et al. Rapid metabolic shifts occur during the transition between hunger and satiety in Drosophila melanogaster. *Nat. Commun.* **2019**, *10*, 4052. [CrossRef] [PubMed]
70. Mangge, H.; Summers, K.L.; Meinitzer, A.; Zelzer, S.; Almer, G.; Prassl, R.; Schnedl, W.J.; Reininghaus, E.; Paulmichl, K.; Weghuber, D.; et al. Obesity-related dysregulation of the tryptophan-kynurenine metabolism: Role of age and parameters of the metabolic syndrome. *Obesity (Silver Spring)* **2014**, *22*, 195–201. [CrossRef]
71. Connick, J.; Lombardi, G.; Beni, M.; Moroni, F. Decrease in rat cerebral quinolinic acid concentration following chronic hydrocortisone treatment. *Neurosci. Lett.* **1988**, *88*, 216–220. [CrossRef]
72. Yates, J.R.; Gay, E.A.; Heyes, M.P.; Blight, A.R. Effects of methylprednisolone and 4-chloro-3-hydroxyanthranilic acid in experimental spinal cord injury in the guinea pig appear to be mediated by different and potentially complementary mechanisms. *Spinal. Cord.* **2014**, *52*, 662–666. [CrossRef]

73. Saito, K.; Markey, S.P.; Heyes, M.P. Effects of immune activation on quinolinic acid and neuroactive kynurenines in the mouse. *Neuroscience* **1992**, *51*, 25–39. [CrossRef] [PubMed]
74. Laugeray, A.; Launay, J.M.; Callebert, J.; Surget, A.; Belzung, C.; Barone, P.R. Peripheral and cerebral metabolic abnormalities of the tryptophan-kynurenine pathway in a murine model of major depression. *Behav. Brain Res.* **2010**, *210*, 84–91. [CrossRef] [PubMed]
75. Guidetti, P.; Okuno, E.; Schwarcz, R. Characterization of rat brain kynurenine aminotransferases I and II. *J. Neurosci. Res.* **1997**, *50*, 457–465. [CrossRef]
76. Frintrop, L.; Trinh, S.; Liesbrock, J.; Leunissen, C.; Kempermann, J.; Etdöger, S.; Kas, M.J.; Tolba, R.; Heussen, N.; Neulen, J.; et al. The reduction of astrocytes and brain volume loss in anorexia nervosa-the impact of starvation and refeeding in a rodent model. *Transl. Psychiatry* **2019**, *9*, 159. [CrossRef] [PubMed]
77. Reyes-Haro, D. Glial cells in anorexia. *Front. Cell Neurosci.* **2022**, *16*, 983577. [CrossRef]
78. Agudelo, L.Z.; Femenía, T.; Orhan, F.; Porsmyr-Palmertz, M.; Goiny, M.; Martinez-Redondo, V.; Correia, J.C.; Izadi, M.; Bhat, M.; Schuppe-Koistinen, I.; et al. Skeletal muscle PGC-1α1 modulates kynurenine metabolism and mediates resilience to stress-induced depression. *Cell* **2014**, *159*, 33–45. [CrossRef]
79. Gul, S.; Saleem, D.; Haleem, M.A.; Haleem, D.J. Inhibition of hormonal and behavioral effects of stress by tryptophan in rats. *Nutr. Neurosci.* **2019**, *22*, 409–417. [CrossRef] [PubMed]
80. Sato, T.; Laviano, A.; Meguid, M.M.; Chen, C.; Rossi-Fanelli, F.; Hatakeyama, K. Involvement of plasma leptin, insulin and free tryptophan in cytokine-induced anorexia. *Clin. Nutr.* **2003**, *22*, 139–146. [CrossRef]
81. Hernandez, L.; Parada, M.; Baptista, T.; Schwartz, D.; West, H.L.; Mark, G.P.; Hoebel, B.G. Hypothalamic serotonin in treatments for feeding disorders and depression as studied by brain microdialysis. *J. Clin. Psychiatry* **1991**, *52*, 32–40.
82. Saeed, R.; Mahmood, K.; Ali, S.B.; Haleem, D.J. Prevention of diet restriction induced hyperactivity but not body-weight reduction in rats co-treated with tryptophan: Relationship with striatal serotonin and dopamine metabolism and serotonin-1A auto-receptor expression. *Nutr. Neurosci.* **2022**, *25*, 1764–1773. [CrossRef] [PubMed]
83. Silverstone, T.; Goodall, E. Serotoninergic mechanisms in human feeding: The pharmacological evidence. *Appetite* **1986**, *7*, 85–97. [CrossRef] [PubMed]
84. Blundell, J.E.; Hill, A.J. Influence of tryptophan on appetite and food selection in man. In *Amino Acids in Health and Disease: New Perspectives*; Kaufman, S., Alan, R., Eds.; Liss: New York, NY, USA, 1987; Volume 55, pp. 403–419.
85. Poesen, R.; Mutsaers, H.A.; Windey, K.; van den Broek, P.H.; Verweij, V.; Augustijns, P.; Kuypers, D.; Jansen, J.; Evenepoel, P.; Verbeke, K.; et al. The Influence of Dietary Protein Intake on Mammalian Tryptophan and Phenolic Metabolites. *PLoS ONE* **2015**, *10*, e0140820. [CrossRef] [PubMed]
86. Dencker, M.; Björgell, O.; Hlebowicz, J. Effect of food intake on 92 neurological biomarkers in plasma. *Brain Behav.* **2017**, *7*, e00747. [CrossRef]
87. Barbarich, N.C.; McConaha, C.W.; Halmi, K.A.; Gendall, K.; Sunday, S.R.; Gaskill, J.; La Via, M.; Frank, G.K.; Brooks, S.; Plotnicov, K.H.; et al. Use of nutritional supplements to increase the efficacy of fluoxetine in the treatment of anorexia nervosa. *Int. J. Eat. Disord.* **2004**, *35*, 10–15. [CrossRef]
88. Goodwin, G.M.; Shapiro, C.M.; Bennie, J.; Dick, H.; Carroll, S.; Fink, G. The neuroendocrine responses and psychological effects of infusion of L-tryptophan in anorexia nervosa. *Psychol. Med.* **1989**, *19*, 857–864. [CrossRef]
89. Van der Does, A.J. The effects of tryptophan depletion on mood and psychiatric symptoms. *J. Affect Disord* **2001**, *64*, 107–119. [CrossRef]
90. Boehm, I.; Hennig, J.; Ritschel, F.; Geisler, D.; King, J.A.; Lesch, I.; Roessner, V.; Zepf, F.D.; Ehrlich, S. Acute tryptophan depletion balances altered resting-state functional connectivity of the salience network in female patients recovered from anorexia nervosa. *J. Psychiatry Neurosci.* **2022**, *47*, E351–E358. [CrossRef]
91. Weinert, T.; Bernardoni, F.; King, J.; Steding, J.; Boehm, I.; Mannigel, M.; Ritschel, F.; Zepf, F.; Roessner, V.; Ehrlich, S. No effects of acute tryptophan depletion on anxiety or mood in weight-recovered female patients with anorexia nervosa. *Eur. Arch. Psychiatry Clin. Neurosci.* **2022**. [CrossRef]
92. Steding, J.; Ritschel, F.; Boehm, I.; Geisler, D.; King, J.A.; Roessner, V.; Smolka, M.N.; Zepf, F.D.; Ehrlich, S. The effects of acute tryptophan depletion on instrumental reward learning in anorexia nervosa—An fMRI study. *Psychol. Med.* **2022**, *Mar 28*, 1–11. [CrossRef]
93. Kerley-Hamilton, J.S.; Trask, H.W.; Ridley, C.J.; Dufour, E.; Ringelberg, C.S.; Nurinova, N.; Wong, D.; Moodie, K.L.; Shipman, S.L.; Moore, J.H.; et al. Obesity is mediated by differential aryl hydrocarbon receptor signaling in mice fed a Western diet. *Env. Health Perspect.* **2012**, *120*, 1252–1259. [CrossRef] [PubMed]
94. Moyer, B.J.; Rojas, I.Y.; Kerley-Hamilton, J.S.; Hazlett, H.F.; Nemani, K.V.; Trask, H.W.; West, R.J.; Lupien, L.E.; Collins, A.J.; Ringelberg, C.S.; et al. Inhibition of the aryl hydrocarbon receptor prevents Western diet-induced obesity. Model for AHR activation by kynurenine via oxidized-LDL, TLR2/4, TGFβ, and IDO1. *Toxicol. Appl. Pharm.* **2016**, *300*, 13–24. [CrossRef] [PubMed]

nutrients

MDPI

Review

Comparison between Different Groups of Vegetarianism and Its Associations with Body Composition: A Literature Review from 2015 to 2021

Tatiana Fontes, Luis Monteiro Rodrigues and Cíntia Ferreira-Pêgo *

CBIOS—Universidade Lusófona's Research Center for Biosciences and Health Technologies, Av. Campo Grande 376, 1749-024 Lisbon, Portugal; f6776@ulusofona.pt (T.F.); monteiro.rodrigues@ulusofona.pt (L.M.R.)

* Correspondence: cintia.pego@ulusofona.pt (C.F.-P.)

Abstract: Background: Vegetarian and vegan diets have become increasingly popular in the last years for many reasons, including their association with various health benefits when compared to omnivorous diets. The main objective of the study was to collect recent (2015–2021) scientific evidence for potential implications between a vegetarian/vegan diet and an individuals' body composition. Methods: A literature search was conducted in PubMed, with 22 studies selected for inclusion in our collective evaluation. Of the 22 studies included, there were 12 randomized controlled trials, 1 nonrandomized controlled trial, 1 comparative study, and 8 cross-sectional. The overall sample included in this study consists of 436,178 participants, 10,090 of whom were vegetarians, 5044 vegans, and 421,044 omnivores. Results: Most studies, 17 out of 22, reported a significant positive relationship between a plant-based diet and body composition. Conclusion: There is scientifically sound evidence that vegan or vegetarian diets are associated with weight and body mass index reduction and, in some cases, fat mass distribution changes.

Keywords: vegetarian diet; vegan diet; body composition; body mass index; literature review

1. Introduction

A vegetarian diet predominantly consists of foodstuffs of plant origin (cereals, vegetables, root crops, oilseeds, fruit, and nuts) and tends to exclude any type of meat, fish, or animal product or subproduct [1,2]. The vegetarian diet can be further divided into several subgroups: ovo-vegetarian (includes eggs), ovo-lacto-vegetarian (includes eggs and dairy products), and lacto-vegetarian (includes dairy products) [1,2]. Flexitarian diets are another type of vegetarianism, although they are less stringent regarding the consumption of meat and fish [3,4]. The vegan diet is the strictest, as no animal-derived foods (including honey) are consumed [1]. Individuals who follow a vegan diet are normally concerned not only with what they eat but also with the environment and animal protection issues [5]. Vegetarian diets have become increasingly popular, in part because they have been associated with many health benefits when compared to omnivorous diets [5]. Foods in these diets are typically rich in fiber, phytoestrogens, antioxidants, phytochemicals, n-3 fatty acids, and poor in cholesterol and saturated fat, allegedly contributing to a reduction in risk of cardiovascular disease, diabetes, and obesity, among others [2,5,6]. According to the World Health Organization (WHO), about 1.2 billion people in the world were overweight at the turn of the 20th century [2,7]. It is now known that obesity is a complex disease, and its comorbidities are responsible for thousands of deaths worldwide. It is therefore extremely important to find more effective solutions to combat this pandemic [2,8,9]. Recent reports support the claim that a well-balanced vegetarian diet may be associated with a lower body mass index (BMI) compared to other diets [2,10]. These diets have also been linked to a wide range of beneficial nutritional, metabolic, and health outcomes, including lipid metabolism, bone mineral density, body weight, body fat percentage, obesity-related meta-inflammatory profile, and diabetes risk [2,4,10]. Its therapeutical potential to address obesity has been suggested [2]. However, despite these associations, there is still much controversy related to this type of diet and its true efficiency and safety [2,5]. Low levels of vitamin B12 and the increase in serum homocysteine are frequently raised concerns [2,5]. Thus, it has become increasingly important to understand the health benefits that a vegetarian diet might bring, especially in terms of weight loss and fighting obesity. This study aims to review the most recent scientific evidence regarding the potential associations and consequences relating to vegetarian/vegan diets and human body composition.

2. Materials and Methods

2.1. Search Strategy and Inclusion and Exclusion Criteria

According to the PRISMA statement 2020, we identified all potentially relevant articles through a computerized search in PubMed (from April 2021 to September 2021). Search terms included keywords "vegetarians", "vegetarianism", "vegetarian diet", "vegan", "veganism", and "vegan diet" used in combination as MeSH terms and text words such as "body mass index" and "body composition". All manuscripts that did not compare the vegetarian or vegan diet with another diet, studies not performed in humans, studies performed in children or adolescents, as well as review articles, or systematic reviews/meta-analyses were excluded from this review. The manuscripts' inclusion decision was initially based on the title, then on the study abstract, and finally on the complete study manuscript. All studies with body composition-related values from a vegetarian/vegan population and not meeting any of the non-inclusion criteria were included, even if body composition measurements were not the main objective of the study.

2.2. Data Collection

In the first identification phase, 651 articles were found, which was reduced to 592 studies after the exclusion of duplicates. In the second selection phase, 492 articles were excluded after reading the title and abstract, as they did not meet the purpose of the research. This resulted in 100 studies. In the third eligibility phase, from those 100 articles selected for thorough reading, 78 were excluded: 52 were excluded because their publication was prior to 2015, 24 were excluded because their research was not related to the objective of this study and, finally, 2 were excluded because the studied population was children/adolescents. In the fourth inclusion phase, 22 articles that met all the inclusion criteria and the research objective were selected for the present review after detailed evaluation by the authors (Figure 1). Of the 22 studies included, there were 12 randomized controlled trials, 1 nonrandomized controlled trial, 1 comparative study, and 8 cross-sectional. The overall sample included in this study consisted of 436,178 participants, 10,090 of whom were vegetarians, 5044 vegans, and 421,044 omnivores.

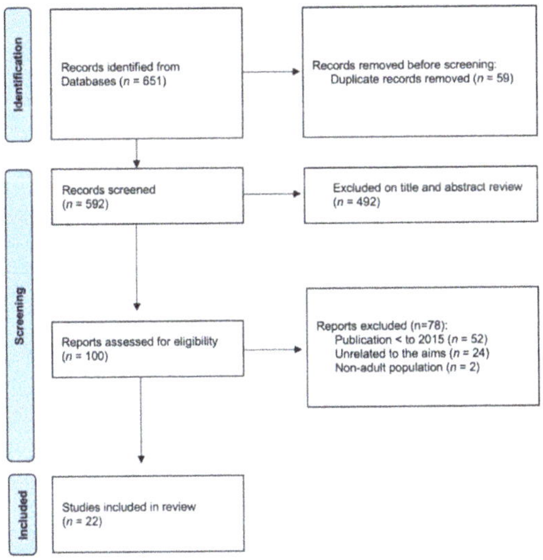

Figure 1. Flowchart for search strategy.

3. Results

In most studies, we found that sociodemographic characteristics were not statistically different. Study participant ages ranged from 18 to 75 years old. Most studies found a significant positive relationship between vegetarian/vegan diet and body composition, as shown in Figure 2.

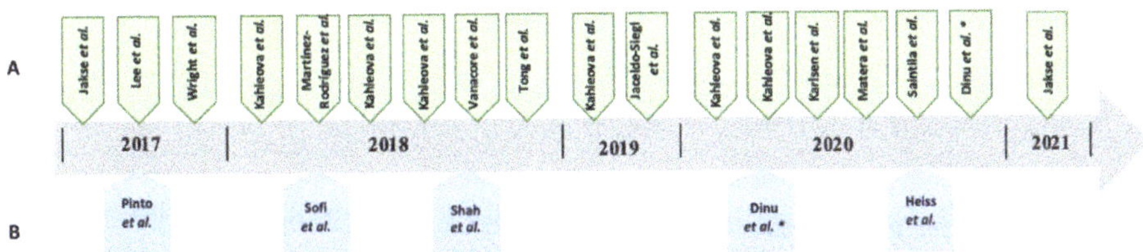

Figure 2. Epidemiological studies included in the review: (**A**) significant positive relationship, and (**B**) no demonstrated effects between vegetarian/vegan diet and body composition. *First intervention no demonstrated effects, between vegetarian/vegan diet and body composition but second interview found a significant positive relation.

3.1. Experimental Studies

Table 1 includes 12 randomized controlled trials and 1 nonrandomized controlled trial. The total sample consisted of 1388 participants, 650 of whom were vegans, 144 vegetarians, and 594 omnivores. At the beginning of each study, the participants in both groups (intervention and control) had identical weight and BMI, with the exception of the study by Jakse [11], where the intervention group started with a higher weight. The vast majority of studies observed a significant decrease in body weight and BMI [11–19] in the intervention groups (vegan or vegetarian diet) compared to the control groups (omnivorous diet). Likewise, some studies also found a significant reduction in visceral fat and fat mass only in the intervention group [11,14,16–18,20]. Martínez-Rodríguez et al. [21] verified that women who suffered from fibromyalgia and consumed an ovo-lacto-vegetarian diet had better results in reducing both pain and body composition, with an increase in muscle mass and a decrease in fat mass. On the other hand, the studies by Sofi et al. [22] and Shah et al. [23] did not observe differences in weight loss and BMI between the diet groups.

Table 1. Summary of the experimental studies included in the present review.

Reference	Type of Study	Population/ Methods	Main Findings
Jakse et al., 2017 [24]	Nonrandomized Controlled Trial	325 participants: control group (n = 84) and intervention group (n = 241).	"The intervention group lost a significantly larger amount of weight, body fat, and visceral fat. The relative proportion of muscle mass and total body water increased relative to the control group."
Lee et al., 2017 [12]	Randomized Controlled Trial	30 women: intervention group (vegetarian diet, n = 16) and control group (normal diet of participant, n = 14). Duration: 10 days	"Bodyweight and BMI decreased significantly in the intervention group compared with that in the control group."
Wright et al., 2017 [13]	Randomized Controlled Trial	49 participants: intervention group (n = 25) and control group (n = 24). Duration: 6 months to 1 year	"At 6 months mean intervention BMI reduction was 4.4 kg/m^2 and from 6 to 12 months intervention BMI increased non-significantly by 0.4 kg/m^2. For weight, intervention reduction at 6 months was 12.1 kg, and at 12 months was 11.5 kg."
Kahleova et al., 2018 [14]	Randomized Controlled Trial	75 participants: intervention group (n = 38) or a control group (n = 37). The intervention followed a low-fat vegan diet and the control group made no diet changes. Duration: 16 weeks.	"Parameters such as BMI, fat mass and especially visceral fat volume were significantly reduced in the intervention group."
Kahleova et al., 2018 [15]	Randomized Controlled Trial	75 Participants: intervention group (plant-based high-carbohydrate, low-fat (vegan) diet; n = 38) or control group (current diet; n = 37). Duration: 16 weeks.	"In vegan group, there was a decrease in weight and in fat."
Martínez-Rodríguez et al., 2018 [21]	Randomized Controlled Trial	21 women with fibromyalgia: Group A (core stabilization exercises + Lacto-vegetarian diet, n = 7); group B (stabilization exercises with ultrasound turned off and without the use of conductive gel + Lacto-vegetarian diet, n = 7) and group C (control, n = 7). Duration: 4 weeks.	"Group A, compared to groups B and C, showed significant changes, at the end of the intervention, in pain reduction and body composition. There was an increased muscle mass and decreasing fat mass."
Sofi et al., 2018 [22]	Randomized Controlled Trial	118 participants: ovolactovegetarians group (n = 60) and Mediterranean diet group (n = 58). Duration: 2 periods of $\geq$3 months.	Weight loss was identical in both groups (vegetarians: −1.88 kg; Mediterranean diet: −1.77 kg). Similar results were observed for BMI and fat mass.
Kahleova et al., 2018 [14]	Randomized Controlled Trial	75 overweight participants: vegan diet (n = 38) or a control diet (n = 37). Duration: 16 weeks.	"Reductions in BMI, body weight, fat mass, and visceral fat volume in the vegan group."
Shah et al., 2018 [23]	Randomized Controlled Trial	100 participants with angiographically: vegan diet (n = 50) or American Heart Association recommended diet (n = 50).	"No differences were observed in weight loss, BMI, and waist circumference reduction."
Kahleova et al., 2019 [20]	Randomized Controlled Trial	75 overweight participants: low-fat vegan (n = 38) or control diet (n = 37). Duration: 16 weeks.	"A low-fat vegan diet was associated with decreased fat mass, insulin resistance, and enhanced insulin secretion."
Kahleova et al., 2020 [17]	Randomized Controlled Trial	115 participants overweight: vegan group (n = 65) and control group (n = 50). Duration: 16 weeks	"Bodyweight decreased in the vegan group, mainly due to a reduction in fat mass and visceral fat."

Table 1. *Cont.*

Reference	Type of Study	Population/ Methods	Main Findings
Kahleova et al., 2020 [18]	Randomized Clinical Trial	Overweight or obese participants: intervention group (n = 117), following a low-fat vegan diet, and control group (n = 106). Duration: 16 weeks.	"Mean body weight, fat mass and visceral fat volume decreased in the intervention group."
Dinu et al., 2020 [19]	Randomized Controlled Trial	107 participants: vegetarian diet (n = 54), and Mediterranean diet (n = 53). Duration: 2 periods of ≥3 months.	"Reduction in body weight, BMI, and fat mass was observed in both groups, with no difference between the two diets."

Abbreviations: body mass index (BMI), body fat percentage (%BF).

3.2. Descriptive Studies

Table 2 summarizes eight cross-sectional studies and one comparative study. The total sample consisted of 434,790 participants, 4394 of whom were vegans, 9946 vegetarians, and 420,450 omnivores. The majority of studies observed a significant decrease in body weight and BMI in individuals who consumed a vegetable-based diet [5,25–29]. The study by Tong et al. [30] found that white individuals who did not consume meat had lower values for body weight, BMI, waist circumference, and fat percentage. However, the same study found that these values were not as pronounced in the Indian population, although those who did not consume meat continued to present lower values for all parameters. Our research also found that some studies [31,32] did not observe statistically significant differences between diet groups, either for BMI or for other markers of body composition.

Table 2. Summary of the descriptive studies included in the present review.

Reference	Type of Study	Population/ Methods	Main Findings
Pinto et al., 2017 [31]	Comparative Study	23 participants following a vegan diet for ≥2 years compared with 24 omnivorous participants.	"No significant differences in mean BMI or other markers of body composition (%BF)."
Vanacore et al., 2018 [5]	Cross-sectional	30 participnats: vegetarians (n = 10); vegans (n = 10) and omnivores (n = 10).	"Decrease in muscle mass index and lean body mass between vegan vs. omnivorous groups."
Tong et al., 2018 [30]	Cross-sectional	Data from UK Biobank cohort participants. Caucasian individuals: 6 diet groups (regular meat-eaters, low meat-eaters, poultry eaters, fish eaters, vegetarians, and vegans). British Indian population: 2 diet groups (meat-eaters and vegetarians).	"White population who were poultry eaters, fish eaters, vegetarians, or vegans generally weighed less and had a lower BMI, waist and hip circumference and body fat percentage than the regular meat-eaters. British Indian vegetarian women had a slightly lower body weight and lower lean mass than meat-eaters."

Table 2. *Cont.*

Reference	Type of Study	Population/ Methods	Main Findings
Jaceldo-Siegl et al., 2019 [25]	Cross-sectional	3475 Hispanic/Latino adults: vegan (*n* = 202), vegetarian (*n* = 664), pesco-vegetarian (*n* = 409), semi-vegetarian (*n* = 227) and nonvegetarian (*n* = 1973).	"Compared to the nonvegetarian, estimated BMI were lower among vegans, vegetarians, pesco-vegetarians, and semi-vegetarians. Plant-based diets were associated with lower BMI."
Karlsen et al., 2020 [26]	Cross-sectional	8226 participants: whole food plant-based (*n* = 2141), vegan (*n* = 1584), Paleo (*n* = 1202), try to eat healthy (*n* = 968), vegetarian and pescatarian (*n* = 814), whole food (*n* = 690), Weston A. Price (*n* = 458) and low-carb (*n* = 369).	"BMI was lower among longer-term followers (≥1 year) of whole food, plant-based, vegan, whole food, and low-carb diets compared with shorter-term followers. Among those following their diet for 1–5 years, BMI were lower for all groups compared with try to eat healthy group."
Matera, 2020 [27]	Cross-sectional	370 participants: 188 vegetarian and 182 omnivorous.	"Vegetarians had a lower BMI."
Heiss et al., 2020 [32]	Cross-sectional	124 Participants: 72 omnivores, 27 meat-reducers, 20 vegetarians, and 5 vegans.	"Vegetarians reported lower BMI compared to meat-reducers."
Saintila et al., 2020 [28]	Cross-sectional	149 participants: vegetarians (*n* = 62) and nonvegetarians (*n* = 87).	"Vegetarian males had a lower weight, waist circumference and BMI than nonvegetarian males."
Jakse et al., 2021 [29]	Cross-sectional	Two groups: vegan (*n* = 51) and non-vegan (*n* = 29).	"All anthropometric and body composition variables were significantly lower in the vegans than non-vegans, except for body height."

Abbreviations: body mass index (BMI), body fat percentage (%BF).

4. Discussion

This review aimed to collect recently published scientific evidence related to vegetarian/vegan diet and body composition. The 22 included studies, published from 2017 to 2021, included a total of 436,178 participants, which corresponds to a large sample size and wide geographic coverage. Several interventional and cross-section studies directly or indirectly assessed the effect of vegetarian/vegan diets on the body composition compared to omnivorous diets. The study by Jakse et al., involved an intervention with a low-fat vegetable-based diet and vegetable meal replacement (intervention group) and an omnivorous diet. These authors observed that the intervention group lost a significantly larger amount of weight, body fat, and visceral fat. Similar studies [13–18,20] choosing low-fat plant-based diets for the intervention group observed statistically significant reductions in body weight, BMI, and, in some cases, fat mass. These findings reinforce this potential association between low-fat diets and significant weight loss [33]. Other cross-sectional studies [5,25–30] also observed a significantly greater reduction in weight and BMI in individuals consuming plant-based diets. Karlsen et al. [34] found that the BMI reduction is more pronounced in individuals who followed this type of diet for more than one year. These results are in line with the EPIC-Oxford cohort study reporting that vegans and vegetarians lost weight after a 5-year follow-up trial. Lee et al. [12] performed a 10-day intensive health promotion study where individuals frequently performed physical activity and consumed a vegetarian or an omnivorous diet. At the end of the intervention, weight and BMI was found to be significantly reduced in the vegetarian diet group. However, psychological variables were not assessed, meaning that other factors beyond diet might contribute to the reported results. Recently Dinu et al. [19] compared the Mediterranean and vegetarian diets and suggested that statistically significant differences between these two regimens could not be detected in a first intervention. This study reported that after a second intervention, significant reductions in body weight, BMI, and fat mass were detected in both groups. Low caloric density and reduced levels of saturated fatty acids have been reported to explain these impacts of vegetarian/vegan diets on body weight and BMI [35]. The involvement of other nutrients such as higher mono- and polyunsaturated fat or fiber content has also been reported [35]. The lack of statistically significant differences between individuals consuming plant-based and omnivorous diets in body composition was found in four studies. The study by Sofi et al. [22] used a low-calorie diet intervention to reduce weight and cardiovascular risk. No statistically significant differences could be found for weight loss, BMI, and fat mass between the two groups. Shah et al. [23] found no differences in weight loss, BMI, and waist circumference between the vegan diet and the American Heart Association recommended diet in individuals with coronary artery disease. However, the American Heart Association recommended diet was created specifically for individuals with cardiovascular diseases [36], while the same does not apply to the vegan diet. The studies by Pinto et al. [31] and Heiss et al. [32] found no statistically significant differences regarding body composition between vegetable-based and omnivorous diets. However, it is not possible to establish a causal relationship with the results obtained due to the type of study conducted. One explanation for no statistical differences observed in different studies between vegetarian diets and body composition may be that they originate from developing countries where the diet is plant-based, or are those reliant on the Mediterranean diet for the obvious reason. However, in the present review, the five papers that did not find any statistically significant positive association all originate from developed countries. It is also important to understand that there is no clear consensus on the effects of plant-based diets on body composition. A recent study reported a relationship between being vegetarian/vegan and higher levels of fat mass and visceral adipose tissue, although these were non-statistically significant differences [37]. It is also noteworthy that all these studies presented various limitations. As an example, although the vast majority of studies have assessed body composition through dual-energy X-ray absorptiometry, some studies used self-reported measurements [25,27], normal scales [5,28], or the bioimpedance method [11,19,21,22,28,30,31]. Physical activity and lifestyle are not included as determinants in most of the studies. In these conditions, any comparisons involve significant bias. Other limitations are related to cross-sectional studies, which do not allow for establishing a causal relationship. In these same studies, there was a greater discrepancy in the sample (population) size, with some samples being very small [5,31] and others with significant heterogeneity between the dietary groups [25,26,30]. However, the fact that most of the studies included in this review were randomized clinical trials is a strong point in support of the scientific evidence presented.

5. Conclusions

Results gathered in this review suggest that vegetarian/vegan diets are associated with weight loss and BMI reduction and, in a few cases, with fat mass modifications. Our results also suggest that research on these matters should aim for larger and more representative numbers of vegetarians and vegans regarding the general population. It is also necessary to assess not only the effect of plant-based diets on body composition but the positive or negative contribution of each food group and nutrients within these same diets.

Author Contributions: Conceptualization, L.M.R. and C.F.-P.; methodology, T.F.; software, T.F. and C.F.-P.; validation, L.M.R. and C.F.-P.; formal analysis, C.F.-P.; investigation, T.F.; resources, L.M.R. and C.F.-P.; data curation, T.F.; writing—original draft preparation, T.F.; writing—review and editing, L.M.R. and C.F.-P.; visualization, T.F. and C.F.-P.; supervision, L.M.R. and C.F.-P.; project administration, L.M.R. and C.F.-P.; funding acquisition, L.M.R. and C.F.-P. All authors have read and agreed to the published version of the manuscript.

Funding: This research was funded by national funds through FCT—Foundation for Science and Technology, I.P. (Portugal), under the [UIDB/04567/2020] and [UIDP/04567/2020] projects. C.F.-P. is funded by the FCT—Foundation for Science and Technology, I.P. (Portugal) Scientific Employment Stimulus contract [reference number CEEC/CBIOS/NUT/2018].

Institutional Review Board Statement: Not applicable.

Informed Consent Statement: Not applicable.

Data Availability Statement: Not applicable.

Conflicts of Interest: The authors declare no conflict of interest.

References

1. Hauner, H. Vegetarian/vegan diet: Reasonable or dangerous? *MMW-Fortschritte der Medizin* **2015**, *157*, 41–43. [CrossRef] [PubMed]
2. Pilis, W.; Stec, K.; Zych, M.; Pilis, A. Health benefits and risk associated with adopting a vegetarian diet. *Rocz. Państwowego Zakładu Hig.* **2014**, *65*, 9–14.
3. Derbyshire, E.J. Flexitarian Diets and Health: A Review of the Evidence-Based Literature. *Front. Nutr.* **2017**, *3*, 1–8. [CrossRef] [PubMed]
4. Oussalah, A.; Levy, J.; Berthezène, C.; Alpers, D.H.; Guéant, J.L. Health outcomes associated with vegetarian diets: An umbrella review of systematic reviews and meta-analyses. *Clin. Nutr.* **2020**, *39*, 3283–3307. [CrossRef]
5. Vanacore, D.; Messina, G.; Lama, S.; Bitti, G.; Ambrosio, P.; Tenore, G.; Messina, A.; Monda, V.; Zappavigna, S.; Boccellino, M.; et al. Effect of restriction vegan diet's on muscle mass, oxidative status, and myocytes differentiation: A pilot study. *J. Cell. Physiol.* **2018**, *233*, 9345–9353. [CrossRef]
6. Crowe, F.L.; Appleby, P.N.; Travis, R.C.; Key, T.J. Risk of hospitalization or death from ischemic heart disease among British vegetarians and nonvegetarians: Results from the EPIC-Oxford cohort study1-3. *Am. J. Clin. Nutr.* **2013**, *97*, 597–603. [CrossRef]
7. Berkow, S.E.; Barnard, N. Vegetarian diets and weight status. *Nutr. Rev.* **2006**, *64*, 175–188. [CrossRef]
8. Conway, B.; Rene, A. Obesity as a disease: No lightweight matter. *Obes. Rev.* **2004**, *5*, 145–151. [CrossRef]
9. Duncan, B.B.; Chor, D.; Aquino, E.M.L.; Bensenor, I.M.; Mill, J.G.; Schmidt, M.I.; Lotufo, P.A.; Vigo, Á.; Barreto, S.M. Doenças Crônicas Não Transmissíveis no Brasil: Prioridade para enfrentament e investigação. *Rev. Saude Publica* **2012**, *46*, 126–134. [CrossRef]
10. Bakaloudi, D.R.; Halloran, A.; Rippin, H.L.; Oikonomidou, A.C.; Dardavesis, T.I.; Williams, J.; Wickramasinghe, K.; Breda, J.; Chourdakis, M. Intake and adequacy of the vegan diet. A systematic review of the evidence. *Clin. Nutr.* **2021**, *40*, 3503–3521. [CrossRef]
11. Jakše, B.; Jakše, B.; Pajek, J.; Pajek, M. Effects of an Ad Libitum Consumed Low-Fat Plant-Based Diet Supplemented with Plant-Based Meal Replacements on Body Composition Indices. *Food Nutr. Res.* **2019**, *63*, 1560. [CrossRef]
12. Lee, K.S.; Lee, J.K.; Yeun, Y.R. Effects of a 10-day intensive health promotion program combining diet and physical activity on body composition, physical fitness, and blood factors of young adults: A randomized pilot study. *Med. Sci. Monit.* **2017**, *23*, 1759–1767. [CrossRef]
13. Wright, N.; Wilson, L.; Smith, M.; Duncan, B.; McHugh, P. The BROAD study: A randomised controlled trial using a whole food plant-based diet in the community for obesity, ischaemic heart disease or diabetes. *Nutr. Diabetes* **2017**, *7*, e256. [CrossRef]
14. Kahleova, H.; Tura, A.; Hill, M.; Holubkov, R.; Barnard, N.D. A plant-based dietary intervention improves beta-cell function and insulin resistance in overweight adults: A 16-week randomized clinical trial. *Nutrients* **2018**, *10*, 189. [CrossRef]
15. Kahleova, H.; Dort, S.; Holubkov, R.; Barnard, N.D. A plant-based high-carbohydrate, low-fat diet in overweight individuals in a 16-week randomized clinical trial: The role of carbohydrates. *Nutrients* **2018**, *10*, 1302. [CrossRef]
16. Kahleova, H.; Fleeman, R.; Hlozkova, A.; Holubkov, R.; Barnard, N.D. A plant-based diet in overweight individuals in a 16-week randomized clinical trial: Metabolic benefits of plant protein. *Nutr. Diabetes* **2018**, *8*, 58. [CrossRef]
17. Kahleova, H.; Rembert, E.; Alwarith, J.; Yonas, W.N.; Tura, A.; Holubkov, R.; Agnello, M.; Chutkan, R.; Barnard, N.D. Effects of a low-fat vegan diet on gut microbiota in overweight individuals and relationships with body weight, body composition, and insulin sensitivity. A randomized clinical trial. *Nutrients* **2020**, *12*, 2917. [CrossRef]
18. Kahleova, H.; Petersen, K.F.; Shulman, G.I.; Alwarith, J.; Rembert, E.; Tura, A.; Hill, M.; Holubkov, R.; Barnard, N.D. Effect of a Low-Fat Vegan Diet on Body Weight, Insulin Sensitivity, Postprandial Metabolism, and Intramyocellular and Hepatocellular Lipid Levels in Overweight Adults: A Randomized Clinical Trial. *JAMA Netw. Open* **2020**, *3*, e2025454. [CrossRef]
19. Dinu, M.; Colombini, B.; Pagliai, G.; Cesari, F.; Gori, A.; Giusti, B.; Marcucci, R.; Sofi, F. Effects of a dietary intervention with Mediterranean and vegetarian diets on hormones that influence energy balance: Results from the CARDIVEG study. *Int. J. Food Sci. Nutr.* **2020**, *71*, 362–369. [CrossRef]

20. Kahleova, H.; Hlozkova, A.; Fleeman, R.; Fletcher, K.; Holubkov, R.; Barnard, N.D. Fat quantity and quality, as part of a low-fat, vegan diet, are associated with changes in body composition, insulin resistance, and insulin secretion. A 16-week randomized controlled trial. *Nutrients* **2019**, *11*, 615. [CrossRef]
21. Martínez-Rodríguez, A.; Leyva-Vela, B.; Martínez-García, A.; Nadal-Nicolás, Y. Efectos de la dieta lacto-vegetariana y ejercicios de estabilización del core sobre la composición corporal y el dolor en mujeres con fibromialgia: Ensayo controlado aleatorizado. *Nutr. Hosp.* **2018**, *35*, 392–399. [CrossRef]
22. Sofi, F.; Dinu, M.; Pagliai, G.; Cesari, F.; Gori, A.M.; Sereni, A.; Becatti, M.; Fiorillo, C.; Marcucci, R.; Casini, A. Low-calorie vegetarian versus mediterranean diets for reducing body weight and improving cardiovascular risk profile. *Circulation* **2018**, *137*, 1103–1113. [CrossRef]
23. Shah, B.; Newman, J.D.; Woolf, K.; Ganguzza, L.; Guo, Y.; Allen, N.; Zhong, J.; Fisher, E.A.; Slater, J. Anti-inflammatory effects of a vegan diet versus the american heart association–recommended diet in coronary artery disease trial. *J. Am. Heart Assoc.* **2018**, *7*, 1–14. [CrossRef]
24. Jakše, B.; Pinter, S.; Jakše, B.; Bučar Pajek, M.; Pajek, J. Effects of an Ad Libitum Consumed Low-Fat Plant-Based Diet Supplemented with Plant-Based Meal Replacements on Body Composition Indices. *Biomed Res. Int.* **2017**, *2017*, 9626390. [CrossRef]
25. Jaceldo-Siegl, K.; Estevez, D.; Fraser, G.E.; Hayes-Bautista, D.E.; Flores, H.; Jordan, M.; Singh, P.N. Plant-Based Diets in Hispanic/Latino Adult Adventists in the United States and Their Association With Body Mass Index. *Am. J. Heal. Promot.* **2019**, *33*, 869–875. [CrossRef]
26. Karlsen, M.C.; Lichtenstein, A.H.; Economos, C.D.; Folta, S.C.; Chang, R.; Rogers, G.; Jacques, P.F.; Livingston, K.A.; McKeown, N.M. Participant characteristics and self-reported weight status in a cross-sectional pilot survey of self-identified followers of popular diets: Adhering to Dietary Approaches for Personal Taste (ADAPT) Feasibility Survey. *Public Health Nutr.* **2020**, *23*, 2717–2727. [CrossRef]
27. Brytek-Matera, A. Interaction between vegetarian versus omnivorous diet and unhealthy eating patterns (Orthorexia nervosa, cognitive restraint) and body mass index in adults. *Nutrients* **2020**, *12*, 646. [CrossRef]
28. Saintila, J.; Lozano López, T.E.; Ruiz Mamani, P.G.; White, M.; Huancahuire-Vega, S. Health-Related Quality of Life, Blood Pressure, and Biochemical and Anthropometric Profile in Vegetarians and Nonvegetarians. *J. Nutr. Metab.* **2020**, *2020*, 3629742. [CrossRef] [PubMed]
29. Jakše, B.; Jakše, B.; Godnov, U.; Pinter, S. Nutritional, cardiovascular health and lifestyle status of 'health conscious' adult vegans and non-vegans from slovenia: A cross-sectional self-reported survey. *Int. J. Environ. Res. Public Health* **2021**, *18*, 5968. [CrossRef] [PubMed]
30. Tong, T.Y.N.; Key, T.J.; Sobiecki, J.G.; Bradbury, K.E. Anthropometric and physiologic characteristics in white and British Indian vegetarians and nonvegetarians in the UK Biobank. *Am. J. Clin. Nutr.* **2018**, *107*, 909–920. [CrossRef] [PubMed]
31. Pinto, A.M.; Sanders, T.A.B.; Kendall, A.C.; Nicolaou, A.; Gray, R.; Al-Khatib, H.; Hall, W.L. A comparison of heart rate variability, n-3 PUFA status and lipid mediator profile in age- and BMI-matched middle-aged vegans and omnivores. *Br. J. Nutr.* **2017**, *117*, 669–685. [CrossRef]
32. Heiss, S.; Walker, D.C.; Anderson, D.A.; Morison, J.N.; Hormes, J.M. Vegetarians and omnivores with diagnosed eating disorders exhibit no difference in symptomology: A retrospective clinical chart review. *Eat. Weight Disord.* **2021**, *26*, 1007–1012. [CrossRef]
33. Sackner-Bernstein, J.; Kanter, D.; Kaul, S. Dietary intervention for overweight and obese adults: Comparison of low- carbohydrate and low-fat diets. a meta- analysis. *PLoS ONE* **2015**, *10*, e0139817. [CrossRef]
34. Rosell, M.; Appleby, P.; Spencer, E.; Key, T. Weight gain over 5 years in 21 966 meat-eating, fish-eating, vegetarian, and vegan men and women in EPIC-Oxford. *Int. J. Obes.* **2006**, *30*, 1389–1396. [CrossRef]
35. Pieters, M.; Swanepoel, A.C. The effect of plant-based diets on thrombotic risk factors. *Polish Arch. Intern. Med.* **2021**, *131*, 16123. [CrossRef]
36. Eckel, R.H.; Jakicic, J.M.; Ard, J.D.; De Jesus, J.M.; Houston Miller, N.; Hubbard, V.S.; Lee, I.M.; Lichtenstein, A.H.; Loria, C.M.; Millen, B.E.; et al. 2013 AHA/ACC guideline on lifestyle management to reduce cardiovascular risk: A report of the American College of cardiology/American Heart Association task force on practice guidelines. *Circulation* **2014**, *129*, 76–99. [CrossRef]
37. Ferreira-Pêgo, C.; Tavares, R.G.; Lopes, S.; Fontes, T.; Rodrigues, L.M. Body composition assessment of vegetarian-vegan and omnivore young women—An exploratory study. *Biomed. Biopharm. Res.* **2021**, *18*, 15–24. [CrossRef]

MDPI AG
Grosspeteranlage 5
4052 Basel
Switzerland
Tel.: +41 61 683 77 34

Nutrients Editorial Office
E-mail: nutrients@mdpi.com
www.mdpi.com/journal/nutrients

www.ingramcontent.com/pod-product-compliance
Lightning Source LLC
Chambersburg PA
CBHW040743250926
51850CB00007BB/1389
9783725853656